These medicines all had a common point, a vision not piecemeal approach to the human being, but on the contrary a holistic vision. Live in harmony with nature, put the emphasis on prevention as much as the curative, request to his patient to take charge. It is Hippocrates who at the ^{Ve} century av. J.-C. said in his book The medical art, science and doctrine : "Art is long, the short life, the opportunity passes quickly. The test is misleading. The judgment difficult. Not only the doctor must do what it takes, but the sick as well. "

The MTC is a total medicine where body and mind are not separated. Holistic medicine by excellence, it considers that the man and nature are one. Ecologist medicine well before the hour, it highlights the existing interference between our environment and the functioning of the Organization. But it is also a medicine of the soul, capable of treating the root of the dysfunction of the human body.

In the West, we have a very narrow vision of this traditional medicine in reducing it to a symptomatic acupuncture.

A practitioner in MTC must be an excellent "detective" capable thanks to the observation, interrogation, the taking of pulse and the study of the language, to discover the origin of the imbalance, to know where is his patient and what will be its fate.

Once all these investigations have resulted, it must be a multicard practitioner. It is also well acupuncturist, pharmacologist, chiropractor, professor of gymnastics, psychotherapist, masseur, dietician. He must know to juggle with all of these therapeutic approaches specific to the MTC. It must be able to find the proper key which corresponds to his patient.

The Western medicine, in some respects, could be qualified of Emergency Medicine. It gets very interesting results on the symptoms or acute diseases. But as soon as it comes to chronicity, she often loses foot fault to apprehend the exact genesis of the pathology. This medicine has been built on a mechanistic model, where each component is a component of the human body. If one of them comes to fail, it is "sufficient"

1

to repair it for that the machine finds its normal operation. It is this vision that fact that modern medicine has a tendency to turn solely toward the treatment of symptoms, to deal more often the effect that the cause, some evils returning then in a recurring way.

The MTC on the contrary puts the emphasis on the interdependence of all the bodies. It considers that the energy is located upstream of the material. As soon as a dysregulation of energy appears, a symptom alarm signal informs the practitioner or the patient that an imbalance installs. Most of the time, this symptom will not be any of following targeted. It will disappear by itself when the root cause of the disruption will have been processed. If the imbalance is not corrected, little by little, this will be the physical bodies, vital, which will be achieved.

One of the major features of the MTC is not to differentiate the psychological balance, the overall balance of the human body. Physical, mental and emotion are in very close relationship. Since more than 3 000 years, the MTC explains that each component is a body "thinking". We will see that the emotional imbalances are the root causes of almost all the internal pathologies.

Another salient feature, not to say essential to this medicine, is not to be confined only to the remedies, techniques to combat the disease. It advocates before all a certain quality of life which takes the place of prevention. "Prevention is better than cure" is the basic axiom of the MTC. We will see that all the curative techniques taught in this book may also become elements of prevention.

About This Book

The traditional Chinese medicine, old of its 3 000 years, remains a modern medicine and young which has more and more followers with the dawn of the twenty -first century. Although very complex by its many theories and schools, it often stems of the good sense and the observation of our environment. It allows you to refocus on itself and to be listening to our body.

"The body has not been built for fall ill, but to autoguérir continuously. "Yet should he in back the means! That is the whole object of this book.

In this book, written in the manner of a oral teaching, I wanted to demystify the traditional Chinese medicine and make it affordable to everyone. This book is therefore directed to a very wide public.

"The layperson who has the more often than a piecemeal vision of this medicine. Throughout these pages, the pieces of the puzzle will be reconstituted. It will be between the hands all the tools necessary to put in place a genuine policy of prevention. The health and longevity are the states that deserve. In a society that encourages us continuously to become assisted, learn to self-determination request of efforts, certainly, but they will be quickly rewarded. The practical implementation of technical, all described in this book, as the digitoponcture, moxibustion, massage, dietetics, respiration, gymnastics of long life through the Qi Gong, psychotherapy will enable him to find this balance both sought on the "Cable of life".

"To the student or the future student who wants to start in such studies. He will find there a reference book on the whole of the facets of the MTC, drawn from the same source of the Tradition. He will very soon realize that the MTC is not confined to a few recipes or acupuncture. It is a medicine of a lifetime. He will not stop until the end of his days, learn again and again. This multifaceted book will be as many doors to open for its own evolution.

"To the practitioner confirmed. It contained in particular in annexs of the lessons rarely given in the West. Among other things, the ancestral techniques of acupuncture and digitoponcture, and the "grid of choice of points", applicable to all pathologies. All this learned the lessons of one of the greatest modern masters in MTC, the pr Leung Kok Yuen.

3

The Conventions

"Rather than repeat each time "Traditional Chinese Medicine", it will be used the abbreviation MTC throughout this book.

"When we are talking about a body, it must be before any to apprehend the energy that underlies the functioning of the body. It is for this reason that all the organs such as the liver, heart, etc. will be preceded by a capital letter.

How This Book Is Organized

The traditional Chinese medicine for Dummies consists of five thematic parts more the sixth part of the ten well known to the collection.

First part: the fundamentals of traditional Chinese medicine

This part allows you first of all to apprehend the very sources of this medicine, far from the Modern drifts. It will give you a holistic vision of the human body. An entire chapter will allow you to trim the field and have a profound vision of the MTC. To this title, chapitre 2 is inescapable: It may be read in priority. You will then have the exact definition and understanding of the concepts specific to the MTC, such as the concepts of Yin-Yang, Qi (Energy), Hun (spiritual soul), Po (soul and body) and many others. This part also teaches us the very close relationship between the Man and the Universe, real ecology before the hour. All this is leading to the concept of the five elements, the concept of meridians and energy points.

Second part: The diagnostic methods

This part explains in detail the different methods of observation in MTC. The study of the morphotype, of the face with its shape and its colors, eyes, hands... Allows you very quickly to have a clear idea about the past and the become pathological of an individual.

You get great benefit to soak the chapter on the examination and the "Song of the ten questions": it will allow you to analyze and understand the origin of all your evils (headache , pain, insomnia...), and to consider at the outset as the symptoms alarm signals and not as pathologies with whole share.

And to go further, you will become unbeatable (or almost) in the techniques of decision-pulse and the study of the language. In practice, a practitioner "sees" his patient, has already a few intuitions, asking him precise questions after s be inquired about his CV. Then, it strengthens his diagnosis by the taking of the pulse and the study of the language. A practitioner of high level, after having seen, taken the pulse and "studied the language," will already asked the diagnosis. The patient may not then that answer "yes" to questions which are asked.

Third Part: The major causes of illness

You can not to not create a disease called "internal" by ignorance of the functioning of our body energy. Ignore the alarm signals that emits the body, not to practice on a daily basis the methods Yang Sheng Fa, prevention, can make that an energy imbalance at the outset is transformed into organic pathology at the end of the chain. Do not forget that the energy is upstream of the matter.

But this weakness of the internal will also facilitate the penetration of the "perverse agents "vectors of diseases (virus, microbe, wind, cold, humidity...). It is this that the MTC calls the external diseases.

This part is essential to understand that we are most of the time at the origin of the emergence of our ills. You will no longer be able to say: It is the fault" to no chance," or that of "other".

Fourth part: The major methods of treatment

In this part will be addressed the very wide range of therapeutic techniques and preventive measures taught by the MTC. There are methods reserved for the Practitioner as acupuncture or the use of plants in the traditional pharmacopoeia. At least, you will know the why and how when you made a meeting of acupuncture!

As a bonus, you will find a very simple method to learn in a few minutes the localization and the journey global of 12 meridians of energy.

But this part is directed mainly to all "null" that we are: How to really deal with his health, "without fear and without reproach ", avoiding any radicalism and any excess? You will learn in effect to breathe, to sleep, to relax, to you automasser, to move your body, to meditate. A broad place will be given to the ancestral technique of digitoponcture, with a few large formulas of passable points by everyone.

Fifth part: the dietetics of long life

This part dedicated to the dietetics of the middle you will learn to become the leader of the orchestra of your power supply, with food of the season and region. Not a question of "if enchinoiser" in addition to measure. And this, through "Nine unbreakable rules" that well understood and applied the more regularly as possible, will not only of "make you lose large and swell the meager," but especially to stop tired unnecessarily your organization and to find a state of balance, good health on your cable of life. A chapter will be devoted to the problem if controversial issue of the hydration of the body. The data of the MTC in the material will help you to dispose of the errors conveyed in our modern world.

Sixth part: part of the ten

The life may not be that if we breathe, if we eat and if we believe. These are the three main pillars of the Vitality. We are therefore going to divide this part in three times ten commandments, advice or rules which will help you to find a new balance and a new impetus on your cable of life. We will begin by a charter in ten points to learn to manage our emotions. Then what must be put in place in the morning and evening to recharge continuously the battery of the kidney. As to the Dietetics, we will see an essential aspect, namely the ten reasons why it should be to learn to chew. You can have the best of the dietary, but if you do not chew your food bowl, she ends up losing all its value.

Seventh part: Annexs

The beginning of this part is reserved for practitioners, or future practitioners of the MTC. The Pr Leung Kok Yuen has bequeathed to his students his technique of poncture closest to the tradition. Let us not forget that it was Grand Master in acupuncture and regarded as such in China, and then in the United States. But also the grid of choice of points which will allow you to deal with a few pathological situations which are. If you have the profound vision, you will see that this education is a real treasure.

You will also find in this part of the Useful addresses and a lexicon.

The icons used in this book

You will find in the margin of the text of the icons that signpost you in your reading and allow you to easily locate the information that you are looking for in priority. Follow the guide!!!!

Often, certain misunderstandings come from the lack of understanding of concepts fundamental yet. This icon will respond to your questions.

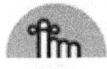
If you have only one thing to remember, it is well that point: put the finger on the essential.

It is the transition from theory to practice. Nothing serves to have a encyclopedic brain to the "ten thousand knowledge", we still need to go to **En pratique** the Act.

Some of the data in the MTC go well beyond the current materialism. More than a philosophy, this medicine affects the essence of the "why". Some **Spiritualité** aspects do the pure metaphysics.

This icon warns you against certain abuses, certain practices or received ideas that may, in the more or less long term, endanger your own **Attention** health. Therefore, "attention".

Part 1
The Fundamentals
Of Medicine
Traditional
In China

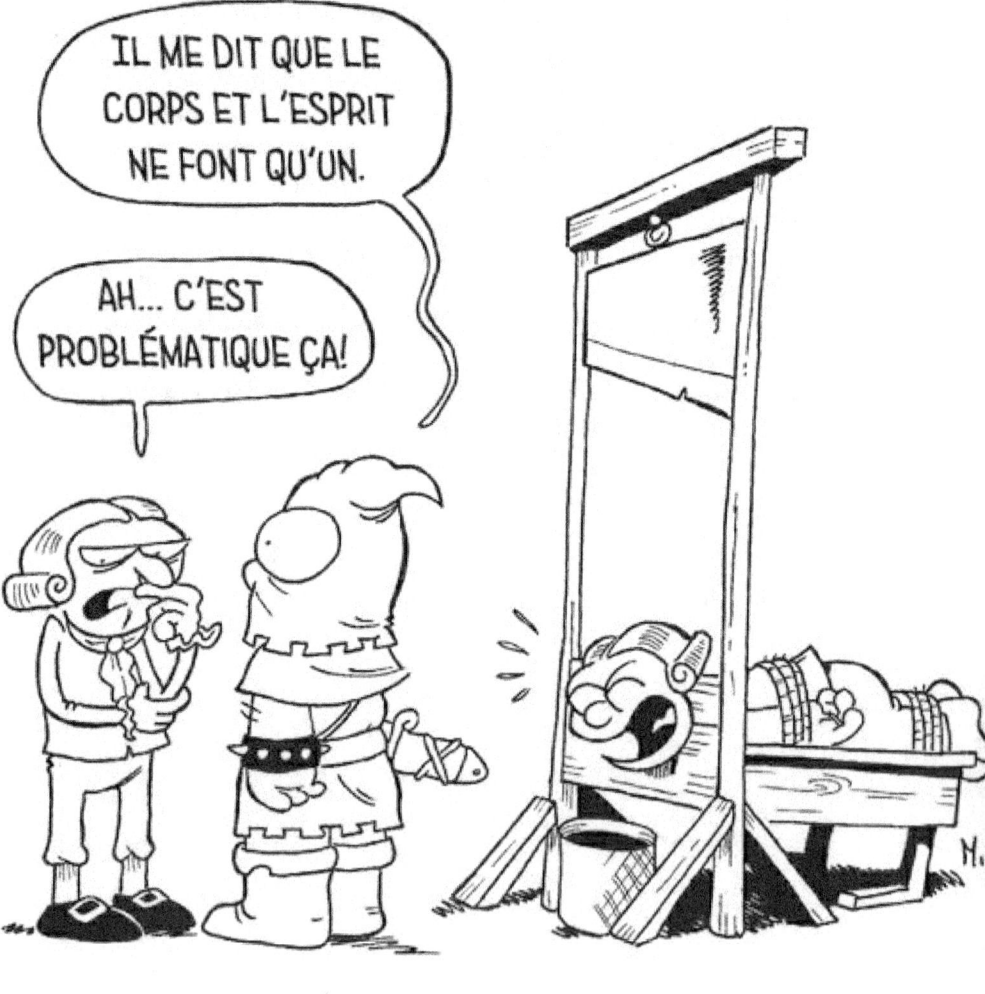

In this part...

This first part covers the fundamentals of the MTC. We cannot understand this holistic medicine without a few basic notions on the metaphysical principles that underlie it. It is this that addresses the chapitre 1. However, if you do not hang any of suite, you can book the reading at the end of this book.

If you have no knowledge of the MTC, it is by THE chapitre 2 that it is appropriate to begin. It will give you all the ins and outs of this medicine.

In the chapitre 3, it is time to go further and to apprehend all the major concepts which are the richness of this medicine.

And if you want to know what your practitioner made during a consultation, or if you want to start in the study of the MTC, go to chapitre 4 to deepen, with different methods of diagnostics, not detailed to not.

Chapter 1

The origins

In this chapter:

" Books The founders of the traditional Chinese medicine

" The principle of the DAO and the uniqueness

" Why are there both of theories?

" At the meeting of the Pr Leung Kok Yuen, the father of the modern MTC

The founding books

The true Chinese medicine dates back to the night of the time. We have already addressed the subject in the preface: it is far to summarize only to the acupuncture. It is a total medicine, as well preventive and curative which affects all areas of life.

The Huangdi NEIJING, 黄帝内经, or Classic of Internal Medicine

It is attributed to the Yellow Emperor (Huang, 黄 wanting to say yellow). It is the oldest manual of Chinese medicine which has served as the theoretical basis for all subsequent developments in the MTC. It goes back to more than 2 500 years. It consists of 19 chapters divided into two parties, the su wen and the **LING Shu.**

The book is in the form of a dialog between the Yellow Emperor and his Minister Qi Bo. The first usually ask questions and the second issues responses which are in reality of lengthy developments. The cosmology, the philosophy, the moral are discussed in relationship with the Chinese medicine.

We will see that the theoretical developments from these writings and developed under the HAN are based on the theory of Yin, 阴 and Yang, 阳, the two elements antithetical to known to all, and the famous theory of the five elements and the digital elements that correspond to them. We will come back at length of course.

Le saviez-vous

The first traces of this holistic approach to the human body dating back to more than 5 000 years, and it is the emergence of the Yi King which is perhaps the first book founder of this medicine.

2 500 years later, the **Nei Jing** which in reality bears the name of Huangdi **Nei Jing** or "Internal classic of the Yellow Emperor" made its appearance. It consists of two parts, the **su wen** and the **LING Shu.**

The major points of reference

To better understand everything that will be said by the suite, it is important to have some points of reference which will allow us to apprehend the very foundations of the MTC.

We could thus from this famous phrase of the Dao de Jing, written in 600 BC by Lao Tseu, Founder of Taoism: "The Dao generates a. A generates two. Two creates three. Three breeds 10 000 beings. "

The Dao

Some people say that the Dao, symbol of the zero, is only a recent invention of mathematicians. In reality, this notion of zero has always been present, in an informal manner. In a sentence, it was simply represented by a vacuum. This is neither a symbol or a concept. It is the metaphysical pure and cannot be apprehended by the intuition that embraces all the words which would serve to define it. In modern cosmology, it is located in front of the wall of Planck which is the border between the physical world and the mathematical world pure. It is located in front of the departure of the Bing Bang. The zero is still called the wu ji, the "non-be". To make it short, too short, perhaps, it is he who is at the origin of the a.

The one is represented by the symbol of Tai Ji, known to all, but too often poorly interpreted.

It is still in the Metaphysics pure. It is the principle from which everything can appear, but it is also the affirmation of the zero, the wu ji. In the theory of the Big Bang, the one represents an extraordinary concentration of energy, infinitely small, who will be at the origin of the "10 000 things," at all.

I remind you that when one employs the aphorism that "10 000", this means that it can no longer count, a bit like the "10 000 grains of sand" on a beach. If one were to make a parallel with the human being, it is the ovule penetrated the spermatozoon: The program is not yet in operation. Everything is in the process of becoming.

11

Then, just the two: it is the explosion of paramount importance, the first cell division, the emergence of the Duality Yin-Yang (see chapitre 3). Let us put aside for the moment the three, the trilogy sky-man-land, the San Bao, namely the "Three Treasures". And the farther away the uniqueness, more the assertion takes shape. It goes very quickly to the 8 trigrams, to 64 hexagrams of The Yi King and then to the symbolic number "10 000".

The big-bang proceeds in the same symbolic. After the explosion paramount, there is expansion of the universe with the appearance of the "10 000 galaxies" which deviate more and more quickly of the One.

And as we live in symbiosis with our environment, we are in the image of the Big Bang. Our modern societies are moving away more and more quickly from one, of the origin.

It is important to understand these concepts of base, because we are at the present time in the phase of "the explosion of the yang." We have lost the overall vision of the Organization, the unit it form, in symbiosis with its environment. The

À retenir

more we move, the more we are losing in the "10 000 Details" and more medicine bursts in "10 000 disciplines". And for the topic of interest to us here, namely the MTC, it is the same. It ends up losing foot face to an incredible amount of techniques, which put end-to-end, eventually contradict between them.

The Tradition

He must know that the Taoism, current of thought from the tradition, which is at the origin of the traditional Chinese medicine, with a capital T is to the pure base metaphysics and not as one hears it said too often a philosophy.

The metaphysics is unique, common to all traditions. It is not to be discussed, but is digested at the discretion of the evolution of our soul. It is like this and not otherwise. By nature, it can hardly be expressed in words. Perhaps by ideographs, but still. These words are compulsorily reducers and are in some way that "lands", not to say crumbs of the metaphysics pure.

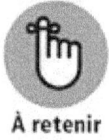

À retenir

The metaphysical proceeded by what might be called the intuition, the "profound vision". And we will see that the intuition and the inner experience play the leading role in the approach of the practitioner who practice some techniques as the digitoponcture or acupuncture.

But with the explosion of the Yang, the multiplicity of "ego", the gradual loss of the oral teaching which in essence is the domain of the anonymity, have arisen" the philosophies". A definition of course reductive of this word: it is, at the departure of the metaphysics in which we add a zest, when this is not a spray of sentimentality.

?

Le saviez-vous

Difference between an ideogram and the alphabetic writing

When you read a word, your brain will apprehend the letters of the alphabet. Taken out of context or as an unknown word, this word doesn't tell you large-thing. While a character is an image, a concept intuitive. In our modern language, we could say that the first type of writing done before any work our left brain, the brain analytical, the one who dissects, husks, peeling, list. A contrario, the reading of an ideogram active rather our brain right, the brain of the conceptualization, of the setback vis-a-vis the event. It treats the information in a holistic manner. It embraces more than it dissects. An example: the ideogram meaning the shaft, the wood is 木, branches at the top, roots down and the vertical line, roots, turning into branch. And do you know by what we ideogram represents a Grove: 林. And the forest? 森林. We, we read f.o.r.Ê.t: this represents nothing. While several trees together are well a forest.

That there is no mistake about it. When we speak of mythical characters, as Shen Nong, the "Divine Laboreur," or Huang Di" the Yellow Emperor," we are in the Metaphysics without ego, we are in the uniqueness. Shen Nong has no importance as a person. It is also very often of a current of thought, of a set of individuals who had plots of Revelation, who spoke of the same subject at the same time. It must be aware of the following fact: as soon as an idea, a theory, a postulate is of an individual in flesh and bones and which is more, gives it its name, it is of the philosophy. We could go as far as to say that there is only one metaphysics and as many philosophers that of people who have questions on the meaning of life.

And what happens when one moves away from the Uniqueness? We then attend to a multiplicity of theories, and as it is said above, techniques which eventually become totally contradictory.

The multiplicity of Theories

If we take for example the theory of acupuncture given by the **Nei Jing, it is very simple. Perhaps even too simple. We have of course the opportunity to revert to them (see** chapitre 13**).** It is clearly said that when one wants to make a toning for example, the insertion of the needle must be slow. It is done at the time where the patient expires. And the withdrawal to the inspired is done quickly. It is also said that this puncture, regardless of the point chosen, must be perpendicular to the plane of the skin. For the sedation, it is the reverse: the insertion is quick and the withdrawal slow, always in perpendicular insertion and still rhythmic on the respiration of the patient.

A few hundred years later appeared the Nan Jing, 'classic difficulties" which is a comment The **Nei Jing. This book has attempted to bring its stone to the building. Some passages are consistent, but others are beginning to enter into contradiction with the founding text. From the 12th** to the 16th century, there are more then the quantity of new theories. Without speak of course of the modern times where we have gone to the hyper multiplicity. It is located in front of a plurality of theories of more and more complex and even the most scholars end up by losing their Latin.

We will be used throughout this book of the theory of the Shaver of Occam who considers that the simple explanation of a fact has a greater chance to be true that a complicated explanation.

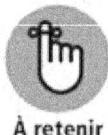

Yes, but this simplicity is only apparent, because it goes under-HEAR A total change of point of view and behavior of a practitioner. In effect the **À retenir** practitioner will be fully invest, but also to give itself the means of this investment to avoid itself be unbalanced on its cable of life. In the trilogy sky-man-land, it will little by little become a mediator, and at the same time a transmitter and regulator of energy to treat his patient.

There is another difficulty and not least with regard to the understanding of the acupuncture, and by extension of the digitoponcture. Even if it is in refer exclusively to the **Nis Jing, this manuscript, to strength to be recopied by of the copyists who had not necessarily the knowledge, these same copyists eventually introduce errors. Some of these errors for a scholar were flagrant, but by respect vis-a-vis the ancestors, Confucianism helping, these errors were corrected in the orality. My master, the pr** Leung Kok Yuen was part of these masters capable of pointing the finger, at the beginning of each course, such errors of copyist. However, the Western non notified, it eventually make these errors of the theories with whole share and sometimes even to give their name to these erroneous theories. It is of course away at great not the truth paramount.

And to complicate the case, most of the component ideograms The Nei Jing are at three levels of reading, which range from a plan the horizontal for the layman to the metaphysical verticality pure for the matched by passing through a medium level. In short, all this is a little complicated, and Happy are those who have had the chance to have access to the true oral tradition with respect to the teaching of the Chinese medicine given by the owners of this medicine, namely the former Chinese.

Throughout this book, we will strive to return to what we could call the "uniqueness", to return to the real ancestral techniques before it has been "perverted" by the explosion of the surrounding materialism.

In the pure tradition of oral transmission?

A special feature of the MTC is to have as a transmission belt the orality. To the origin, there is the sacred texts retranscribed on media very varied (tortoise shell, tissue paper, strips of bamboo, Pierre, jade...). This are phrases, or rather ideograms, meanings very concise much closer to the symbolism that an explanation of text.

The founding texts, their teachings being very airtight, only one master, through the orality could explain that to its students. As well, in the Nei Jing, you find the following sentence: "The water of the Kidney nourishes the wood of the liver and calm the fire of the heart. "Only on this concentrate of sentence, a master is able to teach you whole days to make you understand the contents metaphysical such remarks and everything that follows in the practice of the MTC.

In the initiation, what a difference there is between listen and read?

In MTC, the ears are the opening of the kidney and the energy of the kidney (the "sea of marrow") has a direct link with the central memory of the computer, the brain. When you listen to a course, on condition that you are concentrated, all data will be stored in the central memory which is also under the dependence of the Spirit, the shen. We will also see that the energy of the spleen has a direct relationship with the concentration, but it is at the same time the "railway yard of the information". The eyes are the opening of the liver, and the liver is the "Logis of the Hun", of the spiritual soul. When you read a text which is in adequacy with your felt the deeper, you "Feed in some way your soul". Of course not a text of a magazine, but a text which brings you back to the essence of a concept. What more beautiful example that the reading of a poetry which creates a direct funnel between conscious and subconscious the deeper! Therefore a complete teaching should proceed in the orality, but also to have a written support to allow you to leisure to meditate above.

Who was the Pr Leung Kok Yuen?
The Pr Leung Kok Yuen was one of the first to teach the real traditional medicine in the West. Whereas in the 1950s, Chinese medicine was known in the West that through the work of ethnologists of renown (include among others the Reverend Father Claude Larre and many others to its suite) we are witnessing a reversal of situation. This was one of the first Chinese masters to teach the true MTC origins in

correcting all errors from a misunderstanding of the founding texts.

Portrait

He was born in China in 1922. From 13 generations of doctors from father to son, he was part of the greatest current Masters of traditional Chinese medicine still in life. He held the title of "Shih I" attributed to the Chinese physicians whose family perpetuates a medical tradition since several generations. He began the study of traditional medicine at the age of 5 years in accompanying his father in its long tours of care among the capita, south of Canton. During these hikes, he learned by heart of nursery rhymes and songs in which are placed the keys of the traditional Chinese medicine (mnemonic method very efficient: study in a fun...).

Later, her father explained that these songs and nursery rhymes meant in medical terms. At the age of 11 years, he was able to recite two books written by Zhang Zhongjing by heart: the Jin Kui Yao Lüe and the **Shang Han Lun. He began to make his first care at the age of 16 years! He** was able to observe all the practices that his father used and the way to address the ill and the disease. When he became major, he was directed to another master to perfect his medical education.

From 1952 to 1970, he taught acupuncture in the following schools: Modern Chinese Medical Research Institute and Kowloon Association of Chinese medical practitioners in Hong Kong. From 1956 to 1970, he is president of the Chinese Acupuncture Institute in Hong Kong and the Chinese Acupuncture Association. In 1970, he immigrated to Canada and founded the North American College of acupuncture in Vancouver. From there and thanks, among other things, to the European University of traditional Chinese medicine, he has passed his knowledge to its students Western, which I had the chance to be a part.

Work

His work of learning is considered by far as the most complete. Acupuncture, moxibustion, pharmacopoeia, psychotherapy, massage, preventive medicine, Qi Gong, are as much of disciplines that its students have worked and depth. The Pr Leung Kok Yuen said himself that this knowledge was universal, that it was only the belt transmission of a know dating back to thousands of years. He has ceased his activity as a teacher since he took his retirement in 1992 and has left us with a symbolic age, 90 years, 11 May 2013. The whole basis of his teaching very rigorous was the result of the explanation not to not The **Nei Jing. That is what he called the Orthodox teaching. And in all his teaching, he was able to put in before the methods Yang Sheng Fa, to know how to "cultivate and nourish the life".**

It was one of the greatest of the exegetes **Huang Di Nei Jing. Its other reference books were:**

" The **Nan Jing** (難經), Classical difficulties (220-280), which deals with the classical theories of fundamental and sets out the main points of the **Nei Jing.**

" **Jin Kui Yao** (金匮要略), Breviary of the luggage compartment of gold of Zhang Zhongjing (early iiird century) which deals mainly with various diseases of the internal medicine, of a part of the surgical medicine and diseases of the woman. There are 25 chapters, including 262 requirements.

" **Shang Han Za Bing** (傷寒雜病論), Treaty febrile diseases of Zhang Zhongjing (Year 160): This book explains how a perversity can cross the six "energy layers" of the Organization.

" **Qian Jin Fang** (千金方), prescription worth a thousand pieces of gold of Sun If Miao (late 7th century) in 30 volumes, with a general introduction, varied requirements such as dietetics, the pulsologie, acupuncture, etc.

Chapter 2
A holistic vision
The human body
**CE Chapter has for vocation of "trim" the field. Enter too
quickly in the details might make us lose the immense
scope of this medicine.**
The BODY COMPUTER
Before studying at the magnifying glass the different
elements that underpin the functioning of the body in the
MTC, so let a little back and compare the human body to a
computer. Comparison of as much more easily than we
invented this machine to make up for the inadequacies of our
mental capacities to calculate and store. The Chinese have
the Abacus, we have our kilos bits of data.
In a computer, we have a central memory where are stored
all the data. Software for access and act on this hard drive. A
processor that is behind to direct all this. And a power outlet
for the machine to operate. Finally a battery for that our
computer operates in autonomy. Our organization is quite
comparable to this mode of operation.
The central memory, c is the brain with its billions of
connections and its infinite possibilities which it uses only a
very small part.
The software components
To access this central memory, we have five
software that are the liver, heart, spleen, lung, and
kidney. The term software we arrange here. In
À retenir effect, when we talk of the liver by example, it
must not be immediately see the liver as a physical
body, but the energy that underlies the functioning of this
body. Do not lose sight of the fact that Chinese medicine is
foremost a energy medicine.

19

These five bodies software cannot operate independently of one another. We will see as well that there are specific cycles which link between them these different software and all the art of the diagnosis is to discover the one who has been unbalanced in first.

 The strength of this medicine, which differentiates it from all the others, is to be able to link the appearance of a symptom or an illness must be in

À retenir one of these software five bodies, that this is a physical symptom, mental or emotional. There are no symptoms orphans.

It was thus about 900 symptoms" alarm signals" possible : a headache to such or such place, insomnia, a pain, a nervous condition, etc. Let us repeat: this is not yet a disease, but a symptom in energy first, then physics through the suite that emits the organization. To us, thanks to the knowledge that will follow to learn to recognize, especially not to obscure any of suite and take adequate measures of prevention to regain its balance on its cable of life.

The Chinese medicine is not to treat the Crown of the disease, the symptom, but the cause deep. The symptom will then disappear from itself, having no more reason to be.

The Qi, energy

To operate, this machine has need of energy. The energy, the Qi as we will see in the chapitre 3. To make it short we can split it into two parts:

" An innate energy that the Chinese call "the previous sky";

" Energy acquired, or "the posterior sky".

Each of these energies is divided also in several parties.

The innate energy

As well, energy innate first conducts of the legacy of our ancestors, of the genetic heritage. The MTC goes back as a general rule to three previous generations. Example: If you are from three generations rather brought on the bottle, there are great chances that you héritiez of an energy of the Liver "tense", and therefore of a temperament innate

20

nervous, angry, table that can easily lead later on of the hypertension. However, the Chinese Medicine considers that these are predispositions, and if they are known in time (c was the role of the physician to inform the parents), they are not going to go "back to the surface". The second part is called Ling in Chinese. It takes into account for example of the position of the stars at the time of the birth.

The innate energy is also an energy infinitely more subtle, which will be developed further, namely the soul which will break up at the time of his Incarnation in "spiritual soul," the Hun "housed" in the liver and the soul of the body, the Po, housed in the lung (see chapitre 3).

Le saviez-vous
This innate energy can be compared to an oil lamp (the microprocessor of the computer). This "oil energy" allows us as a human being to live theoretically 120 years. This is our vital potential of birth which wears more or less quickly in the light of the combustion of the wick. There is a direct relationship with our way of life, our physical health and mental health. This small drill has a name in Chinese, it is the "Fire of Ming men". The oil that is the Yuan Qi, the original energy.

The energy gained

This are taken of current that we connect directly to our environment. It can be divided into three parts:

"*The energy of the air* is a direct contact with our environment and in the immediacy, the more vital energies. The Pr Leung Kok Yuen (see chapitre 1) said: "If mit end-to-end, you do not breathe in full conscience throughout the day two to three hundred times, all other practices do not serve almost to nothing. "

"*The energy of the food. Still it is necessary that our food are loaded energetically, and especially that the software Spleen, conductor of the digestion of the food bowl is able to give the right directives to digest this food bowl. One of the causes of depression is a collapse of the energy of the spleen. The Depression promotes the accumulation of food waste in the body.*

"*Emotional energy. We will see later that each emotion affects directly the circulation of blood and energy in the organization.*

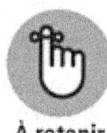

The importance of breathing

The three pillars of the vitality are breathing, power and our mental states and emotional. Our

À retenir Unbalanced emotions can shorten our life expectancy, but this request of months or even years to create not to not a cancer, or throw themselves voluntarily to its cable of life. Stop eating and especially to drink it, we still live a dozen days. Stop to breathe, it is three minutes that it remains for us to live!

The battery of the body

Outside of these "Power Outlets" which makes us live in symbiosis with our environment, our body-computer has a certain autonomy of operation that we can assimilate to a battery. We will see that it is located virtually in the lower abdomen," between the two kidneys". In the West, one begins to understand the importance of the immune defenses. The MTC goes much further.

This battery represents the immense capacity to self-healing of the body, but also its capacity totally unsuspected of adaptation. On the condition of

À retenir course that this battery either daily recharged to its maximum by the practice of the methods Yang Sheng Fa, prevention, that we will see throughout this book.

We can say that, in a certain way, your organization will become its own Referring Doctor:

"

A poison comes to penetrate your food bowl in your stomach? If it is too violent, your

En pratique organization will use one of the seven therapeutic methods available to her, namely the "vomification". You will immediately or in the hours following the reject. If this are poisons at low noise as of pesticides or other chemicals, our organization rejects

22

the following day by the stool. They do not have the time to return to the organization. This is only true if the battery is fully charged. Certainly, it should be the most possible to "eat Own", but we do not control everything. This vision of things allows us to remove some of our fears.

"*An extreme emotion comes to arise on your cable of life.* Your organization must be able to put very quickly in place what is called "the resilience", a yoke of lead to avoid that this emotion does disrupts the functioning of your body. In a second time, it the phagocyte permanently, thus avoiding that it does not become "waste emotional" able to resurface at any moment of your life.

How it works?

This is the battery that will be able to send you the "Symptoms alarm signals" when one of the five software begins to be unbalanced.

In the event of abrupt climate change, in the epidemic periods, it will give orders adequate to protect you from all attacks say external.

We will see that each emotion is to put in a relationship with a component software specific. The emotion the more devastating to which we are faced is the fear. It "draining" literally the battery. It also plays a role of magnet: it draws the object of our own fear. The battery recharged to block, the emotions are regulated and the fear disappears.

This battery daily recharged allows us not to draw in our ancestral oil. We avoid as well of aging early. It is the great teaching of the MTC as to the durability and the fact to be able to die at an age certain "in good health".

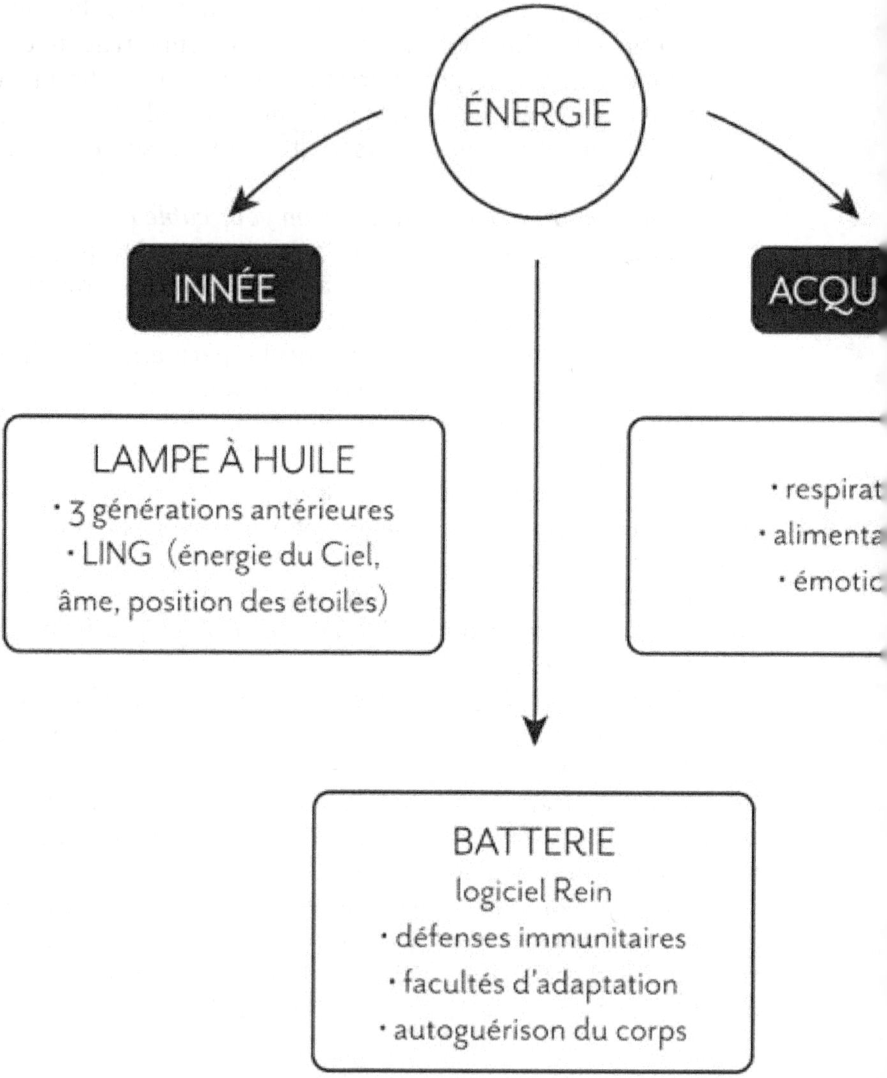

ÉNERGIE

INNÉE

ACQU

LAMPE À HUILE
· 3 générations antérieures
· LING (énergie du Ciel,
âme, position des étoiles)

· respirat
· alimenta
· émotic

BATTERIE
logiciel Rein
· défenses immunitaires
· facultés d'adaptation
· autoguérison du corps

Figure 2-1 The energies of the body.

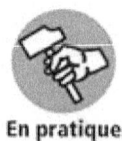

En pratique

He wakes up in the morning at the end of a night more or less remedial. Nobody has obliged to run: his mental energy is there and the aid to recharge its battery. He has followed the advice of dietetics (mixture of slow sugars and sugars fast) to give him the fuel. In short, it starts with its "energy of the day". The race begins. It feels strong and powerful. But at the end of a few kilometers, its machine begins to give signs of failure. An alarm signal is issued: fatigue. A wise Taoist would then have taken a little of rest for leave. Impracticable under penalty to become the laughing stock of the flock. It continues. That made his body? It is branch on its battery, not necessarily fully recharged. It feels again in form. But this battery was soon to completely discharge. A large signal of alarm appears: Grosse fatigue. Its Formatting Media, its small daemon slipped her in the hollow of the ear: "continues, bangs-thee, proves that thou art a man my son. "As it is said in some countries " there is no problem. "He continues. But at that time, her organization puts in direct contact with its oil lamp, its essence vital, that which allows him to live more than centenary. Not only this oil runs out, but his energy of the liver, which secretes of endotoxins akin to a drug participates in the following state: the great past fatigue, he will feel a Superman and could continue even after the line of arrival. Yes, but at what price! He just draw unnecessarily in its reserves. He just run... to its loss. A very wise Taoist would not have participated in this race...

The five bodies software

We will examine in detail in chapitre 3 the links of these five "Software organs" with different functions, symptoms or malfunctions. We will here simply knowledge with these bodies.

We have five software bodies, namely those of the liver, heart, spleen-pancreas, of the lung and kidney. A very important Convention: when we are talking about a body, we are talking about the

À retenir energy of this body, energy foregoing let the matter, the structure.

Each component software includes within it two bodies:

"*A body "full", that we call Yin body. It is he who, as a vital organ, will be reached last in the evolution of a pathology. We cannot live without heart, liver, Rate-Pancréas, kidney, lung. And if a pathology comes to directly reach one of these bodies, it can become very quickly a deadly pathology.*

"*A body "hollow,", Stacker, which in the light of the body Yin will be called Yang. "The Yang protects the Yin": it has the role of protecting the body Yin vital. And it is he who will be at the source of the first symptoms alarm signals. A special feature: you can remove all or part of this body as the gall bladder, stomach, bladder... and continue to live.*

What are these bodies? Three couples are easy to remember:

"

The Liver (yin) coupled with the gallbladder (yang);

À retenir **" The spleen-pancreas (yin) coupled with the stomach (yang);**

" The Kidney (yin) coupled with the bladder (yang).

It is appropriate to make an effort of memorization with the two other software components that are:

"*The Lung (yin) coupled with the large intestine (yang): as well for the problems of constipation, we will be brought to take points on the meridian of the lung, the reverse is equally true.*

"*The Heart (yin) is coupled to the small intestine (yang). It is said that the energy of the small intestine is leading the "Track of the waters". A lack of the energy of the heart to easily lead to a PAO, an acute edema of the lung.*

For the moment, we are at ten organs. However, the energy of the heart is regarded as the master of the organs, the Heart Emperor. If your heart stops beating, you will die. It is he who must have a maximum of protections. He will have two bodies of additional protection, not having real anatomical media. It is located here on a purely energy. This are:

"*The pericardium, still called the constrictor of the Heart (avoid the call as it is too often the master heart, because the heart does not have a master), which will be the side yin.*

" *The three households, considered as a body of energy in whole share which is the side Yang. We will come back to in the* chapitre 3.

We are therefore in the presence of 12 bodies, six bodies Yin and six bodies Yang. These 12 bodies such as we are now going to see are put in relationship with the surface of the body through the system of meridians.

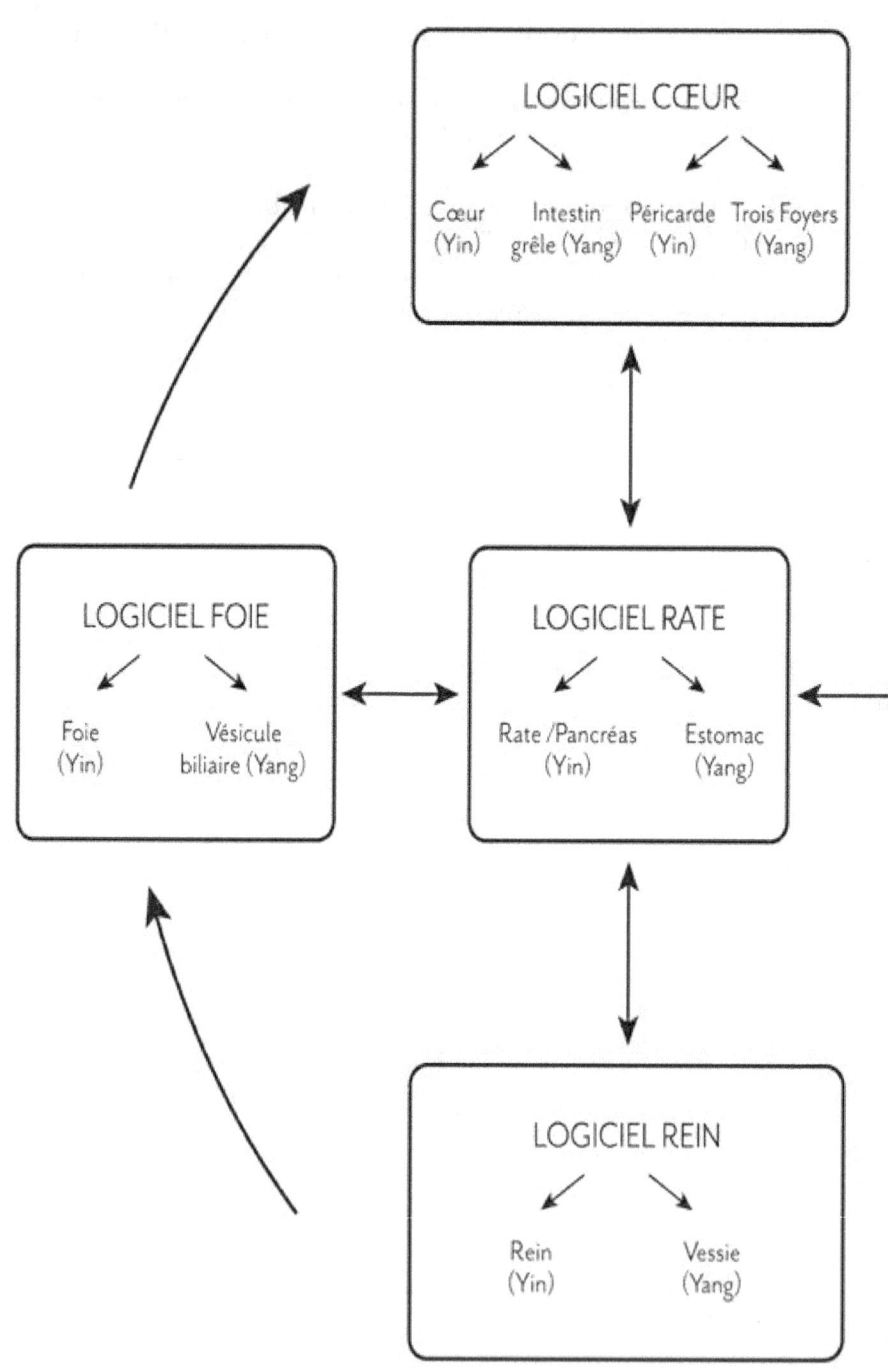

Figure 2-2 The five software bodies.

The concept of the meridians

It is the flagship of the Chinese medicine. It is of journeys, of channels where flows an energy very subtle well beyond the materiality. Our master insisted on the fact that no device, no detector had the possibility of the highlight. It cannot measure while a potential difference, coarse aspect of the energy.

From where the energy?

It is a mixture very subtle between the quintessence of the energy of the air and the quintessence of energy in the digestion of food bowl. The aspect "rude" of this mixture is represented by the atom of oxygen (air) which is fixed on the Globule rouge (supply) to give the hemoglobin, which allows the transport of energy in the body. We stand here in below, at the level of the pure energy, which circulates therefore in the meridians.

What is the role of a Meridian?

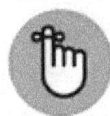

Put the relationship between the surface of the body with the internal organs. Given that there are 12 bodies fundamental energy, we will have 12 meridians:

À retenir

"Six meridians at the level of the Legs (three meridians Yin and three meridians Yang);

"Six meridians at the level of the arm (Three Yin and three Yang).

In the chapter on the acupuncture, you will have a mnemonic unstoppable to learn how to retain without difficulty the journey of 12 meridians In a few minutes.

There is a symmetry axis in the body supported by the vertebral column: the meridians will be double compared to this axis. We will thus have two meridians of the large intestine, the heart, the stomach, etc. These meridians form a continuous cycle. They are driven by wells, nodes, energy concentrations: this are the famous points of acupuncture or digitoponcture. I refer you to the chapters on acupuncture and digitoponcture (see chapters 13 and 14).

There are two other meridians which will be very useful in our treatments: It is the vessel of design or REN May and the vessel governor or the May. These meridians thanks to their specific points are directly related to the six bodies Yin and six bodies Yang and by that same to 12 meridians of the body. Located on the median axis anterior and posterior of the trunk, they will be unique. As well we will have a single point 4WD or 14DM.

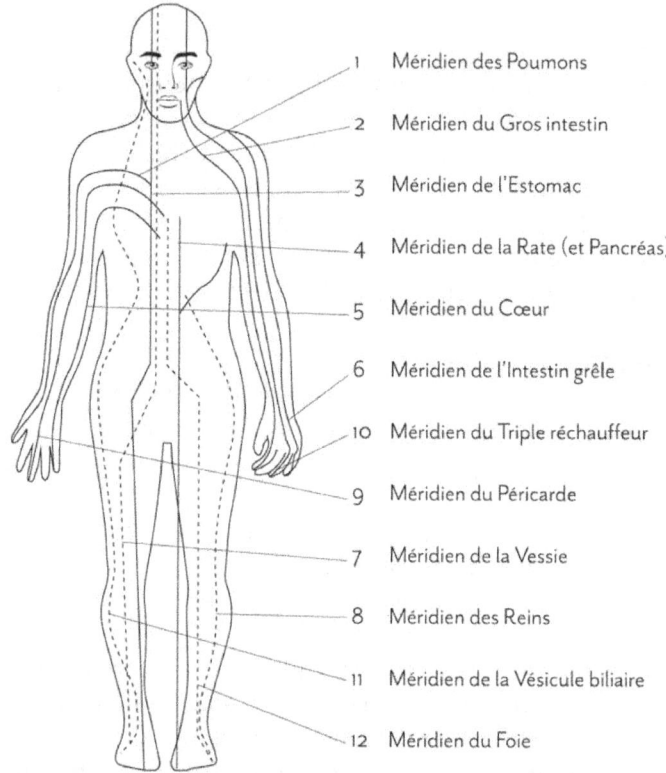

1	Méridien des Poumons
2	Méridien du Gros intestin
3	Méridien de l'Estomac
4	Méridien de la Rate (et Pancréas)
5	Méridien du Cœur
6	Méridien de l'Intestin grêle
10	Méridien du Triple réchauffeur
9	Méridien du Péricarde
7	Méridien de la Vessie
8	Méridien des Reins
11	Méridien de la Vésicule biliaire
12	Méridien du Foie

Figure 2-3 The 12 systems meridians.

The theory of the meridians

The meridians, their action and their localization are the result of thousands of years of observation and experience. Of our days, despite all the research, the nature of these meridians and the mode of transmission of the energy of the external to the internal and vice versa still remains a mystery. But it works! It should be the study in their practical applications, through their relationship with the organs and their interest in pathology.

The system of the meridians

The system of the meridians consists of two lanes of traffic fundamental:
" The main traffic routes called Jing;
" The Luo, vessels linking the Jing between them and the vessels used to "capillaries" for the main meridians.
They form a seamless network that reaches all parts of the body. Among them, 12 Jing main which are to put with the 12 bodies are the most important.
The names of the meridians are derivatives of the old divisions of the Yin-Yang. The wise, since antiquity, have observed the interference between the Yin and the Yang. They have distinguished in any evolution three phases Yin and three phases Yang called successively Shao Yin, Tai Yin, Jue Yin and Shao Yang Yang Ming and Tai Yang.

 They observed that the Jing ranging from hands toward the trunk are yang. Those who are going in the opposite direction are Yin. On the contrary, on

À retenir the lower limbs the meridians Yin depart the feet and join the chest while the meridians Yang depart from the head and join the feet.
The meridians Yin correspond to the solid organs, vital and the meridians Yang to hollow organs, receptacles.
It has six meridians at the level of hand (lung, large intestine, heart, small intestine, pericardium, three homes) and six meridians at the level of the feet (kidney, bladder, spleen, stomach, liver, gallbladder).

Classification of meridians

We have:

The meridians Jing
" 12 meridians Jing, the Jing May, between the OS and the muscle very in depth.

"12 Jing IBE, internal branches of Jing, leading toward the inside of the body and the different organs.

"8 Jing "individuals," or Qi Jing Ba may, in relation more random with the Jing Main.

"15 Luo vessels linking between them the Jing main which are divided into superficial Luo crossing the members and the body transversely to feed the tissues and the Luo capillaries, tiny vessels forming a complete network through the entire body.

"This network very complex is in connection with the internal, 12 bodies which are at the origin of the Jing May by 12 Jing Jin or 12 meridians tendino-muscle and with the external, the skin areas or Pi Bu.

We should remember the essential point:

Table 2-1 The 12 main meridians.

Zu Tai Yang or meridian of bladder	Shou Tai Yang or meridian of the small intestine
Zu Shao Yang or meridian of V.B.	Shou Shao Yang or meridian of three households
Zu Yang Ming or meridian of bladder	Shou Yang Ming or meridian of large intestine
Zu Tai yin or meridian of spleen	Shou Tai yin or meridian of the lung
Zu Shao or meridian Yin of kidney	Shou Shao yin or meridian of Heart
Zu Jue yin or meridian of liver	Shou Jue yin or meridian of the Pericardium

Table 2-2 The eight meridians individuals.

Ren May, vessel design	Governs the Yin and the blood
The May, vessel Governor	Governs the meridians Yang
Chong May, vital vessel	Sea of 12 meridians. Governs

	the blood
Dai May, vessel of Belt	Connects all the meridians of the trunk
Yang Wei May, relative to the Yang	Governs the protection
Yin Wei May, relative to the Yin	Governs the emotions, connects the Yin
Yang Qiao May, relative to the Yang	Control neuromuscular chains Yin
Yin Qiao May, Movement Yin	Control neuromuscular chains Yang

The 12 main meridians, as well as the vessels Governor and design have their own points. It brings them together under the name: "The fourteen meridians". The other six meridians do not have own points. They borrow their points to the fourteen meridians.

The Circadian Cycle

The circulation of the flow of energy through the meridians undergoes a tidal phenomenon in the course of 24 hours of the day. This characteristic is sometimes used in the treatment of diseases rebels. Each meridian undergoes an intensification of energy flow which lasts two hours. This can be used in the diagnosis. For example heart disease usually gets worse toward noon, those of the lungs before dawn...

The movement begins at the meridian of the diaphragm, then it was successively P - IM

- E - RTE - C - IG - V - R - MC - tr - VB - F - p.

Table 2-3 slots.

LUNG	3-5 hours
Large intestine	5-7 hours
STOMACH	7-9 hours
Rate-Pancréas	9-11 hours

Heart	11-13 hours
Small intestine	13-15 hours
BLADDER	15-17 hours
KIDNEY	17-19 hours
Pericardium	19-21 hours
Three households	21-23 hours
Gallbladder	23-1 hour
LIVER	1-3 hours

If your practitioner gives you rendez-vous at 3 hours of the morning to treat your liver, beware when same. It is a little seedy…

Attention

The acupuncture points

And what is there on the journey of the meridians? The famous acupuncture points. In the antiquity, they were all of the names highly symbolic explaining their properties and characteristics. Of our days, it was assigned numbers to the points, and this, taking into account the direction of the circulation of energy in each meridian.

In the classical texts, the total number of points was 365. Of our days, it adds very many points expressed outside meridian, which greatly increases the number. But the return to the Uniqueness is required. Is it not said that well chosen, and especially well pitted or Massé, a single point is sufficient to treat a patient?

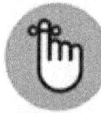

In reality, a 60 points are largely enough to treat and prevent a few pathologies that this either. We will come back to in the chapter on the acupuncture (see chapitre 13).

À retenir

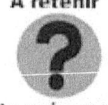

Le saviez-vous

What is a point?

Called Xue Wei, c is the place where the practitioner plant its needle, mass or heat with a stick of sagebrush. We can consider that it is a place of poses in a continual flow of energy. It is a place where converges and emerges the energy.

And as we are microcosm in the macrocosm which surrounds us, these are the same characteristics of the point that you will find in the Feng Shui. These points allow therefore to harmonize the energy. A beautiful definition of Cyrille Javary, in the speech of the Turtle (Albin Michel, 2003): " It is a place of exchange subtle does not exist by itself. It is as Station Exchange, a little in the manner of the eyes in a network of pipes, in the framework of a mesh vectorized by the flow of the breath-energy to the inside of the human body. "

The three strata of energy

Comparable to a water pipe in a building, where the big arrivals at high pressure are located in depth, to reduce then to the water that comes out of the TAP, we have three levels of energy circuit on the surface of our Organization:

"

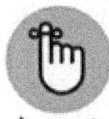

À retenir

The Meridien to strictly speaking, the big energy pipe, located very in depth between the OS and the muscle. It is one of the reasons for which the acupuncturist uses very thin needles to act on the points located on this "LED".

" *A medium level, between the flesh and the muscle. What are the ramifications of the principal meridian, pipes much smaller that are accessible by the digitoponcture (see* chapitre 14*), or the spot massage deep.*

" *A superficial level. This are, like the blood vessels, of energy capillaries located on the surface of the skin. There is no more talk of meridians, but of zone Yin or Yang. On the surface of skin, we are witnessing a tangle of the meridians Yin and Yang meridians. We gain access to this area through all the techniques of superficial massage of the body.*

En pratique

It is enough to put themselves in the four legs, hands turned toward the outside. All the hidden areas, located inside (abdomen, chest, internal face of the lower limbs and senior members) are the areas Yin. They are directed toward the inside or toward the earth which is yin. In contrast, the back, the external face of the senior members, where are located the hairs, the face posterior external of the legs are called "zones Yang." These areas are therefore directed toward the outside or toward the sky which is itself of Yang polarity.

A basic axiom in MTC: " The Yang protects the Yin". In the practice of martial arts, when succumbs to the number, one learns to ball and to create a kind of energy armor, by binding all of its muscles. This are the areas Yang who are reached by the blows, among other the DOS, but the side Yin where are the vital organs is preserved, protected. In contrast, a blow on the chest or stomach can be fatal.

Le saviez-vous

The fragility of the human being
While most of the Celestial animals terrestrial or have their side Yang of the body turned toward the sky, their side Yin is toward the earth. We restated, outlining our side Yin, chest-abdomen, where are our 12 vital organs, our organs" thinking "toward the front, open to the other. It is a double-edged sword.

As be emotional, we receive in "full belly" negative emotions of others. But we can also more easily give this same emotional energy to heal another. It is our weakness, but also our strength.

Predict the evolution of a pathology

An internal pathology may not unexpectedly appear, "the knowledge of its voluntarily". When we chutons, receive a shock, we know why we have evil. But before triggering a rheumatism, diabetes, cardiovascular disease, depression, cancer, we have had, several months or even years before very many alarm signals that it will agree not to conceal.

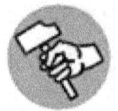
En pratique

The MTC will allow us to predict the evolution of a pathology through knowledge of these symptoms.

In an ideal case, a pathology will begin to issue these signals:
" On the meridian Yin or Yang at the opposite of the component concerned. For example a Breast cancer linked to emotional blockages, doing stagnate energy at the level of the liver, will begin on the left breast external side, where passes the meridian of the gallbladder.
" On the meridian Yang before the meridian Yin (Yang protects the Yin). When a meridian Yang is reached, the symptom appears rather at the top of the body, side Sky, Yang for progress then toward the bottom of the body, on the land side, yin. This will be the reverse for the meridians Yin.

If we do not change anything to our habits of life, the pathology will progress and achieve the body Yang that protects the body Yin.

Finally, it is only in the last place that the body Yin, vital, is reached.

Chapter 3
The major concepts
Of Medicine
Chinese Traditional
In this chapter:
" The concept of the Yin-Yang
" The Qi, energy
" The Great Hun-Po triad-Shen
" The three households, San Jiao

NOu will see that in MTC, each element of the nature is to be put in relation with a software component.

The doctor Chinese: a detective in power or history of a simple fungus

For example, the energy of the Rate-Pancréas is to put in relationship with the earth. In nature, when the Earth is hot and humid, there is multiplication of small creatures and manufacturing of manure. In our organization, we are seeing the same phenomenon. It is said: "The Spleen hates the moisture". What are the factors that promote this state: the excess of rapid sugars, saturated fat, milk, butter, cheese, beverages, exposure to the external moisture and..., the excess of the thoughts and reflections! All causes, when this state installs in the body, it will "export" to distance of symptoms alarm signals. On the foot of a patient, we observe "mushrooms" under the nail of the big toe. We will see that the yin meridians of the liver and spleen begin at this level. We anticipate a problem related to the moisture. It is looking for a few additional indices (brand teeth on a thick language, weight gain by the retention of liquids, Menton darker than the rest of the face, etc.). The diagnosis is made: excess moisture at the level of the spleen. If the practitioner has not this profound vision of the symptom, it prescribes an antifungal (or, anecdotiquement, a special varnished to hide the mycosis). We just to conceal a symptom alarm signal. The patient is released in the nature and persists in its imbalances, in the absence of having been "educated". The pathology will move toward the internal Of Month to Month: vaginal secretions White, sensation of heaviness, fatigue, lack of taste, presence of pinworms, Anal itching, etc.

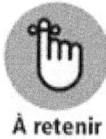

À retenir

If it does that deal with these various symptoms, the pathologies will eventually reach the stomach (component Yang) and last the pancreas (component Yin) vital. Then settled gradually the different stages of diabetes, and in the case ultimate, pancreatitis or cancer of the pancreas. With the knowledge and the practical implementation of the methods of prevention, all of this could have been avoided!

The concept of the Yin-Yang

What the Yin-Yang is not!

Attention

The Yin-Yang is not summarized especially not, as we have seen too often in two lists that face where we will see a white side, the other black, yes-no, top-down, etc. This type of risk vision to make us believe that the MTC is Manichean. The yes or no well disposed of our language does not exist in the Chinese vision. The ideogram means "Yes, But..." or "No, but...".

Attempted definition

Outcome of the One, of Tai Ji, c is the duality which is the basis of all possible aspects of life, such that we grasp. A concept, whatever it may be, cannot exist without that its complementary opposite does not exist. Thus, it could not know that the day exists if the night do it, was not associated. The yes without the non, the top without the bottom, the man without the woman, the love without hatred... we could make to the Prévert throughout the remainder of this book.

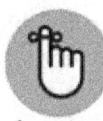

À retenir

One of the major features of this duality is the ability to be at the same time in opposition (while knowing that each of them carries in himself the germ of the other), in interdependence (one could not conceive without the other) and in a relationship of begetting (the night leaves little by little the place in the day).

The origins of the concept

We have seen that the **Nei Jing,** medical book by excellence, was old of 2 500 years (see chapitre 1). But, it is necessary to know that before the **Nei Jing, 2 500 years before, existed the Yi Jing, i.e. there are 5 000 years. This book is the foundation, the beginning of the whole of the Chinese culture. The Yi Jing** processes before any of the astrology, the cosmogony, of what is happening between the sky and the earth. But also of Feng Shui, of biology and of Medicine. This is the part which is recovery in the **Nei Jing.**

In the **Yi Jing, there is this fundamental sentence which is divided into three parts: "Tai Ji is the source of the two opposed who are themselves the source of the four phenomena, which generate the eight Gua, Ba Gua. "**

The head to the Toward

Le saviez-vous

It is fundamental to appreciate the differences that exist between the Chinese Thought and The Western thought. If we take for example the writing, it is done from the left to the right for the westerners, while in China, she makes the right to the left. That is why the orients, points of guidance are different. In the West, the east is to the right, the west to the left, the North at the top and the south at the bottom. While in China, the West will be on the right, the is to the left, the North at the bottom and the south at the top. If you do not know these differences, it can make serious errors of interpretation of ancient texts.

If we take the case of the man. The man lives between the sky and the earth. Since its birth, it will observe above his head the sky and below him, he will see the earth. The light and the darkness, the sky and the earth, in Chinese Thought represent two opposed and are supposed to be contained in any thing. We are witnessing here in the elaboration of the concept of the Yin-Yang. At the beginning of the day, we see that the sky is clear. As the sun disappears, the sky darkens, the sun declines. At sunset, the universe is plunged in darkness. The moon rises in the sky dark and the man realized that the sun is really the source of light.

Furthermore, we can see that the sun is at the origin of the appearance of the shadow. If we take the example of a tree, when the sun darde its rays, the tree produces a shadow. The night after the sunset, it can also be observed that the moon spreads a light and that it can also project a slight shadow. But it is obvious that the Moon is much less luminous than the sun and the one often sees the clouds go before it and the obscure.

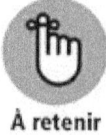

40

À retenir

All these phenomena are used to understand that Tai Ji, one, the vacuum is at the origin of the duality. Between the sky and the earth, there was nothing, then the two opposed have emerged. The first is called Yang, which is therefore the light that spreading the sun and that illuminates the earth. The night belongs to the Yin. These contrasting phenomena, this opposition is called Yin-Yang. Where the first sentence: "The A PRODUCT Two. "

The Tai Ji, the A encloses in him all the possibilities

To make it simple, the Tai Ji, the A encloses in him all the possibilities of achievement.

"To the left, "the comma Yang," it is the vitality under the emblem of the fire, the rise, acceleration, the functions that generate heat, the extroversion, the male principle, the centrifugal force. Symbolically, it is represented by a continuous line: _____

"To the right, the Yin He represents the vitality under the emblem of the water: it is the descent, the introversion, the slowdown, the Feminine Principle, the centripetal force. It is represented by a dashed line: __ __ __ __

However, as nothing is all white or all black, in part Yang, we will have a small sphere Yin and vice versa the side Yin where we will have a little bit of Yang. If such was not the case, everything would be set on this earth.

A track of Meditation: What is the time?

Before the birth, there is no time, even after death. In humans, we can say that the time appears only **En pratique** at the time of the first cell division, the first duality, within the matrix. The time exists because there is a before and an after. By convention, which is before will be called Yin and which is after, Yang. However, as there is a little bit of Yang in the Yin and a little Yin in the Yang, this makes the time "flexible": a minute can seem to us eternity and vice versa.

Is there a non-time in our earthly life? Neurobiologists define the time as a permanent succession of thoughts. But they cannot overlap. Between two thoughts, there are a few milliseconds. The meditators confirmed try to increase this time between two thoughts: it is the non-time. And if they arrive to enter in the breach, c is the awakening.

Do not get lost in the maze of the Yin-Yang

To force to make excessive work our left brain, to classify in the extreme, Lister, we do not understand that the same concept can be sometimes Yin, sometimes Yang. Everything is a question of referent and refer, from the point of view which it is located. As well, we will say that all Chinese teas are Yin, since they come from the earth. But if it is attached to the study of the different categories, green teas, Oolong or black, we will say that the black tea is Yang in the light of the green tea that will be rather Yin.

In the texts, it is said that "The Yin pure, and the pure Yang are not part of the field of the realization". It is said when the Yin becomes extreme, it transforms into Yang: When you tap an ice cube (yin), it eventually you burn your fingers (yang).

Le saviez-vous

Why do we say yin-yang AND NOT Yang-yin? It is said that everything begins with a time Yin. The first demonstration at the output of the womb of our mother, it is the inspiration that is characterized by the return, a centripetal force, a concentration of air to the interior. It is an act of Yin. The opposite will occur elsewhere at the time of the Passage. It is the last expiry, the leak of the Yang.

The Qi, energy

The Qi, energy, is the basis of the understanding of the MTC. Nothing in the organization could not operate if there was not this energy underlying it. In studying the ideogram that defines, we may already have a profound vision as to its meaning:

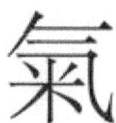

It breaks down into three parts: top, the aroma, steam, in the middle, the processing and in the bottom a bunch of rice. This character therefore presents a vapor escaping from a cereal that cooked.

Where it comes from?

In the human body, the Qi which maintains the vitality is called Zhen Qi, the original Qi, the original energy. It comes from the energy which we inherit (one goes back to the three previous generations), but also of the energy of the sky and the earth, called Ling Qi. As soon as the birth, these two energies are an innate capital which will be housed in the kidney. This energy capital is then called the Yuan Qi, the fundamental Qi, the qi of start in life (what we called the "oil lamp" earlier).

After the design, the lungs begin to breathe. We receive the energy of the air, the air of heaven called Yang Qi. We also need the energy of food. In Chinese we are talking about Shui Gu, term meaning "the water and cereals". This is the energy of the spleen, which has the function to absorb the essence of food, called Ku Qi. The Yang Qi of the air and the Ku Qi blend to form Zhong Qi, the IQ of the Center still called Qi of the average household.

How foods are transformed-they energy?

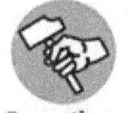 The transformation of the Qi of cereals is done under the Action réchauffante of Yuan Qi stored in the kidney. This fire warming is called fire of Ming

En pratique Men (The small flame of the oil lamp). It is the presence of this fire which triggers the action of the spleen (a digestion begins to 38 degrees!!!). We could compare this to the nightlight of a boiler. From there, the rate begins to transform the food bowl in Ku Qi for the send to the lung. It is at this place that Ku Qi, the energy of the food and the IQ of the air assemble to form Zhong Qi.

What is the energy right?

When the Zhong Qi unites the Yuan Qi, the Qi fundamental, it is going to form the Zhen Qi, the right energy, the energy of defense. This energy will reach all areas of the organization, even the most remote areas. It crosses all Organs and meridians and their ramifications. It has as remarkable property to be permanently renewed, because it dissipates continuously in the body. That is why we regularly hunger and thirst and all the time need to breathe.

One aspect more equipment that energy has found in the famous white blood cells that protect the body and we find in all regions of the body.

It must be continuously that the Organization has at its disposal a sufficient quantity of energy right, Zhen Qi. That which is not used any of suite is put in reserve in the kidney (battery of the body). It is then called Jing Qi which is the surplus of Zhen Qi, energy right. Do not forget: we are here in the pure Energy!

What are the most important organs in the production of the Qi?

The Qi comes mainly the software kidney, spleen and lung, the share the most important being ensured by the kidney. In effect, they contain two energies, the Yuan Qi innate and the Jing Qi acquis (what the Chinese call "energy of the previous Sky" and "energy of the Posterior sky").

We will come back on this concept of IQ in the study of the "three homes," later in this chapter.

The great Hun-Po triad-Shen

Spiritualité

The MTC Tire Any its consistency in the existence of a concept beyond the energy, that we can qualify of soul and escapes from our spirit materialistic Western.

We have previously seen that the duality was inherent to life. But that before life and after the passage, we come from and go back to the Uniqueness. The soul is no exception to this rule. When it will "incarnate," it will become vidual fee. We will have as well a soul called "spiritual" or "Ethereal," called Hun and a soul" "Body which will take the name of Po. These two immaterial entities are going to be the "performers" of the VITALITY still called Shen Ming. However, in our time the so-called "modern", it is totally abstraction of these entities. It is a little as if it viewed a film on the big screen. It dissects the images, we think that what one sees is the reality and we do not think that there is a

44

projector by-behind and that before, a Camera has filmed these taken of views. And what about the producer!

The Pr Leung said: "the Hun is the Heavenly principle, heavenly vocation and the Po is the Heavenly principle, to terrestrial vocation. "

The spiritual soul, the Hun

From a medical point of view, it is an entity immaterial which originates in the universe. This is the side intuitive and non-rational of the human nature.

It has no color, no shape, not flavor. It is invisible. It has no link with the matter. To this title, *it assimilates in the Yang.*

It is said that *the Hun is housed in the liver, and* more specifically in the layer of the Yin of the liver.

À retenir

It will play a very important role in the maintenance of our emotional balance, provided that the energy of the liver is well regulated. If for example the layer Yin of the liver is in inadequate, that it does not receive enough blood, it is said that the Hun loses its remains and can be put to wander without purpose. It is a great cause of insomnia where dreams are very numerous.

"If the blood comes to stagnate at the level of the liver, there is what is called a hindrance to the movement of coming and going of the Hun: the person loses its ability to plan, it becomes disoriented. This is the open door to the Depression.

"If, on the contrary, the Yang of the liver is in excess, there is a hyperactivity of the Hun which gives too much information to the heart, the shen. The latter becomes hyperactive. This is at the origin of very many pathologies mental and emotional, as autism, bipolarity, the behavioral disorders and in line of sight Alzheimer's disease, called a half-DEATH IN MTC: the Hun, the spiritual soul, detaches from the body.

It exists independently of the Spirit. It is the depositary of the ideas, the aspirations, creativity, dreams of life, intuitions. The soul knows everything: is it not said "Be listening to his soul".

The spiritual soul does not think, but it feels and she knows.

45

It is the Hun who will be at the origin of the creation of the Spirit, the shen, the ego, the cognitive faculties, the emotions.

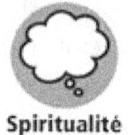

Be listening to his soul

When the body is in perfect harmony, when the Shen, the spirit, our conscious does not permanently the front of the stage, when we are not in "excess of Thoughts", then the Hun can prove to us in the form of dreams, intuition, "psychic glitters". One of the main purposes of the methods Yang Sheng Fa, preservation of life in MTC is to put to rest our Shen, the Spirit, to allow our soul to express themselves. And the purpose of the full conscience is to listen on the whisper" of the soul".

The soul from the body, the po

Po refers to that which exists before the life. It is the support of the living matter. It is something that is not observable.

It is the center of all the automatic functions of the body, "everything that is happening without the knowledge of our voluntarily". It also allows the passage of a step to the other and to create new structures of the body. If we remove the half of the liver, it is the PO which the aid to "push". It is him which also governs the stem cells.

It has under its dependence all primary instincts, suction, swallowing, but also the instinct of conservation.

It is the part of the soul which is inseparably attached to the body and returns to the earth (Yin in the light of the sky which is yang) after death. It is in this that it will have the polarity Yin in face of the Hun which is yang.

In the tradition, it is said that the body soul enters the body three days after the design, while the hun just take place in his house at the time of the rupture of the umbilical cord.

It is similar to a computer program conveyed by the genetic code. If we take the example of a camera, when the film is imaged, we get a negative that, if it is not drawn on paper, does not give a faithful image of the subject. It is a potential image, an image become.

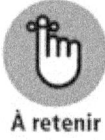

The Po is under the emblem of the lung, this means that the fundamental disorders of the lung will spill on the Po in its vocation in lead the Jing, gasoline.

The skin is therefore part of the software lung by MTC. When emotional tensions affect the lung, such as an excess of sadness, dermatitis "psychosomatic" may appear.

" When the diaphragm is deficient, we say that the Po is poorer. The individual loses his instinct for conservation. The melancholy installs as a bereavement which is never ended. It is the depression and self-destruction which is at the end of the path.

" If it is the PO which takes the governance of the body, it goes any implement for that it returns the more quickly to the earth. It is the explosion of autoimmune diseases, of self-destruction (cancer, rheumatism, diabetes, mental illness and emotional, etc.) which all sign a shortening of the life expectancy.

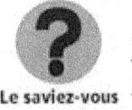

Le saviez-vous

"The breathing is the heartbeat of the po"

The breathing is directly linked to the lung. All meditations which consist to concentrate on the respiration soothe the Po. The Shen, The Spirit becomes quiet and empty. The Hun, the soul ethereal can open and enter in contact with the universal soul.

The spirit, the mind, the shen

The Shen, the Spirit, has an innate part. If you are born of three generations of alcoholics, as all our bodies are thinking people, there are great chances that you have a temperament angry. But it is before any fed continuously by the Hun, the spiritual soul. And as the Hun is housed in the liver, it is said that the "liver is the origin of the emotions and the Heart governs emotions".

The Shen, the spirit and the mental activities are in relationship with the Yang. The heart is said Yang in the Yang.

It includes the innate intelligence, feelings, affectivity, the attraction-repulsion and the innate character. In effect as soon as the birth, we have in us a intelligence, affectivity and a character.

47

Then this Shen will combine the knowledge gained to train our conscience called yi shi in Chinese. When the heart is in contact with an external element, it generates an activity called "thought". And it is this mental activity which will cause an emotion.

The Shen, the spirit manages the receipt of information and the setting in memory. But also the thought, the reflection and the decision. It is in direct relation with our conscience.

À retenir

The Shen is the master of all the emotions. Each emotional excess will therefore be able to touch the spirit.

The "excess of fatigue desire the heart, and by that even the Shen.

"If they are studying and if we think in a reasonable manner and moderate, c is the heart and the Shen who benefit. In contrast, an influx of information eventually injure the Shen.

"It is said when the Yang escapes from the heart (The Shen), the man loses his lucidity. It is also a cause of Alzheimer Disease. But before arriving at this end, there will be many symptoms before-runners. The grand symptom of exhaust of the Yang is the excess of thoughts, therefore the insomnia.

Where is there the Shen? Before everything in the eyes. If these are fixed, if they have lost their mobility (as in a depression), we say that the person has lost his Shen. Similarly, if the complexion of his face is dull or if the movements of the body are slow.

"If it is led by the daemon on the heart, we risk to continue to act in a way aberrant, and deplete our Jing Shen, our vitality, even as our physical force. Our health are then ruin because of this.

Spiritualité

This is the reason for which he must do the exercises often to calm the Shen of the heart so that it is not driven by a demon. As well our spirit in general, our Jing Shen will not be exhausted" (Pr Leung Kok Yuen).

To summarize

Sinking the nail, because all its concepts are fundamental.

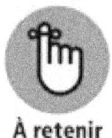

À retenir

The embryo is therefore composed of two entities, the Hun and the Po. The Hun is the Yang original. He is the bearer" of the virtues of the Ancestors", of the innate intelligence.

After the birth, thanks among other things to the education and the experience data by the eyes and ears, we are going to have the training of Shen, of the Spirit. The Po is the yin original. It is the support equipment, the shape of the future man. After the birth, thanks to the food ingested and the air breathed by the nose and mouth and the Po becomes the Jing, gasoline.

The Jing, gasoline, the battery, governs the software five bodies, the three homes, the meridians, blood vessels, and foster liquids. Then, the meeting of the Shen, of the spirit and the Jing, the essence form what is called Zhen Qi, the true energy. This is the energy the body needs to ensure all its functions. Here is the impact of the mind, the emotions on the functioning of the organs.

The example of the spark plug

En pratique

"**The Po, c is the organic matter, the raw material which has served to shape this candle: C is the wax.**

"**The Hun corresponds to the flame, which is yang as the "Fire From Heaven".**

"**The most important part of the spark plug is the point of combustion, the junction between the Hun and the Po. If there is not the candle wax, the flame may not appear. The Hun has need of a anatomical support, the Po, to express themselves, to incarnate.**

"**The Shen, the spirit corresponds to the light, to smoke, which is reached by this flame. That is what we have called Shen Qi, the manifestation of the Spirit.**

"**The Jing, gasoline is the summit of this candle, the point of combustion.**

"**The current of hot air that identifies this flame will be the Qi, energy which contains a force of ascension, expansion.**

The San Jiao, the three homes and The Three Treasures

It is also one of the essential concepts when we want to understand the MTC. The Taoists The also call the Three

Treasures, San Bao. These are the three fundamental components of our being that only can work together.

We are therefore in the presence of three entities:
" The Jing, the petrol;
" The Qi, energy;
À retenir " The Shen, the Spirit.

The Shen covers the thought, but also the desires and emotions, two complementary entities which derive from the sense organs. The development of this sixth sense will not be able to do that thanks to specific exercises of meditation. The reaction in return will be the emergence of emotions that are an integral part of the Shen. Therefore, these three functions, thoughts, desires and emotions are the three parts of the Shen, of the Spirit.

? The Sixth Sense

Le saviez-vous There are five senses: hearing, smell, touch, the view and taste. The "sixth sense" is the intellection, the intuitive perception of ideas.

The Jing, gasoline, covers three entities: the protection, nutrition and the evacuation.

This division into three parts follows what is called the three households, San Jiao, The Home Top, Middle, and bottom.

" *The Upper Home contains the software lung that has under its dependence the two lungs, but also the skin.* To this title, the upper home is considered as the first barrier of Defense of the body. This is the part that is protective of the Jing. It controls the reception. It absorbs the energy of the air by the lungs and the mixture to the energy of the earth which originates in the stomach. Its control point in acupuncture is the 17RM, Dan Zhong between the two nipples.

" *The average home contains the spleen-pancreas, stomach, liver and gallbladder.* The primary role of this home is the transformation of the food bowl and nutrition of the body. It crushes, mixes the food in order to allow the digestion. Its control point is the 25E, Tian Shu, on each side of the navel.

" *The Lower furnace that contains mainly the kidney is responsible among other things for the Elimination.* It controls the separation of liquids and solids. **"It separates what is clear and what is** "disorder (Nei Jing). The water will go in the bladder and the "solid" in the small intestine. To adjust this home, it uses the 6RM, Qi Hai.

The Qi, energy, is the engine of the synthesis, the circulation of blood and energy, adaptation, of assimilation, the reproduction and the elimination.

The synthesis to the elimination, it exists for this a generic term: The metabolism. The metabolism sub-hears two concepts, that of the renewal and elimination. One does not go without the other.

We have said that the Qi also had under its cut the adaptation as well the adaptation to the external environment as to the different variations of the indoor environment. All these activities of synthesis, movement, assimilation, adaptation must be transmitted to subsequent generations. The role of the Qi, the Zhen Qi is precisely to transmit life to the next generation. Zhen Qi, the true energy is therefore also the maintenance of the life.

The three homes and Digestion

Home makes us think of a flame. There is the flame of the lower furnace, the fire of Ming Men, the flame of the "Lamp of ALADIN". This flame will turn on the average home: the digestion is only done to 38 degrees. The problem is that this heat will trigger a evaporation, because all foods are wet. It is necessary that the upper home illuminates, where we would end up by s flood in our Liquid: when it expires, even in summer, it is damp heat.

The Ba Gang, or the "eight rules"

It is the classification of diseases according to specific criteria which will be that no disruption may not remain misunderstood in Chinese medicine. This classification goes even further than that. It allows, a little as in the famous table Mendeleev, where there were empty boxes and where we knew that sooner or later we would find out the name of a new element, to understand that no symptom, no disease can long remain unknown. It will inevitably its location in one of these boxes.

When the AIDS has emerged, as will appear later many other diseases, the passage in the sieve of these Ba Gang, has helped to know the origin, but also and especially its evolution and its methods of prevention, and why not curative.

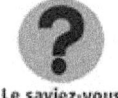

The principle of these eight classifications is a direct application of the theory of the Yin-Yang. It is the tool which allows to distinguish the symptoms, to recognize the pulse and apply methods of treatment.

It is by classifying the signs and symptoms that can decide on the nature of a disease. In effect, when we are in the presence of a symptom or an illness, it can for example be the consequence:

"A Yin excessive or of a Yang excessive, that is to say an imbalance of the Yin and the Yang. Therefore a syndrome may be either Yin or Yang.

"Original internal or external (LI or Biao).

"In nature either hot or cold (Han and Re).

"And finally, it may be the consequence of a lack of or excess (XU or Shi).

For example, we will say in such patient that he will have an imbalance of the energy of the spleen, sub-heard a state of weakness and heat. You will learn that the energy of the spleen hates humidity and that things are starting to deteriorate when this moisture is transformed into heat. However, it is a cause most often external (food imbalance), which is gradually transformed into internal cause.

Table 3-1 The ba gang or the "eight rules".

Yin	Yang
Internal, Li	External, Biao
Cold, Han	Hot, Re
Weakness, Xu	Fullness, Shi

Chapter 4
The relations of
The Man and the Universe
In this chapter:
" The Man, inseparable from the Nature
" The five elements, Wu Xing

TheA Chinese medicine, holistic medicine by gasoline, has put in before, since a very long time, the theory called "signatures" to understand what is happening to the inside of our body. Everything that we is external works on the same mode that our interiorité and vice versa. To us to be quite "intuitive" to establish these relationships. A few tracks:

" In the Nei Jing, it is said: "The man, the sky and the earth is similar. "The man is active the day and sleeps the night in the same way that the sun rises in the morning and layer in the evening.

" The life of the man is settled by the four seasons. It undergoes the influence of spring, summer, fall and winter that occur in a cyclic manner.

" It is said in the Nei Jing: "The man cannot evade the natural laws": it is the ancestor of our modern ecology.

The five energies of the sky and the earth
That brings the sky to the man? The energy of the five climates :
" The wind;
" The heat;
" The humidity;
" The drought;
" The cold.

That brings the earth to man? The energy of the five flavors:
" The acid;
" The gentle;
" The Bitter;
" The Spice or the acrid;
" The salted.

The Five Flavors, generic term meaning "all foods" come from the earth: the man the ingest. The five climates of the sky are the foundations of our vitality. We will see that there is a sixth climate according to the Nei Jing, the fire, which is in reality that a transformation in internal to external heat (see chapitre 11).

If the man is in harmony with the five energies of the sky and the earth, it preserves its life.

The sky will produce the sun and fire (Yang original). The earth produces the mountains and the plains, the sea, rivers and the water (Yin original). The Yang descends on the earth (heat of the sun) and the Yin rises toward the sky (evaporation of the water). This movement of ascent and descent product the air: this movement of air is at the origin of the four seasons. In effect, this movement is never identical: it may be soft, warm, fresh, cold. It is said in the Nei Jing that "this movement of air is at the origin of the six phenomena that are wind and thunder, clouds, rain, dew, snow".

The five elements of nature

The combination of the four seasons and the six phenomena will give the different elements of the nature that are:
" The wood;
" The fire;
" The Earth;
" The metal;
" The water.

These five elements represent all the elements which constitute the universe and are used to represent the production, life and death. These five elements are not static. They will evolve according to a cycle which represents the five stages of any evolution:
" The birth;
" The growth;
" The maturation;
" The harvest;
" The conservation.

Each of these five elements knows itself, individually the same steps in its evolution.

These five elements are used to the MTC to systematize all medical knowledge. In effect, the

À retenir

54

man, as we have seen, corresponds to the sky and the earth and will follow the same cycles.

The meaning and emotions at the pace of the nature

The human being also includes a original Yang, the spiritual soul, the Hun and the Po, the soul of the body, the Yin original. It is identical to the sky and the earth. The Hun will produce the Shen, the Spirit, and the PO will produce Jing, gasoline.

The sky had produced the sun and the fire, the Spirit produced the wisdom and emotions.

The Po, the soul body (the earth) Product successively:
" The five solid organs, the Zang;
" The six hollow organs, the FU;
" The three households, San Jiao;
" The meridians, Jing Luo;
" The Foster liquids, Jin Ye.

Everything that is formed by the Meeting of the Spirit (SHEN) and gasoline, Jing form what is called the Qi, energy.

Whereas in the Universe we speak of air and different climates, in the body This corresponds to the energy that it also flows through the whole body and product:
" The view;
" The hearing;
" The smell;
" The taste;
" The touch.

 These different sensory perceptions will produce an effect that will manifest itself to the outside by emotional energies, the "Seven emotions" or "Seven feelings" that are:

À retenir

" The joy;
" The anger;
" The concern;
" The reminiscence;
" The fear;
" Sadness;
" The fear.

The Man therefore has the ability to perceive what surrounds it and therefore of the transform in the form of emotions.

These emotions can be used in a beneficial way or on the contrary to misuse. It is this interaction between receive and produce which is the life of the man.

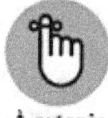

The six the wishes of the MAN

À retenir This are the desires to see the nice things to decorate his house: it is a desire of the view. Others prefer to listen to beautiful music or hear of compliments. It is the desire of the hearing. Others are gourmets. All pleasant sensations for the nose, mouth, ears, eyes, the body are the first five desires. The sixth, the Thought (IF) corresponding to the intellection, the cognitive faculties, to the activity of the intellect. These six desires which contain the behaviors can we make life happy when the man through his wisdom can control them. But conversely, they can We Rot life.

The seven emotions will give in their turn the six desires, directly related to the sight, hearing, smell, taste and touch. The sixth corresponding to the spirit with the thought. These six desires which condition the behavior are similar to the wind which may be beneficial or negative. Does not speak-t-we not of the "Fire of desire", the "Fire of passions" which will affect the heart-spirit.

The cycle of life

The life of the man will also know a cyclic development as the nature:

" The children (birth);

" Youth (growth);

" The ripe age (maturation);

" The disease (harvest);

" The Old Age (the placing in reserve).

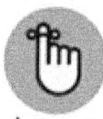

Maturation is a transitional era, a turning point between the beginning and the End. It is this turning point which precedes the harvest in the autumn and the conservation in the winter. It is at

À retenir this time that it should be to avoid squandering our ancestral energy, but on the contrary to amass to prepare for our second part of life.

In nature, an alteration of climates can affect the smooth functioning of the entire chain of causality of the different stages of the life. Thus, a storm will be able to destroy the flower which will not be able to mount in seed and therefore by there, will destroy its future evolution. It is a abnormal intervention of the universe on the five stages of evolution.

In our body, the disease can occur in childhood, youth, middle age. What is the cause? It is the alteration of the real energy, Zhen Qi, by lack of knowledge of the rules for the preservation of life.

Why me and not him!!!

If two people go out and face the same climate, return home, one of the two will have taken cold,

Le saviez-vous while the other will have nothing. That which has nothing shows that she has a faculty of correct adaptation to its environment. The other person, perhaps did she not enough sleep, it may be a bad digestion or is under the influence of the emotions. When it is exposed to the wind, it can adapt and this wind the attack. Therefore, all these single wickedness will not reach us if we are in good health, if our vital energy, Zhen qi, is correct. It is in this that the man is in very close relationship with his environment, with the sky and the earth.

The five elements, Wu Xing

This concept will we serve as a referent for the understanding of any Chinese medicine. The Pr Leung said that a whole life was not sufficient to understand all the subtleties and the symbolic of these five elements.

The four elements and the Man in the center

What is the origin of this theory? Let us start by tracer mentally a cross, and place By convention the is to the left of the horizontal axis (the sun rises in the East) and the West on the right. From there, we can define two additional directions: on the vertical axis, it will position the south and the North to bottom.

However, it is found only in the spring, it is the wind of IS which Breath priority, while in autumn, it is the wind from the west, the wind from the south in the summer and the north wind in winter. In addition, there are a maximum of heat in the summer solstice and a maximum of cold weather in the winter solstice. Between the two opposed heat and cold is the spring: before the spring it is cold, after the spring it is hot. The fall is also an intermediate season, but in the autumn, it is hot before the fall and then cold. The growth of vegetation is carried out in the spring. This is the time where the trees and the whole plants begin to grow, to germinate, come out of the ground.

The cycle of the four seasons

"*Fire corresponds to the SUMMER:* In summer, the trees are already large and the Heat becomes intense. In the same way that the forest fires.

"*The fall is represented by the metal:* in autumn, the time refreshes and this freshness is comparable to the freshness of the metal when the key. It is not really cold, it is fresh. In the same way that the metal, the freshness is hiding in the soil.

"*The winter is symbolized by the water.* After the fall, cool season, comes the cold. When the cold approach, the Yang is sinking deeply into the water. That is why in winter the air is cold, but in depth, in the water, it is warmer. It is because the Yang is pressed deeply into the water. The water always flows to the bottom. It flows also deeply that it is possible to do so, to the deeper parts of the earth. That is the nature of the water.

"*The Spring corresponds to the element earth.* After the winter, the Yang content in the water begins to climb and pushes the water toward the surface of the earth. Then, the earth starts to cause the germination; plants germinate.

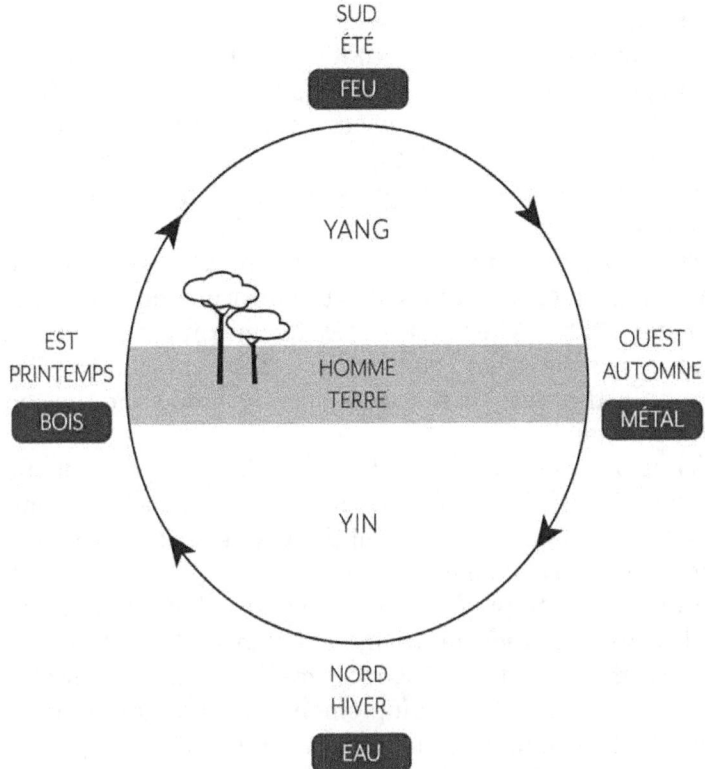

Figure 4-1 The origin of the five elements.

And the man in all of this?

The man remains on the earth. It is in the middle. Let us look at the Diagram: The metal is sinking under earth, also water. The fire is above the earth as well as the wood, although the roots of the vegetation are always in the earth, wood, the vegetation grows toward the top. The metal is at the same level as the Earth, but it has a tendency to push there. He may not raise. If you drop a piece of metal, it falls to the ground. The wood, him, is different. It always rises. The wood and metal are on the median line that corresponds to the earth.

The earth is thus at the root of any thing. It is for this reason that it is the located in the center of the "wheel" events.

À retenir

The pentagram

Another possibility of representation is the pentagram. We can integrate the earth in a cycle, the cycle of the five elements or the successive periods of human life. In MTC, it uses to understand the evolution of any disease. This cycle is not frozen, but on the contrary a permanent transformation. As well we have:

"*The cycle of begetting, Shen,* the fundamental relationship mother-son: each item creates the next in a movement of constant flux. When it reaches its maximum potential, energy overflows and gives birth to the next element. For example, the water is the mother of the wood and the son of the metal.

"*The control cycle, Ke.* Indeed, the balance may not be maintained if the growth is uncontrolled. Each element must control another. As well the water controls the fire, the Fire Controls the metal, etc.

In the diagram below (figure 4-2) we see that growth and control are maintained mutually in balance. As well, water nourishes the wood and wood fire, but the water also controls the fire and thus complements a triad autonomous. This is called "production and mutual conquest".

In the human body, these transformations also occur and when the cycle is disrupted, diseases and disorders appear. Instead of control and to assist each other, the five elements are insulting and destroy themselves reciprocally.

It ends by dialysis!

Le saviez-vous

When the water, in this case the energy of the kidney, is deficient, it can no longer control the fire (the heart). The fire will prevail and an insult to the water. At the same time, the control of the land (rate) on the water becomes excessive, the water is no longer strong enough for the bear. The earth destroyed water, because the control has exceeded its limits. It is the typical example of the self-destruction. And it is the dialysis by renal impairment...

60

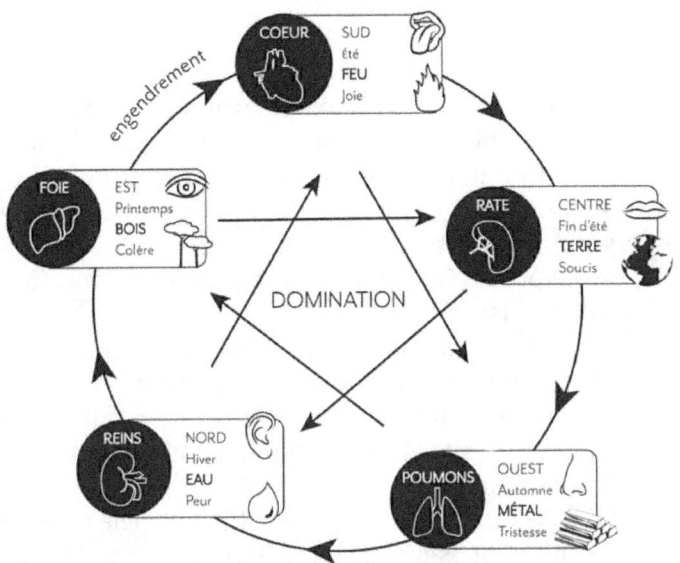

Figure 4-2 **The five movements of elements.**

Classification of five elements

We have seen that the man and nature are in perfect harmony. It is then possible to establish a link between the physiological activities internal to the Man and the natural phenomena that correspond to them. This relationship can be done by using the five elements.

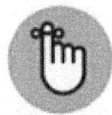

À retenir

Similarly, the pathological changes can be put in relation with the disruption of nature and the treatments are inspired by the natural process of recovery of the balance.

It is the intuitive knowledge of the elders who can put in place such tables. For example, the heat, the red, the summer, the South, the heart, it holds the road. But other relationships are still obscure to our modern minds and can only be entered by a sudden revelation.

This table is necessarily limiting, because everything that exists on this earth can enter in this classification.

Why this table and the cycle of the five elements are they used continuously by a therapist?

The example of the liver

The focus is on the following example to enter the scope of this cycle of the five elements. We find very often in our regions of pathologies linked to the imbalance of the energy of the liver. The main symptoms of the liver are headache and dizziness caused by the upward movement Yang of the liver. But several cases may arise:

" 1St case: it may be a disease called "positive", which takes birth in the body itself. The main symptoms will be headache, dizziness; the face and red eyes, a pulse end and fast. The excessive Yang of the liver may be served directly by a simple treatment and fast.

" 2Nd case: the water in the kidney is insufficient. The disease is: "The mother makes him sick the Son". The wood of the liver is not enough fed, the Branches are then too heavy to bear to the roots. The symptoms are headache, dizziness, syncope, the patient is low and warm. According to the theory of the five elements, the Yang of the Liver rises, but if the practitioner does fact that try to delete the Yang of the liver, the situation will worsen. To treat, we must strengthen the water in the kidney so that the wood in the liver to be encouraged to take root and become stable. It is a fundamental method of treatment that "to help the mother and to support his son".

" 3e case: "The mutual insult". When the metal in the lung is low and can no longer control the wood of the liver, the latter becomes excessive. The following symptoms appear: headache, dizziness, syncope, phlegm and phlegm in the throat, the patient coughs and spits constantly, its chest movements are slow and painful, and there is a loss of appetite. In clinical practice, it is necessary to attend the lung. When the energy of the lung may again circulate, the wood in the liver is controlled and the symptoms disappear.

It is therefore that the headache and dizziness, although symptoms of affection of the liver, may be caused by a malfunction of another body. And all this can only be understood in having in memory the table and the cycle of the five elements with all their relational.

This theory explains in simple terms the effects of components on each other and the mechanisms by which all bodies are working in concert to maintain homeostasis, self-regulation and self-healing of the body and by that same health. In addition, it allows the practitioner to predict the evolution of a disease, thus constituting a valuable method of prognosis.

Table 4-1 The theory of the five elements.

	Wood	Fire	Earth		Water
THE SEASON	SPRING	Been	End Summer / shoulder	FALL	WINTER
ORIENTATION	IS	SOUTH	CENTER	WEST	NORTH
Yin body	LIVER	Heart	STOMACH	LUNG	KIDNEY
Bowels Yang	Gallbladder	Small intestine	Rate-Pancréas	Large intestine	BLADDER
COLOR	Green, Blue-green	RED	YELLOW	WHITE	BLACK
FEELING	Anger	JOY	Reflection, rumination	Grief, sadness	AFRAID
Organ of meaning	EYES	LANGUAGE	MOUTH	Nose, skin	EAR
FUNCTION	VIEW	FLOOR	Taste	Smell, Touch	Hearing

WOVEN FABRICS	The tendons, muscles	The arteries, blood	Flesh, mucous membranes	Skin, hair	Marrow, OS, Hair
FLAVOR	ACIDIC	AMER	SOFT	SPICE	Salé

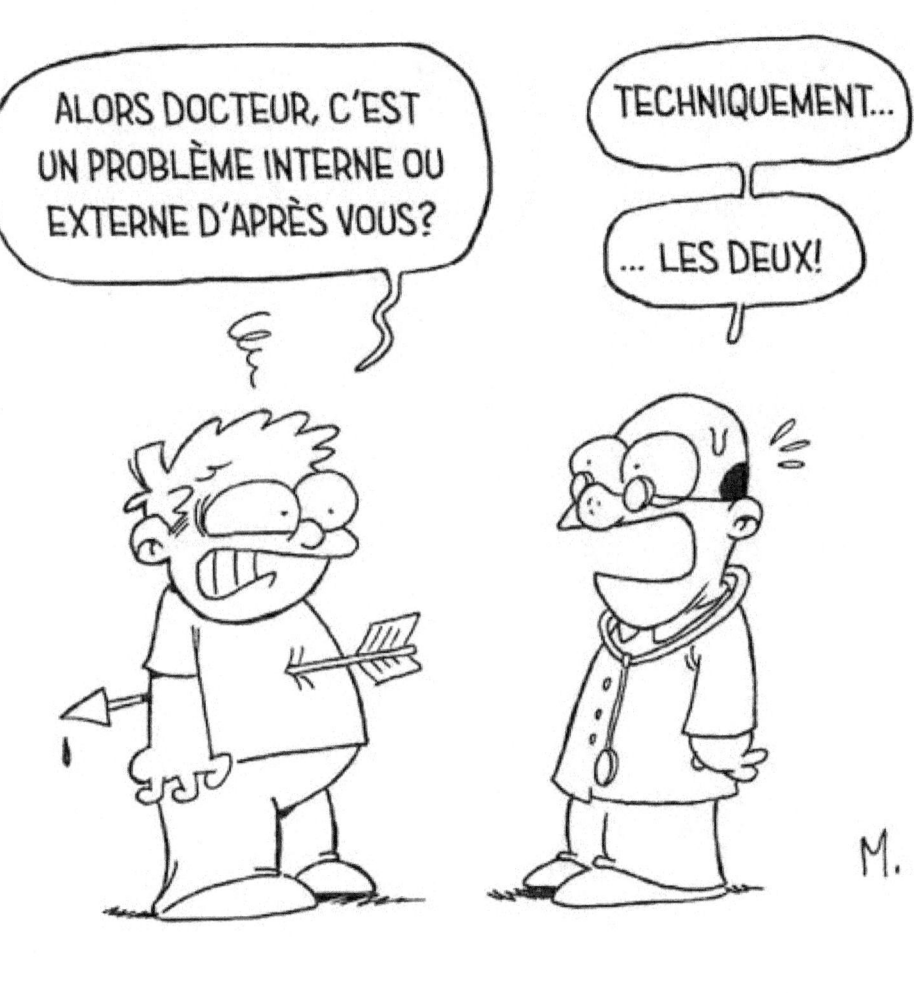

In this part...

This part explains in detail the different methods of observation in MTC. The study of the morphotype, of the face with its shape and its colors, eyes, hands... Allows you very quickly to have a clear idea about the past and the become pathological of an individual.

You get great benefit to soak the chapter on the interrogation and in particular of the "Song of the ten questions": it will allow you to analyze and understand the origin of all your evils (headache, pain, insomnia...), and to consider at the outset as the symptoms alarm signals and not as pathologies with whole share.

And to go further, you will become unbeatable (or almost) in the techniques of decision-pulse and the study of the language. In MTC, a practitioner "sees" his patient, has already a few intuitions, asking him precise questions after s be inquired about his CV. Then, it strengthens his diagnosis by the taking of the pulse and the study of the language. A practitioner of high level, after having seen, taken the pulse and "studied the language," will already asked the diagnosis. The patient may not then that answer "yes" to questions which are asked.

Chapter 5
The four methods

UN practitioner in MTC is a real detective (see chapitre
3**). It should bring together a whole series of symptoms
by of the Exams Only charged to the assistance of its five
senses. Then, it must pass the data collected to the
chaffer Ba Gang, "eight rules" (see** chapitre 3**), to finally
install a diagnosis. This diagnosis will not be definitive
and the practitioner will certain weapons at its
disposal to allow him to follow very regularly The
evolution.**

In the _chapitre 5_ of the su wen, it is said: "The one who has the
experience in the establishment of a diagnosis, when he
observed the colors and that it traces the pulse, distinguishes
first the Yin and the Yang, separates the pure and the impure
and thus recognizes the place of the disease. It notes the
State of the respiration, listening to the sounds and the
timbre of the voice and knows the bitterness of the patient.
The state of the Order and of the balance of pulse, he knows
the organ responsible for the affection. It traces the Radial
pulse and look at whether it is superficial or deep, smooth or
rough and he knows the cause of the disease. In doing so, he
will not erroneous treatments and his judgment will not be
bad. "

The four diagnostic methods
The practitioner has at its disposal four methods to perform
a systematic investigation, and this, thanks to our five senses:
" These Eyes allow him to observe the patient.
" These ears to listen to the voice of the patient.
" His nose allows him to feel the odours by the different
    regions of the body.
" His mouth allows him to question the patient on the
    sensations he feels.
" His hand will allow him to take the pulse.

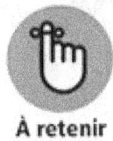

À retenir

These different methods can be Summarized that the MTC called "The Four Reviews":

" The observation;

" The olfaction;

" The Interrogation;

" Palpation.

These various tools of inquiry which has the practitioner will enable him at any time to the information on the different external disturbances or internal to the patient, but also to follow the evolution of the affection and even to ask a prognosis.

A real investigation

It should be however ensure some points. Indeed, the conclusions that can be drawn from the observation, the auscultation, examination and palpation are very complex. The diseases themselves are fairly complicated. It must not only get answers, gather facts, but we need to know how to interpret them. The practitioner is located in front of a real police investigation and his insight, his intuition fruit of his experience, and its logic will not be too much for unravel the threads of the disease.

It is nice to have harvested a whole series of indices, data as to the pathology. But it is going to analyze. This are the ba gang, the "eight principles" (see chapitre 3) which will allow him to order, to classify all these symptoms. Is it that the clinical picture is rather Yin or Yang instead? The pathology is-it of origin whether external or internal? Is it characterized by a state of weakness or on the contrary of fullness? In short, you can see that these four couples allow you to define precisely the state of the patient. It is the indispensable basis of Diagnosis IN MTC.

The four points which must ensure the practitioner

All this is recounted in the **Nei Jing, the bible of the Chinese medicine.**

Assess whether the symptoms are normal

It is necessary to distinguish what are the symptoms normal and abnormal and carefully analyze. It is possible for example that the disease is of such a nature yang, but in part Yin and Xu. This is an abnormal phenomenon that it is appropriate to examine with care. Certain diseases Xu to the extreme resemble a disease Shi or then to a disease Xu apparent. You know the old adage "the extremes Join": a Yang excessive can become yin and vice versa. When you keep for a long time a ice cube in the hands, he can eventually burn you. In the case of a person who has had a heat stroke, one can find weak pulse. Conversely, in some cases of loss of knowledge, one can find pulse very fast. All this thus represents the abnormal phenomena that it is appropriate to analyze with care. It will therefore be necessary to before anything else is to ensure the consistency of the symptomatic table.

Distinguish What are the main symptoms symptoms secondary

For example, if we have determined that the main symptoms were related to the meridian of the lung and that at the same time there had heart palpitations which are symptoms of the meridian of the Heart and of the pericardium, or a bad digestion, a symptom of the meridian of the spleen, to attach to main symptoms will not suffice, it will be necessary to understand why these secondary symptoms are present. Most of the time these secondary symptoms are the consequence, the resultant of the main symptoms. If we only deals The main symptoms and that we leave aside the secondary symptoms, these remain and may cause the appearance of other diseases.

Have a profound vision...
If you are an architect and you want to build a house, but that before it is necessary to destroy

En pratique another: if the House to destroy is independent, this poses no problems. On the other hand, if it is attached, it must ensure that the neighboring houses are strong enough to withstand the demolition. If they are as old as the House to demolish, it is appropriate first to the repair, support in order that they do not suffer damage. It will therefore be very attentive and take precautions. The treatment will have to act on the two types of symptoms.

This is a crucial difference between the traditional Chinese medicine and modern medicine. Modern

À retenir

medicine is essentially concerned with what is called the main symptoms, but not at all to the secondary symptoms. It does not treat the consequences caused by the major symptoms.

Predict the evolution of the disease

Le saviez-vous

In effect, a disease is never stationary. It is evolving in a day on the other and even from morning to evening. Let us not forget that there is a battle, a recovery attempt in hand of the proper functioning of the body by the energy right, the barriers of defense. If your energy right is powerful, the disease moves backwards. If it is low, the disease installs and is sinking deeper in the body.

Whether it is high blood pressure, diabetes, or all other pathologies, we will not necessarily be the same treatment all days, or the same dose. It must follow, is modeled on the evolution of the disease.

" A disease can evolve in a positive or negative. It can for example say that when a disease presents for internal symptoms a day, and that the following day appear of external symptoms, the evolution is positive. The disease goes toward its healing. It is said that "the internal disease manifests itself to the outside."

" Similarly, if a patient presents symptoms of organs Zang, Yin, full, vital and that the next day he presents symptoms of organs Fu, Yang, hollow, it is the sign that the disease evolves favorably for the internal toward the external.

" On the contrary, if the day before, the patient had of external symptoms such as headache, fever, runny nose, and that the following day there are abdominal pain, diarrhea, this shows that the disease is getting worse and will of the external to the internal.

Assess the strength of the combatants in the presence

In a disease whatever it is, in effect there are two forces in the presence:

" The attacker, called Xie IQ, or energy (perverse the microbe, the virus, an emotion exacerbated, abrupt climate change, a food flavor in excess, etc.).

"Opposite, we have several lines of defense, called Zhen Qi. To make it short, this are the immune defenses.

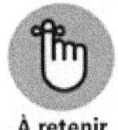

A symptom is that the objectification of this war that is taking place under the eyes of the practitioner. It is one of the reasons for which we should think twice before taking drugs to lower any of following a low grade fever that appears.

À retenir

It is very important to know, at a moment T, which of energy right or of the Perverse energy is the Most High? After each phase of evolution, after each treatment, it must see who takes over, it was necessary to assess and compare the state Xie Qi and Zhen Qi, of the attacker and the defense. This assessment will allow to establish a prognosis, whether a disease is evolving favorably or unfavorably.

Once the disease is cured, it can remain a weakness that affects the functioning of the bodies and that it is necessary to arrive to objectify to avoid relapse.

Chapter 6
The observation

The'Observation is one of the most important methods of diagnosis. Formerly, it was considered that the ultimate in the art of the diagnosis and the sign of a great doctor was to be able to install a diagnosis by simply watch the patient, without the need of the query or the palpate.

Le saviez-vous

It is also by the observation that it Between in contact for the first time with a patient. The observation is therefore the diagnosis by the next, by the view.

The different tools at its disposal are first of all the study of Shen, which is the manifestation of the energy to the outside of the body, then the different colors, the shape and the morphology of the patient, his behavior and his temperament and finally the observation point by point of the body.

Clues given by the study of Shen

We have seen that the Shen designates the Spirit (see chapitre 3), the manifestation of mental activities, but it also refers to the different manifestations, visible from the outside and which reflect the state of the organs and viscera, energy and the blood.

It is said in the **Nei Jing** : " **Those who possess the Shen have a thriving life, those who lose the Shen also lose life.** " It is for this reason that the changes in the Shen represent major indications enabling to judge the importance of the disease and a diagnosis.

It must be based on the principle that everything that lives on this earth has the Qi, of the energy. And when the energy is going, the life is extinguished.

But it is not that easy to observe what is called the shen to a patient. This is a print not quantifiable, and there must be a sense of observation very developed to draw all the subtleties. The qualifications required for a good observation are the qualities expected of an artist and first and the ability to see the details. This ability is however rarely a innate gift and must be developed. These qualities being acquired, this does not automatically confer the doctor a good sense of observation. It must strive to put aside continually its own thoughts, its own mental schemas in order to observe the actual condition of the patient and not the condition assumed.

How to observe the Shen Qi?

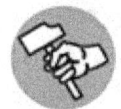

Let us take an example. When a person has slept poorly when she comes to spend a night White, the next morning we can see that his Shen is

En pratique insufficient. From a first glance it realizes that. Is it not said that it has a bad mine? If someone is a natural worried, anxious, sad, if his emotions are constantly being excessive, we can see in observing this person that she does not have a bright appearance, dynamic. It lack of liveliness and liveliness.

The Shen is observed everywhere in nature. When you go to buy fish, by observing its gills and his eyes, you will know immediately if it is a fish caught the standby or a few days ago. The Shen also concerns the plants. In the spring when you observe the plants, flowers, they are full of life. Your eye appreciate all of following the vitality of a rose which comes to hatch and overcomes the leaves tender green. When it is on its decline, this is seen at first glance.

Or observe-t-on the Shen of man?

Mainly by observing the complexion of the face and observing the eyes. If the Shen is missing, the complexion is dull and the muscles are flanges. The observation of the brilliance of the color has a paramount importance.

At the level of the eyes, if someone has the Shen, his eyes are bright, mobile, have the brilliance. Is it not said that such person has eyes sparkling of life? On the other hand, if its Shen is insufficient, the eyes do not rotate quickly, they have slow movements. They can close easily. One has the impression that the person has the desire to sleep. They are dull. His eyes indicate that the vitality is lost.

The gestural, respiration, the manner in which he speaks, any this intuitive observation gives us valuable information on the state of the Shen.

Small story told by my master

One of his pupils who practiced the Chinese Medicine received a day in his cabinet a patient for a consultation. When the latter entered the local, it was hiding a knife behind his back. And a single blow, he wields and threw himself on the practitioner in the purpose of the murder. Fortunately, our practitioner had been trained in the method of observation-diagnosis. As soon as the arrival of his patient, at first glance, it was realized that something was not. His gaze was weird, even that its behavior and gestures. He immediately perceived that his patient was crazy and all its meaning is are instantly put in awakening. When the latter attacked him, he could then easily deal the coup and the control. His mastery of the observation saved his life.

Table 6-1 The observation of the Shen.

Form COLOR	- Firm muscles, tonic - Complexion of the shining face	- Dull complexion - The muscles flanges, meager - Not good colors, bad mine
EYES	- Sharp movements and fast - The Eyes Have the brilliance	- Movements of the eyes slow - Ternes and close more easily
Attitudes GESTURES	- The gestures and coordinated movements - Speak normally	- Confused thoughts
BREATHING	Regular Basis	- Abnormal, sigh

			- Rapid or slow, uneven

Clues given by the study of colors

The colors that appear on the surface area of the body are the different expressions of the Qi, energy and blood Xue of internal organs. They also show the different stages of the evolution of a disease. We already know that there are five colors which are to be put in relation with the five software bodies. As well:

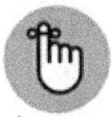

" The green is to be put in relation with the energy of the liver.

" The Red in the relationship with the heart.

" The yellow in relationship with the Spleen-pancreas.

" The White in relationship with the lung.

" And the black, in relation with the kidney.

When color is observed, it must be put in relation the colors with the bodies. If a component is sick and that its color is manifested, for example if the liver is out of adjustment and the green that appears, this is considered normal. If this is not the color of the body which is manifest, it must then determine whether the color is a color beneficial or harmful. In the table below you will already have a vision of the Assembly:

Table 6-2 Components Software and their colors.

Body		The Season		
LIVER	WOOD	SPRING	Bright green as the pen of a bird	Bluish green without the glare
Heart	FIRE	Been	As red as the crest of a rooster	Red as blood clots
RATE	EARTH	End of the	Yellow	Yellow as the

		summer	resembling the inside of a crab	bark dried orange
LUNG	Metal	FALL	White as pork grease	White as a OS dried
KIDNEY	WATER	WINTER	Black as the feathers of a Raven	Black as coal or soot

In addition, a body who falls ill may demonstrate a color that is not that of the body, what is called "a color right, authentic, Normal".

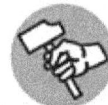

En pratique Let us take the example of the Liver: If the liver is sick and that the black color appears, the black belongs to the water, green wood. In the cycle of generation, the cycle Sheng, water causes the wood, "the mother generates the Son". It is then considered that the color is beneficial and that the disease is not that serious. However, it must not be that the black either as coal or soot. It must be shining bright.

On the contrary, if it is the red which appears, it is known that the red belongs to the fire and the heart, the wood to the liver. The fire attack the wood, it is a bad sign. We are in the face of a difficult disease to treat. In the table below you can have a view of the whole relatively to the emergence of these colors that can be "right, Normal", up to very serious.

Table 6-3 The diagnosis by the colors.

	Liver	Rate	Lung	Kidney	
RIGHT-NORMAL	GREEN	RED	YELLOW	WHITE	BLACK
Favorable-Bénéfique	Black brilliance	Glow green	Glow red	Glow yellow	Bright white
Negative against the current	- RED	YELLOW	WHITE	BLACK	GREEN

Harmful, but not serious	YELLOW	WHITE	BLACK	GREEN	RED
Very serious	WHITE	BLACK	GREEN	RED	YELLOW

Clues given by the study of the morphology

When a patient comes to consult his practitioner, or when we are in the face of an individual who presents a pathology, the observation of his body is very important. The Review allows you to detect the alterations visible on the body of the sick. It is not enough to weigh the patient and to know its size to see if size and weight are in concordance.

Other criteria are very important to take into account to make a good diagnosis. For example, if we see arrive a person lean, large, hairy with a very long neck, we are in the presence of the morphology of the Tb. On the contrary, if a person is strong, small, with a dyed red, everyone knows that this person is subject to the hypertension.

Attention

77

"The energy of the five bodies and of the six viscera serves to make your body strong. The head is the home of the Jing Qi, of the vital energy, because the essence of the zang-fu Monte and focuses on the head. If the head falls, if the patient decline the head and must all look very closely, this means that the Shen is insufficient. The person lack of vitality. The back is the home of the thorax. It is said that it "supports the chest". If the back is arched and that the two shoulders fall in before, this indicates that the Zhong Qi, the energy of the Center is decreased. The arched back promotes a compression of the lungs and it is known that the Lung controls the energy. The lumbar region is the residence of the kidneys. If the lombes are tight, are difficult to move, difficult to move this indicates that the kidneys will soon be sick. The knees are the residence of the tendons. If the flexion or extension of the knees is difficult, the tendons will soon be sick. If the patient cannot be held long standing, or, if its approach lack of stability, this indicates that the OS will soon be sick, wounded. If the body is strong, the patient will live, if it is low, it will become more and more low. "

To what morphotype Am I related?

Le saviez-vous

We can classify the individuals according to five profiles, five temperaments, and this from the theory of the five elements. Do not do a diagnosis with whole share, but just a beam of presumptions in our investigation.

The wood type

These people have a subtle nuance of green in their complexion, a head relatively small and elongated, large shoulders with a dos right, a body large and muscular and hands and feet small.

They are workers, reflect much, with a trend also to worry about easily. They have intelligence developed, but their physical strength is low.

The people of wood type often suffer from perverse diseases in autumn and winter. They are in good health in the spring and summer.

The type fire

The complexion is red, resplendent, a small head often in tip. The chin can be sharp, hair that are either curly, Slightly Abundant. The muscles of the shoulders, the Dos, of the hips and the head are well developed. Hands and feet are relatively small.

They are fast, energetic, active. They walk on a firm and move a lot their body in walking. They can be coléreuses. They think a lot and tend to worry about easily. They have a good sense of observation and analyze things in depth.

They are generally in good health in the spring and summer, but more sensitive to the attack of perverse energies in the fall and winter. The texts say that the people of type fire have a tendency to die of sudden death.

The type earth

They have a yellowish complexion, a round face, a relatively large heads, wide jaws and shoulders and a dos well developed and well proportioned, a important abdomen, thighs and of the muscles of the strong calves, hands and feet not very great, and in general of the muscles strong. They walk with a firm step without raising the feet very high.

They are quiet and generous and have a stable character. They have a temperament altruistic and do not have exaggerated ambitions. It is easy to agree with them.

These people are in relative good health in the fall and winter. In contrast, in the spring and in the summer, they can easily be attacked by the perverse energies.

The Metal Type

They have a relatively Complexion pale, a face square, a head relatively small, shoulders and a dos Small, an abdomen relatively flat and of hands and feet small.

They may have a strong voice and move quickly. Their thoughts are sharp. They are of temperament honest and law, quiet and calm, but may be capable of decisive action in the event of need. They have a natural ability to manage and to order.

In good health in the fall and winter, they can be easily attacked by the perverse energies in the spring and summer.

The type water

They have a relatively Complexion Dark, wrinkles, a relatively large heads, a face and a round body, the cheeks wide, of shoulders Narrow and small, a abdomen important. They have always the body in movement when they walk and have difficulty to stay quiet.

A natural relaxd, they forgive easily. They can be very good negotiators and can easily make them confidence. They are aware and sensitive.

In good health in the fall and winter, they can easily be attacked by the perverse energies in spring in summer.

What is my personality?

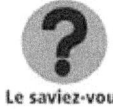

Le saviez-vous

Still according to the **Nei Jing, we can distinguish five types of individuals, five types of personalities established according to the behavior. As well, we are going to have the**

type:
" Tai Yin;
" Shao Yin;
" Tae Yang;
" Shao Yang;
" And the type Yin-Yang balanced.

We will see that there is relatively large differences with respect to the profile of these individuals, both at the level of their health, their personality, their character and their resistance. It will be necessary to take into account when we will have to establish a diagnosis and especially a treatment.

The type "Yin abundant" or Tai Yin

These individuals have as characteristic of having a Yin abundant. In reality, there is not enough of Yang to balance the Yin.

The character of these individuals is marked by the greed, envy, and also by the lack of Friendliness, kindness. This envious side prevents any generosity. The appearance is humble, simple, courteous, polite toward others, but in their heart, internally, they are crafty.

This type of person does not say what it feels, does not say what he feels, does not say what he thinks. It is said that it is versatile, it changes as a weather vane. It can easily become opportunistic although it has difficulties to have specific goals.

They have too much of Yin and the blood is too concentrated in the body. The energy does not flow well. It is for this reason that they have the thick skin and tendons low.

This type of person has not much of Yang, and therefore does not move much, does not a lot of exercise, which explains that the tendons are soft and without force.

Appearance, this person is taciturn, she does not like to talk about, his complexion is dull. It has not of strength, not tone, the head is lowered. One has the impression that the person reflects all the time, the back is arched, the head falls.

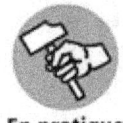

When one treats this type Tai Yin, it must use methods strong and fast, because the blood is disturbed and the energy obstructed in its

En pratique movement. If it is not strong enough, it will not happen to release the energy and restore the blood.

The type "Yin low" or Shao Yin

81

Attention

This type of person is also envious and greedy, but in addition it has a "heart of thief". It can go up to take by force what does not belong to him. He likes to attack the people, it is aggressive. It is constantly in the process of simmer in his head something, or an action which may attack, injure the other. These acts of wickedness may be totally free. It may for example to remove the Chair before that someone sits down, make a croc-in-leg. It does yields nothing and if you ask him why he has done this, it does not know itself.

When he sees someone to happy and who knows a moment of glory, it does not rejoice as much as the person concerned. It can even get angry and become jealous.

It is said that the type Shao Yin will have a small stomach, but that the intestines are large, because there has been too much Yang. It has been seen that he always échafaudait plans in his head, and the fact of ruminating too in his head ends up having an impact on its stomach, a consequence of the disruption of the software spleen-pancreas. It does not happen to eat a lot.

It cannot keep quiet, it walk without stops as if he had cramps, muscle spasms.

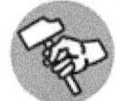 To treat this type Shao Yin, it is first necessary to know where to find the obstruction affecting the blood and energy. But these are patients often
En pratique difficult to treat.

The type "Yang abundant" or Tai Yang

It is the opposite of the types Yin precedents.

The person belonging to this profile likes to talk a lot, tell its affairs. But she likes to talk about important topics and do not like the questions of detail. It has a tendency to inflate its ambitions, likes to talk about politics, economics, of subjects very large.

She likes lie, she likes to give the emphasis to his speech. It does not care about the other, she feels she is the best, the stronger. She knows what she wants. When she wiper a failure, it has no remorse.

It is often said that she is brutal, violent, vulgar, that it is not very fine.

Often she undertakes something when she knows that she does not have the capacity to carry out its business. But this does nothing, she likes to do, is bragging about all the world, tells the whole world what it undertakes in order that the whole world knows what it is doing. Although having boasted, even if the result is bad, she is not afraid of the reproaches of others.

His attitude is very proud. The Chest and Abdomen focuses in front, and even the knees. The knees are so rights that they give the impression to bend to the upside down, for that the feet are even more in before.

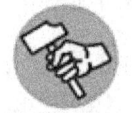

En pratique At the level of treatment, we have seen that the Yang was abundant. But if you use methods to reduce these events for excessive and Yang you may cause very quickly a disability of this Yang who deflates as a bubble. Normally the Yang has for nature to disperse, to resume. If it is reduced too, it will eventually disappear. The element Yin him is already reduced and it is still easier to deplete. Therefore, the treatment should not be too reduce the Yang and in addition to preserve the Yin. It is the principle of treatment for the type Tai Yang.

The type "Yang low" or Shao Yang

It is the megalomaniac. Barely a-t-it a small function that it is already considers as an important character. He likes the worldly life, social activities. He does not like work locked up. In this type Shao Yang, as the previous Tae Yang, there are a lot of Yang, but a little less, and little Yin. Health is not very good. This type of individual has the air very strong, but in reality the health is bad, because the energy of the meridians is low, insufficient.

The Yang is excessive to the outside while it is insufficient in internal. There was thus an imbalance that makes the person more vulnerable to the disease.

At external attitude, he prefers to raise the head, the gaze is directed toward the top. When walking, it is balance without stopping, the two hands are generally in the back.

At the level of treatment, it must above all not reduce the Yang, because the subject is in fact very low in the interior. Externally, it has the air

En pratique Fort and in good health, but inside it is low.

The type balanced Yin-Yang

Those who belong to this category are people calm and balanced. They have an open character and are constant in their behavior. This are beings of peaceful, very friendly, courteous. Everything can make them pleasure.

They are not very active, they are rarely concerned. They have not of great joy not more. There is not a lot of things that can excite them and make them excessively merry nor a lot of things that can make them afraid. They are not anxious, they adapt to all the circumstances, they are very simple in their relations with others.

It is said that "the vessels are in harmony". This type of person is not often sick, his health does not pose problems.

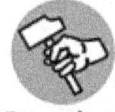

At the level of treatment, we have seen that this type of person fell that very rarely sick. In the case of diseases, it is not generally of diseases due to

En pratique the emotions nor due to digestive disorders, because the operation of the intestines and the stomach is normal. The internal diseases are therefore rare for this case. The more often the disease is external cause due to the attack of a perverse energy and the treatment is often very easy, when it has need of treatment.

The observation of the face

When the practitioner receives a patient, the first thing he must observe in him is his face. What is reviewed before any on the face, it is the complexion. In looking at the complexion, we can determine what meridian is reached. Each disease may be suggested by colorations different. We have already discussed this subject in "Data indices by the study of colors".

Do I have a good complexion?

If the complexion is rather green, this indicates a "cold wind External" or a pain somewhere in the body. It is a sign of stagnation of blood or of energy. Often this sign a serious illness.

" If the complexion is red, it indicates the more often of the heat. When we are in the presence of a heat Xu, weakness, the red has the air to be placed on the white, which gives an aspect rosé, as the fard that are some ladies. For the heat Shi, fullness, there is the red, also, but it is a red much more lively.

" The Crimson face sign a syndrome of excess or fullness, due to hyperactivity of Yang internal.

" The gently cheeks dews are thus due to heat Xu consecutive to a weakness of the Yin. It is the color that can be found during the "puffs of heat". The Chinese call this "the false heat".

" The pale complexion with migratory redness is seen in chronic diseases or serious. This indicates the presence of a State cold with periods of false Chaleur. It is a little as if a State Yin important sporadically released of bouffés of Yang at the level of the face.

" If the complexion is yellowish, it is very often to put in a relationship with a excess moisture at the level of the spleen. We know that the muscles and the chairs are to be put in relation with the Spleen. They are not quite fed by a lack of blood and energy, and by an impairment of the spleen to transport the blood, or an excess internal to tan and humidity.

" The complexion light yellow, dry and dull is called "scrambled complexion". It is due to the vacuum of the IQ of the spleen and stomach and the inadequacy of the Qi and blood encountered, for example in the case of hemorrhage, malnutrition or intestinal worms.

" The yellowish complexion accompanied by a facial edema is called "yellowish obesity". It is frequently caused by a deficiency of energy of the spleen and an internal accumulation of moisture.

˝A dyed yellow frankly as well as the yellow eyes are called "Jaundice". This status is due in modern medicine to the failure of the flow of bile by the common bile duct, with a extravasion thereof at the level of the skin. If the color becomes yellow orange, it is a jaundice of type Yang, due to the heat-accumulated moisture. This is caused by an imbalance at the level Foie-Vésicule bile.

˝A sudden illness with a deep yellow of the face, eyes and the body, and a high fever that can be accompanied by a coma, or simply with vomiting, epistaxis and macules skin, is called acute jaundice or epidemic. Then we are in the presence of an attack of heat-moisture which warms deeply the liver and the gallbladder.

˝A yellow complexion smoked copper and is called jaundice of type Yin caused by the prolonged stagnation of cold and moisture in the liver and the gallbladder.

˝If the complexion is black, it is often an indication of a serious illness. It may appear in the case of extreme cold (the Yang is transformed into Yin), in the case of internal pain very important. Often this black color is the result of internal diseases chronic.

And these "buttons" which disturb

The acne on the face is usually due to a problem of heat-moisture that can appear in a manner Chronicle on a general table of vacuum of Qi, in particular at the level of the kidney.

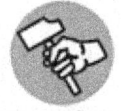

En pratique

Let us take the example of the adolescent. If the latter does not household its battery of the kidney, if it does not recover by a regular sleep, if it is submitted to the stress, if it discovers a little too early sexuality and well of other causes: all this can deplete its reserves. Added to this is a period where he is in full growth. However, the cell multiplication makes contribution of excessive way the battery of the Organization. Therefore on this land of weakness of Qi can supervene a power supply of nature too wet that imbalance the spleen: Excess of sugars fast, of derivatives of dairy products, etc. The Cocktail overall weakness of Energy, excess moisture, weakness of the Yin of the Kidney promotes the transformation of moisture in heat-to-humidity: all the ingredients are there to produce this acne. Golden rule: Never drill a button if it is not ripe. It is not fact while disperse the perversity under the skin and create other buttons to the side.

What to say of wrinkles?

An excess of wrinkles on the face, with a surface area of the skin is very irregular, sign a state of Xue Xu, empty of blood, or of internal heat accompanied by drought. Most often this type of table finds its roots in an inability to properly manage its stress.

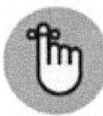

À retenir

The Sun in excess can be concerned. But also a poor hydration of the skin linked to a weakness of the lung. Remember: skin and lungs are part of the same software. Of course the cigarette is not made to arrange the things. And you think you prevent wrinkles by drinking more than it should be. You are all wrong. In reality, you finish by exhausting the Yin of kidney and then the one of the lung. The antidote of wrinkles in the MTC is the Chinese green tea! I refer you to the chapter on the Dietetics relatively to the drinks.

Thou hast beautiful eyes!

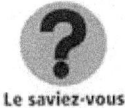

Le saviez-vous

When one observes the eyes, the first thing you see is the Shen, the vitality of the individual. The citations for the ancient texts have made us understand that when one observes the eye, in reality there is the state of the essence of the five organs and the six Viscera, since their Jing Qi, their energies up to the eye and is concentrated there.

The former divided the eye in five parts:

"The eyelids are to be put in relation with the Spleen.

"The two corners of the eye of where emerging lacrimal glands are to be put in relation with the heart.

"The white of the eye with the lung.

"The iris with the liver.

"And the pupil with the kidney.

As well:

"If there is a fire in the heart the two corners of the eye are red.

"If the white of the eye is red on the sclera of the two sides, this indicates that there is a fire in the lung.

"If there is a swelling of the iris, this indicates that the liver is hot, that there is a fire in the liver.

"If the eye is dull and dark and that the patient himself has a poor view, but when you look closely at the eyes are not troubled, it is that the kidneys are low. But if you look at the eyes of the patient, and you see that there is a disorder, like a veil, and that the patient himself does not see, c is the Yang Ming who is ill, it is a disease Shi, in excess of the stomach.

"If the energy is extremely exhausted and that the patient sees evil, that it is almost blind, this indicates that the Yin is exhausted.

"The redness, eyelids swollen or ulcerated indicate the presence of fire in the spleen and the heat-moisture.

"The heat-extreme humidity of the spleen causing a jaundice, gives white yellow eyes.

"The eyelids and the conjunctiva whitish pale and show the inadequacy of blood.

"If the pupil is abnormally dilated, this means a substantial weakening of the Yin of the kidney, the water from the kidney.

"If there are a lot of secretions and crusts in the eye, it is a fire in the liver and the gallbladder.

"The Eyes sunken in their orbits that is also called "hollow eyes" sign or a significant loss of vital energy, such as the it can be found in certain chronic diseases, or a significant loss of organic liquids, for example following an excess of diarrhea or vomiting. The energy is insufficient to maintain the eye. It is a sign of gravity.

"If the globe of the eye is running slowly or by saccades, it is a sign of tan, phlegm which obstructs the meridians. If the movement is made by saccades, it is a problem related to the tan. If the movement is very slow, it is a loss of Shen, of vitality.

"If in the course of a disease the gaze is fixed and oblique toward the top, this indicates an internal disturbance of the wind of the liver.

"If the gaze is fixed and immobile, this denotes a state of severe loss of Jing Qi, gasoline vital.

"The eyes open during sleep are the fact of the weakness of the spleen and stomach.

"The absence of reaction to the light is a critical sign of the exhaustion of the energy of the kidney, that are also to be found in the cases of poisoning, among drug addicts for example.

"If the eyelids are swollen, red and wet, it is a problem related to the presence of fire in the spleen.

"If they are only swollen, this means that it is located in front of a spleen Xu with the presence of moisture.

"If the color is dull, dark, especially if this is beyond the level of the lower eyelid, this sign a problem of stagnant water. The kidneys no more to evacuate the liquids.

And the nose?

Once the nose is called Ming Tang, or even "the entry of light". In effect it is a place where the Yang clear converge. The Yang clear, it is first of all the air we breathe, but also because the vessel Governor, master of all energies Yang, passes through the nose. The nose is located in the middle of the face, we know that the central part of the face corresponds to the spleen. But the lung has also as port nose. Therefore we can say that the surface of the nose is to put in relationship with the spleen and the inside of the nostrils with the lung.

"If the nose is green, it is often because the topic has stomach ache.

"If it is yellow, the person has difficulty to evacuate the stool.

"If it is white, it is known that the energy is low or that the person has lost of the blood.

"If the nose is red, it is a sign of wind-heat which is entered in the spleen.

"If it is black, it is a internal affection due to an excess of fatigue.

"If the black is dull, dark, without shine, if it is not very dark, this indicates that there has of stagnant water.

"The nose expanded, to the thick skin surmounted of outgrowths as of the Acne is called the nose rosacé. This is most commonly due to an accumulation of heat or moisture heat in the Rate-Estomac. As in alcoholics, for example.

The ears do not go unnoticed!

At the level of the five holes, the ears are in relationship with the kidneys. In the chapitre 17 of the **LING Shu, it is said: "The IQ of the Kidney opens to the ears, when the kidney is well balanced, the ears can hear the five sounds. "All the meridians Yang reach the ear or to enter.**

Le saviez-vous

The ears are therefore connected to the whole body and the visceral disorders have an impact on this body auditory. But overall the visual examination of the Ears informs us about the energy state of the kidney, as well as on the pathological states of the gallbladder.

The color of the Ears

"A whitish color of the entire ear is a sign of cold.

"A green color or dark sees himself in the painful symptoms.

"The Ears fine and dry and resembling of dead flowers are a sign of inadequate at the level of the kidney. The right energy, Zhen qi, is low.

"The Ears dry and blackish mark extreme exhaustion of the essence of the kidney. We can find this type of color in the case of diabetes for example.

"If, on the skin of the ears, we distinguish as scales of fish, this is due to an abscess in the intestines.

"When you look at a ear, he must see if there is a red, because it is a good color that shows that the subject is in good health. If the color turns to white, green, black C is very often a bad sign. However if the color is slightly changed, but that it keeps its sparkle, this is not too serious. If on the other hand this color is dull and dry, the disease is serious. But it should be remembered that if the ears are thin, black and dull, this reveals that the kidneys are sick.

And their form?

Outside of the colors, when we observe an ear, you can all result in see its morphology.

Le saviez-vous

"
The ears must be well proportionate in relation to the size of the head, and therefore what represents a large ear in a person can correspond to a normal ear in another.

"A great ear is usually the sign of a good condition hereditary. Even if it is thick, fleshy, well developed, well in the flesh. There will be a tendency to have a lot of blood and energy, and if pathology there is, this will be more symptoms of type fullness.

"Small ears are usually the sign of a bad constitution hereditary, especially if the lobe is very small. This signs a trend constitutional on empty of blood and of energy. Persons with this type of ear will have more chance than others to have of the pathologies of type Xu, empty.

"The Ears swollen are generally caused by heat or heat-moisture which can, among other things, be a problem with the gallbladder.

"The Ears withered, stunted, such as crumpled are usually due to a weakness of organic liquids, or to a vacuum of blood. In very serious cases as of peritoneal carcinomas, when the stagnation of blood and energy is no longer able to feed the muscles and the flesh, we can find this type of ear.

"Buttons on the EAR are always due to the presence of heat, and in particular a heat at the level of the liver and the gallbladder. As well as warts on the ear. The heat at the level of the meridian of the stomach may also be the cause.

The lips without Botox!

According to the theory of the five elements, the mouth and lips are the holes in the spleen, but are in relationship with many other meridians. That teaches us the observation of the lips?

"If the lips are dry, this is due to the heat in the spleen.

"If they are dry and red, it is a normal heat.

"However, if they are dry and black, it is a bad sign. The disease becomes severe.
"

 If the Lips are swollen and red, it indicates a extreme heat of the spleen. Ask when even the patient if it is not passed from the hands of the aesthetic surgeon before install a diagnosis!!!

Attention

"If the lips are red and even violets, this indicates that there is blood clots inside the body, in the stomach or in the duodenum.

"If the color is purple, but that it pulls to the green-black, this indicates the presence of cold to the inside of the body.

"If the lips are pale, almost white, this indicates that the blood is Xu, low, and the stomach cold.

"If the disease is lukewarm, lips become swollen.

"If the disease is due to the wind, the lips tremble.

"If the lips are returned, the disease is due to the cold.

"If there is of wrinkles, if they are wrinkled, is that there is of the heat.

"If they are cracked, rent, the drought is in question.

"If there are itching on the lips, this indicates that there is too much fire.

" If the patient has the impression that his lips are bitten by a multitude of small needles, this indicates a disease of the energy.

" If the lips have not sensation, this indicates a disease of the blood.

" If one finds of the cracking, such as cracks to the corners of the lips, THIS COMES EITHER A heat in the stomach, either of a vacuum of Yin of the stomach with or without heat, Xu.

" A sudden onset of fever blisters on the corners of the mouth or on the edge of the upper lip can originate from a external invasion of wind-heat.

" Buttons of fever chronic or recurrent at the corner of the mouth or on the edge of the lower lip can come from a pathology of the stomach that is the heat-moisture, heat, or a Xu Yin with a vacuum heat. If it is to the upper lip, rather it is a problem of heat-moisture in the large intestine.

The corner of dentists!

À retenir

We already know that the kidney is the mother of the bones of the skeleton, and the Nei Jing said that "the teeth are the surplus, the surplus of the OS, and therefore of the Kidney". The teeth are therefore in close relationship with the OS, and therefore with the kidney.

" If the observation of the teeth reveals major deposits yellow, this indicates a disruption of the functioning of the stomach, the digestion is bad.

" If the teeth are dry, this indicates a lack of organic liquids.

" If the teeth are dry and as covered in dirt, this indicates a fire is very important to the inside of the body.

" If the teeth are dry and bright, they have the appearance of a stone, this shows that the stomach is dry.

" If the upper gums only is dry, not the teeth, but the gum, this indicates the presence of fire in the stomach, excess heat. This can often be a sign of bleeding at the level of the stomach, with possible vomiting of blood. This loss of blood therefore causes the drying of the upper gums.

"If the gum below only is dry, this indicates the heat in the intestines with probable presence of blood in the stool.

"If the patient is squeak its teeth, this is due to the wind in the liver and in the Tan. An excess of Yang at the level of the software Liver may be the cause. In this case, we will soon appear spasms, cramps which will be caused by this internal heat.
"

Le saviez-vous

When there is bleeding from the gums, it is necessary to see if they are painful, very red: In this case, it is an excess of fire in the stomach.

"If, on the contrary, the bleeding occurs without pain and without red coloring excessive, in this case, it is in the presence of a weakness of the Yin of the kidney which will be at the origin of a "false fire " that rises to the top. The hot flushes will have the same origin.

"The cavities are due in Chinese medicine to a problem of heat-moisture in the meridian of the stomach, heat Xu in the stomach and the large intestine, or a weakness of the kidney. On the one hand the heat-moisture in the spleen favors the multiplication of parasites (tartar); on the other, the weakness of the Kidney promotes the embrittlement of the tooth, the teeth being the end of the bone.

"Teeth which move may also have a relationship with the heat in the stomach, or a heat Xu of the spleen or kidney, or both at the same time.

"The Dental plaques are due the more frequently to the heat in the stomach or in the kidney. The vacuum of the Yin of the kidney is another possible cause.

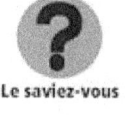

Le saviez-vous

The five areas of the FACE

The Theory The most simple and which allows us to have any information on the internal state of the patient, it is the one of the "Five areas of the face", with respect to the five bodies software. As well:

94

"The heart which is located on the central part of the front, above the eyebrows. The Pr Leung said: "If you must sting a patient while in this area we observe a skin of gray complexion-butternut and which peeling, refrain you, because it is at the edge of the heart attack. "

"The whole of the nose serves to diagnose the software spleen.

"The Menton affects the kidney.

"The left cheekbone, c is the liver.

"The cheekbone right, c is the lung. If you see this cheekbone red in your child, there are great chances that it snaps to cough in the hours which follow.

Very important, the examination of the hand

The first thing that a practitioner before studying the pulse of the patient, it is to take his hand, touch the fingers, examine its skin and muscles. It is important to begin by see if the Palm is thin or thick. For example, a Palm of hands thin, fluette is often a sign of weakness of energy. On the contrary, if the Palm is thick, tonic, this indicates that this same energy is sufficient.

The thenar eminence

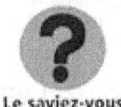
Le saviez-vous

The thenar eminence is this muscle mass which is located at the level of the palm of the hand to the base of the column of the thumb. The muscles the component are called in Chinese " Muscles Fish", because this part inflated of the hand resembles a belly of fish. On these muscles, we can distinguish different colorations, different color variations. The more easy to observe this are the small blood capillaries. As a general rule, we can distinguish a slight redness in this area. This is normal and this indicates that the blood is in good condition. But normally, when a person is in good health, we must not see virtually no capillary.

"If at this place you see of the capillaries in bluish discoloration, this indicates a state of cold in the stomach, weakness. On the contrary, when they are too red, it indicates the heat in the stomach.

95

" If the capillaries are black in color, the circulation of the blood is stagnant.
" If the capillaries appear colored in red, black or blue, depending on the color you can determine if the interior of the body is reached by the cold, heat and this indicates the degree of complexity of the diseases.
" If we can observe the capillaries very small, very short, very purposes, this indicates a lack of energy.
On the palms of the hands, we can still say that:
" If the palms of the hands is dry, chapped, and if in addition it peels, this can sign a vacuum of blood of the liver, heart, or both.
" If the drought is very pronounced and that in addition the hands itch, it is a sign of "Wind in the skin".
" If the hands sweat, it is essentially linked to the meridian of the Heart and the lung. This can come either from a vacuum of QI or Yin, either a heat in one of these two bodies.

The fingers

The morphology of the fingers has its role to play:
" If the fingers are tapered, excessively thin, this signs a lack of movement of Qi in the Jin May. This can also be an important void Qi of the stomach and spleen, or a state of "cold-Moisture" in the spleen.
" On the contrary, if the fingers are pulpy This indicates that the Jin may have a good movement.
" Of the fingers whose end is enlarged, called in to "WAND of Drum", reflect a pathology at the level of the lung, or a Xu Yin, weakness of the kidney and lung cancer. We find this type of fingers in the respiratory diseases chronic.
" Fingers swollen excessively are often due to a syndrome of obstruction that may be painful, or cold-humidity, wind-moisture or heat-moisture. In western medicine, we will talk then of rheumatism.
" But this may also sign a problem of the stasis of blood from the heart and the liver, edema due to a Yang Xu, a weakness, lung and spleen. This state may very often find themselves among the elderly person.

"The Cracked fingers are often due to a vacuum of blood, but also to a stasis of blood.

"You can also find boudinés fingers that resemble the cocoon. This is usually due to a vacuum of blood and IQ.

"Of the fingers stunted and marrowfat show that there is a significant loss of organic liquids that can, among other reasons, be due to the perspirations profuses, significant episodes of diarrhea or vomiting incoercibles.

"A major deformation of the joints of the fingers is most often due to a syndrome of painful obstruction and chronic. This stagnation generates a local inflammation with evaporation of the organic liquids. This heat favors the production of tan. The TAN is therefore the first cause of these deformations. We are going at length to talk about the tan a little further.

What is your type of hand?

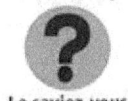
Le saviez-vous

Indeed, in MTC, there are five morphotypes of hand. Each will sign a predisposition to such or such a type of pathology in the light of the theory of the five elements. Let these five hands in review.

The hand of wood type

It is a hand normally well proportionate. It is neither too long nor too short or too narrow or too thick. It is not emaciated. On the other hand, it has the particularity to be nodosa.

It is a hand that at the level of the Palm is particularly streaked. At the level of the fingers, These streaks are parallel, and many furrows dissect the palm. Depending on the hands, the furrows can be more or less deep.

Another particularity, when we look at the back of the hand, it gives the impression to be gnarled especially at the level of the joints inter-phalangeal. The nail is well proportionate, but has particularity as to be convex. If the subject has a tendency Yang, it is hard, solid with a lunule important. Among the subject to trend Yin it may be brittle and fragile.

Le saviez-vous

These nails have particularity as to be often plagued. Let us not forget that the wood and the liver are of the same nature and that in the case of a blockage of the Qi of the liver under the effect of internalized emotions for example, TICS can appear and in particular that of biting nails.

The hand of fire type

This hand is usually long, and fingers appear purposes and agile. These same fingers have the property to depart very widely. This are very fingers laxes, and when stretches, it forms a trough between the thénar Eminences and hypothénars. When the hand is completely extended, it looks like a bracket for chicken.

This hand has a special feature, namely a hyper laxity of the fifth metacarpal and this fifth finger flexes very easily and in a natural way, which gives the person the impression to be a little mannered in its gestures.

The nail of the hand fire is long, quite narrow. When the leaves push, it takes an elongated shape, oval end and very sharp. It is also very domed, much more than the previous one.

The hand of land type

The hand of type Earth is much shorter than the other. When you look at his palmar face, it could enroll in a square, and fingers are short. But what is still the most characteristic feature is that it is thick and chubby.

The fingers are very short and full with a boudiné aspect. Often there is only a single piece in the joints inter-phalangeal. The hand is wide at its attaches to the wrist. The thenar eminence, the thumb and the eminence hypothénar are fleshy. When the person closes his wrist, the whole hand then takes the form of a pear.

The nail of this hand Earth is triangular, the tip toward the bottom. At its root the nail is very distanced himself from the flesh of the Phalanx, this gives the appearance of a net impact strip around the nail. The skin can then easily desquamer and it is often these people who gnaw away their skins because they are easy to reach. The fingernail unlike other hands is not raised, but rather flat.

The metal hand

It has as a characteristic to be long and it is part of a regular oval. The Palm itself is very long and stands out of the fingers who also are long. The fingers themselves, although long are not very purposes.

A special feature: among many hands metal, the Phalanx the more distal, in particular that of the index and the major, has a tendency to tilt on the outer side, or none of the three phalanges is in the axis. With the age, these distortions can be accentuated, and easily give of rheumatoid. The hand will deform then and the fingers will become crooked.

To the palmar face of the fingers, to bending of the joints inter-phalangeal, we see a series of folds features often three in number, and even more. In Chinese medicine, this is called "a triple link".

The nail is rather rectangular with right angles, little arched at their base. Very often one finds of striations in the sense of the length. It is moderately curvature. In some cases, it may be short on this long finger and be convex in both directions, which gives it the appearance of a shell. The last phalange can then expand and take the characteristic appearance of strips of drum.

We know that metal and lung are similar and often among the inadequate chronic respiratory disease, as among people with cystic fibrosis, found these fingers in the shape of the molding of the drum. But this form can also be constitutional, without underlying diseases.

The water hand

The water hand is a hand that has a tendency to be short with fingers short. The skin, as well to the palmar face that dorsal, has a tendency to be soft, released. The fingers often give the impression to be oedématiés, infiltrators.

There is a particular sign that can be found on the dorsal surface of the finger at the level of the articulation of the two first phalanges: when the fingers are strained, instead of a hump, one finds a hollow and if one takes a fold of skin and mounted to the top, it will not resume its original place. The skin keeps the fold.

Another characteristic, always on the dorsal side, the last phalangette is flat and the skin is wrinkled, withered, giving the aspect in fold of Rideau, hand and on the other of the base of the nail. This aspect fadeth darkens the color of the last phalange Who can become downright brownish.

In other cases to the contrary, the phalangette becomes totally smooth, without no fold.

The nail is often in the form of a trapeze, with the small base toward the bottom. The lunule is often flared, and may even have the form of a crescent, a crescent moon. The nail is often soft, fragile and therefore very often cut short by a person who is a carrier. It is a fingernail very flat, it is the less domed of all types of nails, and often it is difficult to see where the flesh ends and where the nail begins, the fact that the phalangette and the nail are if dishes.

The mixed hands

This is for what it is in the study of these five hands. However, it must be understood that we rarely falls on hands with characteristics also trenches. The more often we have to deal with hands that is called "mixed Hands" which are composed of two or even three of the typological elements that we just quoted.

There are for example of hands fire-water. Often a constitution is dominant and it is she who prints the morphopsychologiques characters to the person, the other constitution is secondary.

 Similarly, you can have the hands water-fire, wood-fire or on the contrary fire-wood, etc. This

À retenir

diagnostic approach is exciting in Chinese medicine. Certainly, it request of the time and the experience, but combined with other sources of observation, she can help us very quickly to identify the physical and psychological profile of our patient.

Review of the index in the child

As a general rule, this review is the practice in a child of less than three years. In effect, it is very difficult at this time to have a precise idea of the diagnosis by the Radial pulse, the space between the three fingers are really too small, and there is therefore serves other methods, in other the review of the index, and in particular of the veins of the finger.

The index can be divided into three parts:

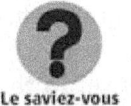
Le saviez-vous

" A first located in the proximal part of the finger, at the level of the first phalanx and that is called "barrier of the wind".

" The second part, located at the level of the second phalanx is called "barrier of the Qi," barrier of the energy.

" Finally the third part located in the distal part, therefore to the third phalanx and that is called "The barrier of life".

This are therefore the three barriers, the "three doors of life, QI and wind". When we are in the presence of a child in good health, the vein of the finger at the level of the barrier of the wind should be pinkish in color or slightly purple. This vein must be very little visible and sometimes even invisible. This vein varies with the external temperature and the age of the baby. Oblique normally and fine, it is more important in the case of heat and more fine and short when it is cold. It is longer in infants of less than one year and shortens with age. So that is as regards the normality.

When one looks at it, it must have adequate lighting and even powerful enough. It holds the hand of the child in one hand and with the thumb on the other, it touches on several occasions by movements of coming and going in order to make this vein more visible.

Let us now look at the information that we can provide the study This vein:

" If during a affection, the vein remains to the barrier of the wind, at the door of the wind This indicates that the achievement is moderate, as the pathology is not very serious. On the other hand, if it extends up to the barrier of the Qi, to the second phalange The disease is more serious. Finally if this vein goes up to the third phalanx, up to the door of life, the disease then is much more serious. If it stretches up to the end of the index, the prognosis is very serious and even unfavorable.

" If the color of this vein is slightly pink or whitish, this indicates a lack of blood and of energy.

" In the case of red color quite pronounced, it is rather in the presence of an attack of cold external.

" If this vein is dark red or purple, this indicates a fullness at the level of the heat.

" A bluish tint may sign the presence of significant pain and even convulsions possible.

" A vein cyanotique or dark purple may reveal a critical state of the baby, a general stagnation of blood.

" If we take the size of the vein, a fine vein will sign a symptom of empty, a State Xu to disability or a state of cold. In contrast, a thick vein indicates a symptom Shi, fullness, or heat.

" If the vein is curved or multiple, this shows that the disease is serious.

If in the course of the evolution of a disease, there is a gradual extension of the vein, this indicates a worsening of the latter. On the other hand, if the vein has a tendency to retract, it is a positive sign: the disease regresses.

Chapter 7
The interrogation
In this chapter:
" Know the Traps
" The conditions of interrogation
" The five errors of the practitioner
" The interrogation on the symptoms or the " Song of the ten
   questions"

HasAlmost have addressed together the diagnosis by the visual examination, we will now see the diagnosis by the examination, namely the fact to interrogate the patient on his felt, on the symptoms that he may submit, understand the history of its symptoms, in short, get an accurate idea of the state of the patient.

The interrogation is said Wen Zhen Chinese. This is obviously a necessary step to identify and understand the pathology. Thanks to this examination, the practitioner will immediately enter in contact, exchange with his patient.

The Chinese have also the habit of saying that the address, tact, the way in which the practitioner led this interrogation deeply influence the result of the treatment.

It may be considered that there is overall two steps in this method of investigation:

"A first part that could be called "the collection of general information". It is a real conversation between the practitioner and the patient that will allow to know the root causes of the disease. Will then be discussed in broken sticks family problems, the environment, the framework of life, the origins, the work, the emotional life, etc.

"A second part which will be a interrogation on the symptoms. This examination will be to identify the tables of imbalance predominant. Each disease has symptoms main and secondary, and this examination also goes well concentrate on the systemic aspect, such as that of the Ba Gong by example (see chapitre 3), that on the analysis of the main symptoms and secondary.

Do not fall into certain traps
"

This should not be a method exclusive. Indeed some practitioners are tempted to use only this method and then apply the treatment types, pre-established. Certainly, in some cases, this may prove to be sufficient. Indeed, some common diseases do not require that a simple treatment. However, it must be remembered that the same symptom may result from different causes, and rely only on this mode of investigation may lead the practitioner to deceive heavily in its diagnosis.

" *The non-cooperation of the patient.* Many patients cannot or do not want to describe exactly their disorder. A sad man who has permanently the need to cry, but whose education the force to remain on its reserve can simply deny the existence of this sign, even himself. Of this fact, it deprives the practitioner of an index is very useful for the location of the disease, here in this case the lungs.

" *The patient who takes himself for a doctor.* Frequently, the patient does not reveal that the symptoms that seem to him to be relevant, giving a table incomplete or incorrect of the situation. Of this fact, in the course of the interrogation, the practitioner must carefully ensure to collect the precise description of all the symptoms as well as the history of the disease. If the interrogation is superficial and lack of interest, the patient will obviously have an unfavorable impression.

" *The examination must be conducted in an orderly and systematic.* We know that the Chinese medicine is based on the unity of the body, its relationship with the environment and especially the impact that can have the emotions on the balance of the organs. Given the interference of several factors, each symptom usually is the natural consequence of a main disturbance. Therefore, the possibility for two different diseases to exist simultaneously in the body is very reduced. The symptoms collected, among others by the interrogation, are useful as an index of the nature or cause of the disturbance. It must never be set aside a symptom which seems without relationship with the problem Present nor accept that the patient tells all his medical history.

These two dangers can be reduced by using a methodical examination that we will now address.

The conditions of the examination

In the **Nei Jing, it is said: "When one wants to examine someone, it is first necessary to close the doors and windows and it is at this time that begins the interrogation".**

An interrogation must be done in good conditions, when it was created a suitable environment. In the contrary case, the patient will not have the necessary concentration to respond precisely to our questions.

The practitioner in this environment must feel in its walls, he must feel at ease. In the same way the patient, when he enters this part must, by the decor and atmosphere which emerges, immediately be put in condition. The decorum, the place must already inspire and generate a feeling of calm and quiet.

À retenir

Patient and Practitioner must be calm all two. And especially, the practitioner must generate a feeling of calm, tranquillity which will promote the future exchanges. And in addition to be calm, the practitioner must be attentive, concentrated.

Let us not forget that the practitioner plays a role of inspector, investigator and that it will have to be concentrated to the maximum for that no symptom, that no sign not to escape it.

Attention

It is also necessary that the practitioner patience and concentration to ask the questions in a very precise way. In our world today, at least during the examination of the first meeting of the session, it would perhaps be advisable not to answer the telephone and be fully to listen to the patient.

This can be complicated in the beginning, but it takes relatively quickly in the habit, during the consultation, it should accept, except in particular cases, no third person. It is important to be alone with the patient. In effect, if the examination focuses on the details of his private life, it is likely that he did not want to talk about, to reveal what he has on the heart before someone else. If another person is present, it is not only probable that the patient does not say everything, but it can even distort the truth.

The five issues of the practitioner

Here are the five critical issues that the practitioner will pose at the outset to his patient. Do not install them, or to omit a, would be an error on his part.

The origin

The first issue outside of his curriculum vitae will concern its origins. Where is he born, what is its cradle family? This type of questions is very important. Indeed, certain pathologies, certain diseases do not develop that in some regions. If we take for example the goitre, it is common to find this type of pathology in the mountainous regions while the rheumatism, especially related to the moisture, will develop, them, in the regions in edge of sea, in the coastal regions.

Le saviez-vous

So when we request to a person his region of origin, not only we can know the most frequent diseases in the said region, but it may also draw some conclusions on the climate, food habits. For example, in some regions, people like to eat spicy, in others, they prefer rather the salted. The food habits influence widely the operation of the digestion.

The Profession

For example if the person must use tremendously its physical force during his work, but that this situation is relatively recent, she can then easily injure his energy, his breath, his IQ. If the person remains permanently Assisi, if it does not do enough to work his body, it is said "it hurts its spleen " it will of the problems related to the digestion of food bowl.

Another example: tinnitus or the emergence of deafness are not necessarily put in relationship with the imbalance of the internal organs. It is the environment where there is excessive noise permanent that may be the cause.

The habits of life

The next step of the interrogation must focus on how to live, the habits of sunrise and sunset and eating habits. All the answers to these questions will be as much of indices for the detective that the practitioner becomes. Here we are always in search of the weapon of the crime.

If in the course of this examination, the person tells you that she likes to eat sweet, this may injure his spleen, if it is drawn by the salt, this will hurt his kidneys. If, on the contrary, it is the acid taste which predominates in his power, it is the liver which will be injured. If it is the tangy flavor that is taken in excess, this will hurt his lungs and too many bitter flavor will eventually injure his heart. It is therefore fundamental to interrogate the patient on its eating habits, see what the person eats the most, inquire about its desires.

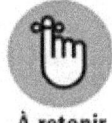 **À retenir** If an individual is perfectly healthy and well adjusted, a transient envy that he sends his organization must indeed be followed. By the dietetics, the body attempts to regularize it. On the other hand, if the imbalances are already present for a long time, if they are entered in the chronicity, follow his desires brings the body to its self-destruction. The renal impairment will be attracted by the salty, and the more he takes, the more it fatigue his kidneys. The person can also drink too much and exceed daily, and often exaggerated way, the liter, sufficient to our fluid intake daily. If it has the habit of drinking tea and that it takes much too much, it can also be transformed into tan-moisture.

If the patient to sunrise and sunset totally unbalanced, it ends up no longer be able to recharge its battery. He then loses the ability to self-regulation of his organization.

The affective state

It is important then to be interested in the emotional state of the patient, his state of mind. It must be very quickly to get an idea of its state sentimental, of its dominant emotions, both by the past that at the present time. This questioning is central. This is the fourth error not to commit. In the contrary case, one would be led to treat the Crown, the surface of the disease and not the root, of this same disease.

A citation of the **Nei Jing**

"If the external appearance of the body gives the impression of a happy person, if it seems quiet, but that his deep feeling that his life is sad, it is a cause of disease.

If the external appearance of the body gives the impression of a happy person, that emotion that dominates is the joy, but if this joy becomes excessive, it can also lead to a disease.

If in appearance the person is quiet, happy, but that his emotions are quite bitter, this leads to a disease in the vessels, May.

If in appearance the person is rather sad on the physical plane, because it has, among other things, a difficult life, but that on the emotional level it is rather of temperament merry, the disease will rather in the tendons.

If in appearance the person is rather sad and also on the emotional level, the disease will focus on the throat.

If the body undergoes often of spawners or fear, it may produce diseases by obstruction of blood vessels in the Jing Luo. "

The origin of the disease

In effect, we must ask the patient in what circumstances he has noticed this evil, how is it appeared? It is the search for the first cause of the disease.

"For example, if the patient returns of a country hot and humid and that it consults for problems of diarrhea and pain in the belly; diagnosis of penetration of heat and humidity will be obvious.

"If it returns of skiing and that on his return he felt he had a fever; we know that it has been attacked by the perversity cold.

"If the patient, before that his illness did not appear, was violently contested and strongly put in anger; the cause of his illness is a pulse emotional.

"If it explains that after a big meal he has not felt very well and that it is then fell ill; his problem is then surely of food origin.

 Inquire also on the medication he takes. He must know that the taking of Pharmacopoeia to the long course, especially in modern chemistry, and in

Attention particular for treatments or hypotensive for treatment of depression promotes the emergence of stagnation of blood and energy accompanied by symptoms of internal cold. These medicines in effect are by nature very cold, and may result in symptoms which will obscure the symptomatology first of the disease. It must take into account this to have an idea of why the current state of the patient.

So, to get a precise idea of the disease, it must be:

" In search for its origin;

" Understanding its evolution;

" And deduct a treatment.

The interrogation on the symptoms or "The Song of the ten questions"

In the first part of the examination, we are interested in the past of the patient, the history and the evolution of the disease. It is a genuine conversation with our patient, which conversation elsewhere may very well take place in the second part of the meeting or in the second session. Everything is a matter of appreciation and contact patient-practitioner.

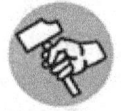

In the second part we will attach to the current situation, to the signs that the patient present at this time. This interrogation symptomatologique, **En pratique** him, will be very targeted, the issues will need to be very quick and we will not let the time the patient to talk for too long and to embark on the answers which, in some way, would eventually drown the fish. This will be almost of the yes or no.

In the work of investigator of the practitioner, the framing of the disease will be to "locked" the patient in the theory of Ba gang, the desired result being to know if the disease or symptom is yin or yang, internal, LI or external, Xu or Shi, i.e. fullness or weakness, and finally if it is hot, Re, or cold, Han. He also wants to know if the disease is located in such or such a meridian, or in such or such a body, that is why the questions must be focused on these various points.

And the practitioner will be used for this in a series of questions and more particularly "the practice of ten questions." This practice has been launched by Zhang Jing Yue (1563-1640). This author is one of the major figures of the Chinese medicine. It is one of the most famous commentators of the Nei Jing and it must numerous

109

clarifications on difficult subjects. The ten questions proposed by Zhang Jing Yue focus on:

" The cold and heat;
" The Sweating;
" The pain;
" The urine and faeces;
" The appetite and buccal flavors;
" The sensations at the level of the chest and abdomen;
" The hearing;
" The thirst ;
" The Sleep and Dreams;
" The gynecological behavior.

That is what is called the song of the "ten questions". Let's now review.

The question on the cold and heat

This question is essential when the diagnosis by the interrogation.

" If he says that he is afraid of the cold and that he has a fever, diseases of external cause often present these symptoms.
" If it was the wind which was in question, he would say simply that he does not like the wind, but as soon as it closes the door, it does the longer fears, then we are saying that he is afraid of the wind.
" On the other hand, if it is the wind and the cold who had attacked the body at the same time, the person would have fear of cold and at the same time fear of wind.
" If after having been covered, the person has no more afraid of the cold weather, it is most certainly a pathology of external cause. But if despite the coverage, it continues to have cold, we can conclude that it is located in front of an insufficiency of Yang of the body and that it has to do to internal cause.
" We will have to have the same type of investigation for fear of the heat. For example for a fever of external cause, the heat rises gradually and when the perversity is eliminated, the heat drops quickly enough. In this case of external pathology, the heat is located on the surface of the skin, on the surface of the body.

The palpation of the hand is important. If it is primarily the back of the hand which presents of the heat, we are surely in the presence of an external cause. On the other hand, if it is the palm of the hand which is hot, surely this is a disease of domestic origin. The chest and the stomach can also be hot.

The question on transpiration

We know that the sweat fate of the pores of the skin. The pores are controlled by the lung. The Lung also controls the breath, the Qi but also the protective energy, Wei Qi. This energy, this Wei Qi allows you to tighten the pores of the skin to protect the body from external attacks of cold and hot. Another very important function of Wei Qi is not to leave the body heat, the Yang, exit to escape.

This is only a excessive sweating which should attract the attention. When the question on transpiration, there are two possible cases, or an excess of sweating or on the contrary a lack of sweating still called anhidrose. And this sweating can originate from an external attack or a internal problem.

Let us take a few examples of transpiration of external origin:

"If there are a lot of heat and not sweating, the protective energy is not sufficient to evacuate the excess of Yang. This will then sign a damage of the lung.
"

À retenir

If the cold perversity enters the body, this cold will have for action to close the pores of the skin. This "confinement of the cold" will then be transformed into fire. The person will be headache, its pulse will be buoyant and tight. There is too much Yang in the body which does not arrive to escape. The person will be evil in the joints, a little everywhere in the body. It is important to ask our patient if it has transpired after having taken cold. If this is not the case, this confirms obviously the diagnosis of the penetration of the cold in the body.

"If, at the time of the attack of the cold your Xie Qi, your barrier of defense is strong enough, at that time there will be sweating. It is a good sign since the body rejects the perversity toward the outside. We will then be in the order temperature before sweating which shows that

111

there is a struggle between the perverse energy and energy right, then sweating and elimination: The cold spell of the body. The patient is then cured.

In practice

Now let us look at a few examples of internal causes that can cause perspiration. The Sweat, transpiration are the liquid of the heart. Gold as the heart controls the blood, the blood controls the transpiration. When you sweat too, liquids, the water in the blood are reduced and therefore the quality of the blood is deteriorating, and by way of consequence the heart can also be affected.

That is why the **Nei Jing** said that he must monitor the heart for all these diseases of internal cause that trigger an excessive sweating. It must not let the person sweating too much.

Attention

The dangers of the sauna to all goes! In the rules of hygiene of life taught by the Pr Leung, there is of course the problem linked to excessive perspiration. It is not used for nothing, and even this can become very harmful, to trigger by excessive efforts, sweating too abundant. It put us in particular in guard against practices such as the sauna.

A dozen minutes may actually allow the skin to release its toxins. On the other hand when the practice too often, or a fortiori too long, we run the risk of exhausting our blood, therefore our heart. All this is therefore to meditate especially for people who already have heart problems.

If the Yang energy in the body is not sufficient, this protective energy will not happen to play its role of barrier. This sweating, unlike that of external cause, has no taste or smell, nor of the flavor and the body does not present with fever even when you sweat. It even has a tendency to be rather cold.

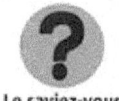

Le saviez-vous

The sweating due to a lack of Yin is a nocturnal sweating only. In the day, there will be no episode of transpiration. It is only the night when the

112

person is sleeping that it occurs. When it wakes up, the body is all wet. This is called a "transpiration stealth".

There are locations with respect to the sweating.

"A perspiration of the Hands Only often comes from a vacuum of Qi of the lung or the heart, or the heat of the lung or heart.

"A transpiration of the chest sign the case of a syndrome of Yin.

"If the patient presents the fatigue, that it is more or less anorexic, he has palpitations and insomnia, it is a vacuum of spleen and of the heart. But it can also be a problem Kidney heart if in addition to the palpitations and insomnia, he dreams a lot and that it suffers from the loin and knees.

Therefore in the interrogation on transpiration there will be a need to consult on his schedule, its location, its quantity, its taste and on the main signs associated.

The question on the Pain

The pain is a subjective symptom frequently encountered in clinic. It can occur in any area of the body.

Since each part of the body is in relationship with one of the "five solid organs or six hollow organs", the "Five Zang six Fu," a meridian or a collateral branch, by distinguishing the localization of pain, it is possible to know precisely what is the body or the Meridien concerned by this disease manifestation.

The example of the headache

Let us take the example of the headache, symptom, more than common in our Western societies. When, in the course of the Interrogation a person says suffer from headache, it should be to differentiate the pain of external origin, those internal in origin.

The headache of external cause are primarily due to the cold perversity.

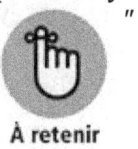
"

À retenir

If it is the wind which is in issue, the person has rarely bad all of suite, this only comes after.

"The summer heat can also be the cause. You know of course what is called the "heat stroke". If such is the case, in addition to the headache that may be important, the person will be thirsty and it transpirera spontaneously.

"There may also be a fire in the body that Monte, even that of the Tan which obstructs the Jing Luo, the meridians, and which causes of the fire that Monte.

With regard to the headache of internal cause, there is often a concept of chronicity which between in game.

"If the cause is an internal heat, headache can be accompanied by symptoms related to the eyes, the ears, nose or throat.

"If the heat is in the lung, outside the headache, often at the inside of the nose there are buttons.

"If the cause is related to a excessive Yang of the kidney, outside of the evil of head there will be problems at the level of the ears.

"If the fire is in the liver, this is accompanied then of sclera red with an inflammation of the eye.

"The headache of internal cause may also be the consequence of a lack of Yin, a Yin Xu.

"An excessive absorption of alcohol will excite the Yang. This excitation of the Yang will injure the Yin of the body.

"You can find a similar problem in the case of excessive sex activity, or at least in the case of ejaculation to repetition. In this case, there is a loss of Jing Ye, the water of the kidney becomes inadequate and the Yang Monte, which can cause headache.

"In the event of overwork, the Zhong Qi, "The energy of the Center", is not enough, and in this case the spleen is injured. The Yang will then fit and cause these pains.

 Another case of headache which is often found in women, more than in man, it is when the blood circulates evil. He must know that the starter of the À retenir rules in Chinese medicine is found to be the energy of the liver. It is the Yang of the liver that pushes the blood to exit. But if there is a state of stagnation of energy

114

at the level of the liver under the effect for example, emotional lock, emotions internalized, there is not enough of Yang mobilizable to trigger the rules and especially there is not enough of Yang at the level of the head. Too of Yin by lack of Yang at the level of the head promotes the stagnation which triggers the headache.

The diagnosis by the examination will need to focus also on the intensity of the pain and its location.

In the case of external attack, the evil of head appears very quickly, as soon as the body is attacked by the perversity and c is a violent pain, acute. It lasts just the time of the external attack and the battle that the body is in the process to deliver. Another special feature, it is not repetitive, except if another attack occurs.

Case of a internal pathology

Le saviez-vous

On the other hand, when it comes to a internal pathology, for example if we take the example of our Yin Xu of women during its menses, these headaches can be repetitive and their repetition can become chronic, last for years sometimes with periods of remission. The headache can then be very violent. With regard to the location, she will follow often the journey of the meridians. For example a temporal pain, where passes the meridian of the gallbladder, will very often to put in relationship with a stagnation in the level of the energy of the liver.

For a pain in the body in general, it must therefore already establish differences between external symptoms and symptoms internal. Then see if these pains are related to hot or cold. This is not as easy as that. It cannot be considered a single symptom to draw conclusions too fast on the disease.

Case of a pain caused by an external element

In the case of the pain caused by an external element as the cold or the wind, they are not frozen to a place; they can

115

move in the whole body. For example, if a pain begins to the shoulder, it can move in the back, in the chest, in the hands or feet. The pain is there, but there is no external signs such as swelling or redness.

An excess of heat to the inside of the body can produce this type of pain. The organization tries to eliminate this heat, and this can cause pain in the body and in the OS. Symptoms such as the fear of heat, of spontaneous transpirations can then appear.

This heat can also come from the moisture that has remained too long to the inside of the body. We said then that the humidity is transformed into heat.

There may also be the production of what is called "a perverse fire". The Tan present at the inside of the body under the effect of stagnation has been able to transform into fire.

Foods that are "remained on the belly", as it is said, a poor digestion after congested The stomach has been able to be at the origin of the production of fire. And this fire can cause pain in the whole body.

You can also find themselves before a case where a person fear neither cold nor hot, it has no fever, but only evil in the OS. This pain has for particularity to be very concentrated. We said then that it is a disease Yin Han, a disease caused by a cold internal. The element Yang is no longer able to balance the Yin. This Yin is become the cold and has stagnated at a specific location of the body. At this location, the pain is transfixiante, acute, it does not move. This pain therefore appears because there is not enough energy Yang. In this regard, the treatment is quite easy. It is sufficient to increase the Yang of heat the needles.

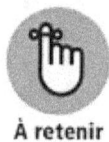

À retenir

A pain can have a emotional support not negligible. If we take as another example the pain of cancers, they can be classified into two groups: a direct pain that appears at the beginning of the disease and which is linked to a compression of a nerve, or a stagnation that generates the inflammation. The second type is Jing Sheng, mental, and is caused by a voltage psychological, by the concern. On the therapeutic plan, the practitioner will deal not only with the direct pain that they are real. But it also requires the implementation of psychological methods designed to cope with the pains of type Jing Sheng for well happen to eliminate them. If we do not put to implement these methods, it will not happen to heal these pain.

The question on faeces and urine

Urination and scats are two methods used by man to evacuate the excess accumulated in the body. According to the Nei Jing, c is the kidney that controls the Urination and defecation. It is known that the stools are evacuated by the large intestine and the urine by the bladder, two bodies located at the household level lower. These two bodies are all two of the Fu, that is to say of the organs Yang, hollow, receptacles. These bodies operate only when they receive orders, they do not have the power to autocontrôler. It is for this reason that the Nei Jing said that "the kidney has the power to control the two, because the lower furnace is controlled by the kidney".

The problems associated with stool

The defecation, although directly led by the large intestine, is intimately linked also to the functions of the spleen and stomach that digest, transporting, transformed. But also to the functions of the liver that transmits and disperses, by the fire of Ming Men content in the kidney, which warms the body. But also by the energy of the lung that cleans and brings down the energy, the Qi. Let us not forget the existence of the torque Poumon-Gros intestine. By querying

117

the patient on his stools, the practitioner may very often obtain very valuable information about his illness.

"When there is too much heat in the lung, the liquids are evaporated. This triggers a drought at the level of the large intestine, and therefore of the constipation. (Attention to smokers).

"Another case to consider is the case where the lung is Xu, low. If it has not enough energy, if the energy in the upper home does not flow well, is not free, the energy in the lower furnace is not free not more. This will have an impact also on the stool.

"In the case of lung Xu, the stools are either normal or soft, but not of diarrhea for as much. The belly is not inflated, the stools are rare, little bulky. There is only a manufacture abnormally low of stools.

"On the other hand, in the lung Shi, the belly is inflated, the stool are dry and hard. There is stagnation of stool volume with poor progression in the terminal part of the tube.

"Another situation is linked to the spleen. If there is heat in the spleen and if there is not enough fluids that come in the large intestine, they are too dry to evacuate. In the ancient texts, we talk about heat in the Yang Ming. At that time he will be able to have some swelling and pain in the belly.

"If the stools are soft, pasty, this may come from an external cause. At the time, this will be the moisture and the warmth that will be incriminated.

"A collapse of the energy of the spleen can be at the origin of soft stools to repetition.

History of the smoking of cannabis, trapped by his Practitioner

Attention He must know that the cannabis between in many forms of traditional pharmacopoeia, in the aim of toning the energy of the spleen. But as in all, the excess turns against the body and collapsed this same energy.

It is a young, around the twenties. It is rather pale, lean. These eyes are not very mobile. It does not breathe the full health. It consults for a state of fatigue quasi-permanent. The practitioner has already "intuition". Question: "How are you going to the saddle ? "Answer:" normally. "If it does not go further in his questioning, it passes to the side of the problem. Question: "How many times per day? "Response: "Ben, two, three times! "Question: "And your stools are soft or hard? "Answer: "Always soft. "Reaction of the Practitioner: "Good, are going direct to the purpose (it already has the answer in your head): How many seals do you smoke in the day? "The patient is caught short and is obliged to answer in the affirmative. It presents all the symptoms of a depletion of the energy of the spleen.

The problems related to urine

It is important to question the sick on the presence or the absence of urination, to inquire as to the frequency, color and the quantity of the latter, to know if the urine are clear or disorders, if they should normally elapse or not and if they are accompanied by pain. The urine derived from the organic liquids, Jin Ye. The lung is superior source of the water. It has the function to maintain and release the track of the water. The spleen governs the transport and transformation of water and moisture. The kidney is involved in the movement of water and liquids, and is responsible for the faeces and urine. The Bladder stores the urine.

A person normally incorporated urine three to five times per day and to zero and at large a maximum of once per night. The frequency and volume of urine are influenced by factors such as the volume of beverages absorbed, body temperature, physical efforts, transpiration and age.

À retenir It is good to remind here that in the West we consume too much of liquids. If one were to take into account the water contained in the food, the water that penetrates through the air we breathe and by the skin, we should not drink more of a liter in the day, provided to drink in small quantities broken down, without taking a big bowl in a single time and avoiding drinking during meals, under penalty of drowning its food bowl. I refer you to the chapter devoted to this recurring problem in our modern diet (see chapitre 20).

The kidneys are a Machine to filter the waste and not the liquids.

Normally the urine must be slightly yellow, straw

Attention yellow.

"If the color is too yellow, and if a heat emerges from the urine to the urination, this shows that there is heat in the bladder or the fire in the heart.

"If the energy is deficient, the color of the urine may change a urination to another.

"If there is a fire in the heart and the small intestine, the urine may also be dark yellow.

"There is not enough energy Yang in the body, if this energy is not sufficient to evaporate the liquid, at that time the urine will be abnormally clear. It is a disease cold. The urine may then be as clear as the water. At that time, the amount of urine may be much more important, the frequency of urination higher, and there may even be loss of control.

"If the person has a urination incomplete in drip, it is linked to a vacuum of the IQ of the kidney and its inability to control the sphincter of the bladder. This can meet in the event of senility or chronic illness.

"A painful urination and obstructive, with a burning sensation and having a character of emergency corresponds to an accumulation of heat-moisture, as in case of cystitis.

"The bedwetting, or spontaneous urination during sleep, is due to a lack of the Qi of the kidney that cannot control the bladder. This occurs in a context of imbalance between the Yin nightlife and the diurnal Yang especially among the child.

The question on the appetite and buccal flavors
The fifth issue concerns the eating habits and the different tastes are likely to appear in the mouth.

Food Habits

Let us therefore start by eating habits. We know that the food after having been chewing, after s be impregnated with the saliva mouth, a kind of prédigestion, then will penetrate in the stomach. The stomach has a relationship internal-external with the Spleen: by the observation of eating habits, you can obtain information on the operation of the spleen and stomach, as well as several other interesting information.

" If the appetite is reduced during the course of chronic diseases, if it is accompanied by mental depression, a scrambled complexion, a pale language and a weak pulse, this signs a weakness of the Rate-Pancréas and stomach, and this is not a very good prognosis.

" The indigestion, such as the reduced appetite with heaviness of the head, epigastric distension and abdominal, coated yellow and bold on the language is primarily due to an excess of moisture cumbersome the spleen.

" The anorexia, means an aversion vis-a-vis food and their smell. This symptom occurs naturally in food poisoning, but in chronic cases, it may also meet in the case of retention of food. If the disgust of food is accompanied by a coating very thick and sticky, this comes from an excess of moisture in the home means that affects the liver and gall bladder, stomach and spleen.
"

The anorexia and vomiting of the pregnant woman to sign a rise against the current of the energy of the liver.

Le saviez-vous

" Finally, the anorexia nervosa done a little part of the table of the Depression. It is very often an obsessive compulsive disorder linked to the liver and due to a blockage, a nouure thereof consecutive to the emotional blockages.

" Furthermore, during the development of a disease, the gradual restoration of the appetite announces the

121

improvement of IQ of the stomach and therefore a healing next. While the gradual decrease of appetite announces an increase of the weakness of the stomach and spleen and therefore a worsening of the pathology.

"During a chronic disease, if the patient eats little and covers suddenly the appetite and eats abundantly, it is a sign of exhaustion next of the average household, of the spleen and stomach. That is what is called in Chinese "The end of the Center". This are the "last glows before the end", a little the swan song.

Buccal flavors

Then, there is a need for focus on the particular tastes that can appear in the mouth.

"
If a bitter taste appears in the mouth, it is an excess of fire in the liver and the gallbladder, or of

En pratique the escalation against the current of the energy of the gallbladder.

"A salty taste may be due to a disease of cold nature, or to a vacuum of Qi of the kidney with reference of cold-moisture to the top.

"A Taste acid is often due to food. This can be a acid regurgitation most often caused by the attack of the IQ of the liver on the stomach and the inability of the IQ of the stomach to descend.

"A sweet taste translated from the heat moisture resulting from an excess absorption of sweets and put too rich. There is accumulation of heat-moisture at the level of the spleen and stomach, and it is "the energy of grain which has just invade the mouth".

"A Taste fade is linked to a state Xu of the liver and the stomach or during a cold syndrome.

Therefore, the taste that the patient is feeling in the mouth can give valuable information to the practitioner.

The question on the sensations at the level of the chest and abdomen

If the person feels that his chest is inflated, full, oppressed, this shows that the energy does not flow well. In this case, the practitioner in the methods of treatment it implements, will avoid toning not to aggravate the case. This poor circulation, this congestion may be due to the weakness of the energy or the obstruction by the tan.

Thoracic oppression

A thoracic oppression with sputum is caused by a stagnation of Tan-moisture and an obstruction of the Qi of the lung.

The thoracic oppression with palpitation and short of breath is linked to a state Xu of the Heart and of the IQ of the lung or a Yang Xu, a weakness of Yang of the upper home.

The thoracic oppression accompanied by frequent sighs is due to psycho-emotional and to the qi stagnation of the liver.

When the heart beats quickly, and that this beat is felt from the chest to the navel, and this, during a long period of time, it is really of pathological palpitations which may be the result:

" A vacuum of blood;

" Of a vacuum of Yin which favors the appearance of a fire which disrupts the Shen in the heart.

A vacuum of the QI and the Yang of the heart may also, by depriving the heart of "heat healthy" trigger this type of symptoms.

There is still the state Xu of the spleen and the Yang of the kidney that promotes an invasion of the heart by the water.

And finally, the obstruction of the vessels of the heart, the famous Coronaries, by the Tan which prevents the blood to circulate freely.

Swelling of the abdomen

After the thorax, we need to look at the upper part of the abdomen which corresponds to the liver and spleen.

123

In the case of swelling of the abdomen, there was a distinction between the States Xu, of weakness and the Member Shi of fullness.

As for the thorax, when it is completed, hard, swollen and painful. This is obviously a case Shi.

"If there is a Deaf pain in the abdomen, that it is not hard, this is called PEI, C is a swelling due to gas. There is the presence of water. It is a case Xu."

If the abdominal distension is due to a state Xu of the Rate-Estomac, it is calmed down by the

À retenir pressure, the palpation or a local heat, a hot water bottle for example. It was case to a weakness of the Yang Qi of the spleen.

"On the other hand, if it is due to an excess of heat, the patient will not bear the pressure. This is due, among other things, to the retention of food in the stomach and the intestines to prevent the movement of Qi.

The practitioner may not rely to 100% according to the patient. When the latter said that the belly is inflated, it is necessary to see if it really is. We can see if under the skin, there is water which is stagnating. When traces with the hand, when pressed on the skin, there is a depression. We look at if it persists or not, as well as the speed at which is carried out the escalation. We can then determine if the cause is the weakness of the energy or of stagnant water.

The question on the hearing, the tinnitus, the view and the dizziness

Dizziness

The Vertigo say Tou Yun Chinese. It is a subjective feeling of the patient that his whole body or that the landscape rotates around him. Often the dizziness is accompanied by disorders of the view. Indeed, in case of dizziness. One has the impression of not having the clear vision.

For the Chinese medicine, the main responsible for the dizziness is the liver. The liver, it is of the

wood. The element Yang of the liver must fit in a harmonious manner. If it rises too much, or if he does not rise enough, this gives dizziness. This imbalance Yin-Yang in the liver is caused most often by the kidney. The water of the kidney is not sufficient to feed the wood of the liver. As well:

"The Vertigo by exhaust of the fire of the liver is accompanied by sensations of strains raised at the level of the skull, cheeks and red eyes, of mood disorders ranging from the hyper susceptibility to the anguish, pain on the flanks, routes of the meridian of the Vb, and mouth bitter.

"In case of excess of Yang of the liver, if there is presence of dizziness, there will also be the pains of type distension of the skull, tinnitus, weaknesses at the level of the knees. The Vertigo of Meniere fall within this framework.

"The vertigo may also be due to the TAN and the inability in the Yang to mount. It is accompanied by the heaviness of head, thoracic oppression, nausea and burdens in the legs. That is what is called Vertigo positional.

"The Vertigo by empty of Qi and blood is monitoring of mental fatigue, shortness of breath, lethargy. It is aggravated by the stress.

"Finally, the vertigo by empty of the Jing of The Kidney gives a feeling of emptiness, tinnitus and loss of memory, the weakness of the joints and knees.

"In another case, the person has not dizziness, or headache. She feels simply as a burden on its head, it has the " *heavy head* ". It is often linked to the fact that the upper part of the body is Xu. According to the **Nei Jing, if the upper part of the body has not enough energy, the brain is not enough fed, the head falls, it is heavy. The Yang does not rise enough, it does not provide enough food to the head.**

Tinnitus

The tinnitus is say Ming 1 in Chinese. The practitioner must ask the patient if it intends to distinctly. There are several cases of deafness:

"External causes as too of external noise, external attacks badly treated (repeated ear infections).

"The Internal causes are often related to the kidney, because the kidney was for hole to output the ears. The Yang energy of the kidney is low, this energy does not happen to fit. The ears do not have enough of Acuity. The weakness of other bodies may be at the origin of progressive deafness. The age will contribute of course to the onset of such symptoms.

In addition to deafness, there may be problems of tinnitus, which are noises in the inner ear of type "Song of cicada" or "buzzing as the rising tide and downlink":

"

Le saviez-vous The tinnitus, as the croaking of the toad or the noise of the waves of the tide, which are not reduced by the local pressure of the EAR are due to a fire of the gallbladder which disrupts the upper holes.

"The tinnitus progressive and bottom of type noise of cicadas and which are calmed down by the pressure of the EAR are due to a syndrome of vacuum of the liver and the kidney, to an excess of Yang of the liver or a deficiency of the Jing of the kidney.

The question on the thirst

À retenir The thirst, Kou Ke in Chinese, means the desire to drink, but also the necessary quantity of water to quench his thirst. Normally, when one is in good health, when you drink regularly in small quantities fractionated warm or hot fluids, it should never have thirst. Thirst is a symptom of "too late": we stayed too long without drink, and it plays to the camel. Or then it is a pathological symptoms, most of the time of internal heat.

126

"If the patient has a dry mouth, that it has a thirst, that he has desire to drink or that it wishes to cold drinks, this indicates a heat that damages the Yin. The physiological liquids become insufficient.

"If the patient has a dry mouth, that it has a thirst and that it wishes to hot drinks in small quantities or if he is thirsty, but not want to drink, and that in addition it has difficulties mictionnelles, is that there is a water stagnation internal.

"There is no difficulties mictionnelles, these symptoms are the result of the penetration of the heat, a disease of warmth in the blood. This last evaporates, transforms and Monte as a tide, causing the sensation of thirst without desire to drink.

"In the absence of high fever, a thirst with desire to drink a lot, accompanied by a urinary flow important is a sign of diabetes, Xiao Ke in Chinese.

The question on Sleep and Dreams

Query a patient on his sleep is essentially to ask him if he is subject to the insomnia, Shi mian, or to the hypersomnia, Duo Shui. In general, the elderly need less sleep than young people. It is a physiological aspect normal.

Insomnia

Insomnia is characterized by a sleep time too short, or falling asleep difficult or even an ease to wake up. Let us look at these different cases:

"The patient does not happen to fall asleep. It rotates in his bed, has thousands of ideas parasites. There may be of impatience at the level of the legs. At this time, it is the fire of the heart which rises too much. Either the blood of the heart is inadequate, either the water of the kidney is no longer in control of the fire of the heart that is ablaze.
"

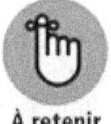

À retenir The patient falls asleep because he is tired, and then he wakes up in the second part of the night without being able to get back to sleep then. It is often a problem linked to a weakness of the Yin of the liver. The Hun content in the liver has a tendency to want to get out. It is said that it loses its anchor, and C is the insomnia that appears. A vacuum of gallbladder will trigger in him a waking up very early in the morning.

"Another case: the person falls asleep, wakes up, falls asleep again... Often at this time, there are pathologies of type fullness. His stomach is never empty. He eats too!

"The insomnia of origin Xu are often due to the heart. This may be the blood of the heart that is insufficient. When there is not enough blood, the Heart lack of food: it is disturbed, disrupted, worried. The Sleep is then intermittent. There is also the fire in the heart that can trigger the insomnia. There is too much fire in the heart, the blood is too abundant, the Yang Monte and sometimes it is not to fall asleep.

"When the person is tense, nervous, it is a sign of voltage of the gallbladder. There is a concentration of fire in the vesicle and if this fire goes up too, the insomnia appears.

"If the person has too many worries, it hurts his spleen. The spleen also produces blood. The person therefore injures his blood and this also causes of insomnia.

"You can also have the temporary insomnia after having eaten too much. In this case, there is also the swelling due to disturbances of digestion.

In MTC, it is not wise to to systematically give sleeping pills in the cases where people do not sleep. For example, if the person has a shortfall in the level of the heart if it gives him of tranquilizers for it to sleep one or two nights, this serves neither arranges nothing. The key here is to restore the balance of the heart for that she redorme.

Hypersomnia

The opposite of the insomnia, we have the hypersomnia, who said Duo Shui, what can also call the somnolence, Shi Shui, which means in Chinese "engage without restraint to sleep".

"The first cause is an excess of fatigue. If the person is too tired, too overworked, it hurts his spleen. If the energy of the spleen is low, the person has always want to sleep. That is what we can call "the blow of pump".

"If the spleen is throttled moisture, this moisture can make the heavy body and it was then always want to sleep. Often the need to sleep appears after a meal.

Nap or not nap?

À retenir

The somnolence after a meal is often linked to a state of "too-full of the Stomach". The organization realizing that he has not enough energy to digest its food bowl (A digestion can deplete of half the battery of the Kidney!) gives you as a symptom alarm signal the need to make the NAP. I am not talking here of the "Siesta crapuleuse" course. At this time, 20-30 minutes of Siesta are quite beneficial. This NAP can be reduced to 10 minutes of relaxation (see the chapter which is dedicated to him), which is equivalent to 3 hours of sleep! But Attention: If you take a siesta of more than 40 minutes; the food bowl will rot in your stomach. You will get the opposite effect to the one expected.

"After a disease, there may be a lot of accumulated fatigue and sleepiness. Then it is a good sign. Sleep much help in this case to restore the element Yin. In this circumstance, the envy of sleep is not a disease. It is a period of convalescence. It is the best medicine of burn-out.

"There is a state of mid-sleep and mid-awakening by extreme mental fatigue, as during the course of a depression. The cause is then a vacuum of blood from the heart and the Yang of the kidney, as well as an excess of cold to the inside of the body. The patient may fall asleep as soon as it closes the eyes and wake up as soon as it is called.

Dreams

That is the dream? The excess of dream is called Ye you in Chinese, which wants to say " walk the night". It is a disturbance very common sleep which is usually due to a factor pathogen that disrupts the Hun content in the liver. It can then be single wickedness as the fire, the TAN, the excess heat, Yang. The cause is often a vacuum of Yin. The dream represents a normal state, physiological sleep. Theoretically, when one is in good health, we must not remember that it was dreamed of.

When the quantity of dreams becomes too important, that these dreams are pleasant or unpleasant, or **a fortiori** when there has dreams to trend excessive emotional as nightmares, at that time the patient can wake up. The questioning on these dreams may then give us valuable information.

" If the dreams of anger and violence are recurring, c is the biliary Foie-Vésicule which is then to incriminate.

" If the dreams are to dominant erotic, and **a fortiori** if there are leaks seminal during the night, then it is a weakness of the kidney.

" If the dreams are of a nature sad, c is the lung that is concerned and so on.

The question on the gynecological behaviors

We conclude this study on the "Ten Questions" by a particular questioning on the gynecological behaviors.

Let us start by menstruation, Yue Jing in Chinese. It is a flow monthly uterine, blood non-coagulated in women of childbearing age.

The interrogation on the menses contains the terms and conditions of the cycle, the duration of the rules, their quantity, their color, their nature and the symptoms escorts.

Women belong to the element Yin. The Yin is in relationship with the moon. That is why there are rules all 28 days.

" If the rules come earlier, if they are in advance, if their cycle is short, one can ask whether there is no heat in the blood or if it is not located before a case of insufficiency of Yin.

" On the other hand, if the cycle is long, but that the rules are normal, this then shows that the blood is not sufficient, or while the person is low. The element Yang is not strong enough to make the blood out.

130

"If a woman has not its rules for months, that there is a judgment of the menstruation, there is obstruction of blood in the meridians. In this case, there may be also the cough, fever, vomiting blood, pain in the stomach.

"But if there is no rules and that all by elsewhere is normal, it should not be forgotten that the woman may already be pregnant. If the pulse as we will see is Hua, slippery, this then sign a pregnancy!

"An increased quantity and abundant of rules is often due to the heat in the blood which injures the meridians Ren May and Zhong may, or the lack of energy that may not retain the blood.

"On the contrary, a blood flow less important than the normal is due to the inadequacy of the production and the processing causing a disability of blood, or then to a stagnation of cold, of blood or Tan.

"The normal color of the Rules is red and their consistency must not be too fluid, neither too thick. There must be no presence of blood clots. The rules of pale red color and consistency fluid are often the result of a "insufficient blood and little prosperous". It is a symptom Xu.

"The menses dark red and thick consistency are a symptom of fullness Shi due to the "internal heat in the blood".

"The Rules of purple color dark with clots are due to a stagnation of cold causing a blockage of the blood.
"

À retenir

If the rules are painful, this often sign a blockage of the Qi of the liver. It must be remembered that the liver in Chinese medicine is considered as the starter of the rules. When, for example, under the effect of emotional blocks we are before a table of nouure of the liver, stagnation of blood and energy at the level of the liver, it may have pain and swelling at the level of the chest and abdominal pain during or before the rules.

"In normal times, the walls of the vagina of the woman are moistened by the secretions of milky white, without smell. If these secretions are excessive and do not stop, it is of vaginal discharge. Losses abundant, of colors white,

131

clear and fluids such as tears, are due to the flow of moisture, consequence of a lack of the spleen.

" Losses yellow, sticky, thick and foul-smelling, accompanied from time to time of itching and pain at the level of the external genitalia are caused by the flow of heat-moisture to the bottom of the body.

" Losses incessant red and odour nauseating slightly correspond to the stagnation of the heat in the meridian of the liver.

" Losses abundant, color dull and dark, consistency fluid, is accompanying a sensation of sluggishness and cold at the level of the lumbar region and abdominal, reflect a lack of the kidney.

Chapter 8
The decision of the PULSE
And the observation
Of the language
<u>In this chapter:</u>
<u>" Location of pulse</u>
<u>" Method of decision -pulse</u>
<u>" The normal pulse and the 27 kinds of pulse</u>
<u>" The final review: the techniques of observation of the</u>
<u>   language</u>

EN Chinese medicine, called this review may Zhen, take the pulse. It is a major step in the clinical examination. It allows you to collect very valuable information on the evolution of a disease, the nature and location of the imbalance, the State organs and viscera, the five Zang six Fu, and the state of the Yin and the Yang.

Let us say at the outset that this is the most difficult of all diagnostics. Excel in this art request not only a great practice, but much rigor, concentration and at the same time a very good theoretical knowledge.

Previously, we took the pulse on nine different arteries, three on the head, three on the hands and three on the legs. We found there, the location of the three homes (see chapitre 3). One finds this description in the description chapitre 20 of the **su wen, the treaty" of the three distinctions and of the nine locations." These locations on which we took the pulse were all of locations of acupuncture points on the Meridians located near the arteries. They** were divided into three main areas making reference to the trilogy earth-sky-man. This first method has been gradually replaced by the socket of the pulse at wrist that is called Cun Kou. We will follow, of course, the oral teachings given by Professor Leung Kok Yuen (see chapitre 1) to study these different forms of pulse.

Location of the PULSE

The main place of the catch of the Pulse in Chinese medicine is therefore at the level of both wrists, in overhang of the radial artery. The meridian of the

À retenir   lung happening precisely in this region. And we

133

know that the energy of the lung, mixture of the quintessence of the energy of the air and energy from the food bowl, therefore flows along the meridian.

In addition, the meridian of the lung begins in the average household and joined that of the spleen. As the spleen and stomach are the source of energy, the Qi, but also of the blood, Radial pulse can reflect the energy states of the spleen and stomach.

Finally, the meridian of the lung is that of the departure and the return of all the meridians on the circulatory Plan, forming the loop of the 12 main meridians, which ends by converge on radial pulse.

For this reason, Radial pulse reflects the state of the five Zang, six Fu, of energy, of the blood and the meridians of the body.

The pulse of the wrist, Kun Kou, is divided into three parts:

" The PULSE Guan, pulse of the Middle still called "barrier". It is located slightly below and next to the Radial styloïde.

" The PULSE Cun, still called "Pulse in front" or pulse of the thumb. It is located just in front of the PULSE Guan, toward the base of the thumb.

" The PULSE Chi, "pulse rear" or pulse of the cubit. It is located in the rear of the PULSE Guan, toward the elbow.

As well each wrist has 3 divisions of pulse, both wrists formed in all 6 divisions of pulse. We will therefore keep for our study the data in the **Nei Jing** to know that on the clinical plan:

" The Pulse of the CUN, of the thumb on the left corresponds to the location of the heart and to the right of the lung.

" The PULSE Guan, of the barrier to the left, corresponds to the liver and to the right of the spleen.

" The PULSE Chi, of the foot on the left, corresponds to the left kidney and right at the right kidney.

There are multiple theories which eventually make us lose foot with the reality and our Master is simply we learn those above.

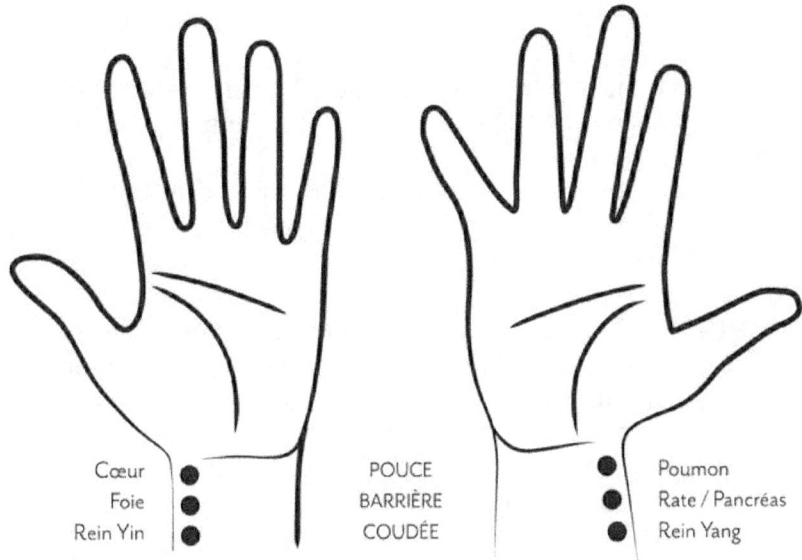

Cœur	POUCE	Poumon
Foie	BARRIÈRE	Rate / Pancréas
Rein Yin	COUDÉE	Rein Yang

Figure 8-1 Location of pulse and the corresponding bodies.

Method of decision of the PULSE

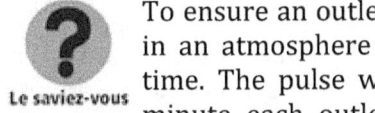

To ensure an outlet for pulse, the patient must be in an atmosphere of tranquillity since already a time. The pulse will be studied at least for one minute each outlet in order to impregnate the best possible of its characteristics.

The practitioner must itself be calm and possess the gift that he must cultivate, that of the "full conscience" of the present moment. Its breath must be quiet. It is a very important point because, as we will see later, it must be able to compare the respiratory rate and heart rate of the patient to his own, knowing that a healthy person and in normal conditions breathes 16 to 18 times per minute in unconscious Breathing and that his pulse bat to 4-5 beats during a respiratory cycle, an inspiration and expiration.

The patient must be in the seated position, the back right, the forearm resting on a flat pad before the practitioner, the palmar face of the hand looking at the sky or the arm in pronosupination. The fingers are flexible and released, leaving the flow of energy, of the Qi and blood flow freely along the Radial pulse.

If the patient is lying, the arms should be elongated along the body, palmar face toward the top. They must not rest on the body of the patient.

Then we come to the most important phase, namely the position of the fingers of the practitioner and the felt that it should have.

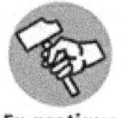
"

En pratique

The three fingers, namely the index, the medius and annular of practitioner, are posed on the same level and slightly arched and come Gently press the pulse of the patient with the pulp.

" The medius press on the pulse Guan, the barrier, the index on the pulse Cun or thumb and the ring finger on the pulse Chi, or foot.

" The position of three fingers must be accorded to the wrist of the patient, without obstacle nor movement of particular torsion.

" Among the child, we can use a single finger to examine the median pulse Guan.

The Practitioner begins to take the pulse of the two arms at the same time, applying a pressure symmetrical with its three fingers, to appreciate the energy state of the three homes. The the most distal point is the position Cun, who wants to say thumb. It is the upper home with, on the left, the pulse of the heart and to the right, the pulse of the lung. The average position is called Guan, " The barrier". C is the average household, with the liver to the left and the spleen to right. Finally, the most distant location of the wrist is the position Chi, foot, with to the right the kidney yang and to the left, the Kidney Yin.

Once it has assessed the overall pulse of two arms, it will work on each wrist and differentiate between the various homes. He studied the pulse at each location, one after the other, in exercising with each finger a surface pressure and then deep.

Before going into the detail of the pulse rate and for the one who does not want to go further, the box below allows you already understand what research the practitioner. Indeed, the traditional texts cite five phases, five movements that must make the fingers at the time of the taking of the pulse.

"**The first maneuver will allow to assess the strength of the pulse at superficial level by lifting the fingers. At that time, the practitioner feels if the pulse is floating, Normal, or empty, at this level.**

"**Then, it must "press", that is to say support very slightly the fingers toward the bottom, to realize the strength of the pulse at the intermediate level and deep. It may, from there, see if the pulse is deep, Normal, or empty, at these different levels. More in-depth, it will be able to see if it is hollow, hidden or empty, without root.**

"**The third phase allows, in some kind of "probe the pulse". That is to say that he will not move the fingers to count the frequency of the pulses. It will thus be able to determine if the pulse is Slow, Fast or Normal.**

"**During the fourth maneuver, the practitioner appreciated with the pulp of the fingers everything that happens around the radial artery. It will thus move very gently the fingers of one side to the other, i.e. perform micro-lateral movements, who do go from the outer edge toward the median side of the forearm. It will thus be able to determine if the pulse is slippery, in drum skin, tight, held, end, rough.**

"**The fifth motion will be to roll the fingers, i.e. to make them move very slightly from top to bottom and from bottom to top. This movement allows us to see if the pulse is long, short, or stirring. It is also the method of decision-pulse of a child of less than a year.**

These five movements allows to get an idea more or less precise of the globality of the pulse. It will then need to go further and consider the pulse at each location in exercising with each finger a surface pressure and then deep to see what home, what body is the most unbalanced by report to another. It may, for example, feel a powerful pulse at the level of the Liver located in the Kuan, to the barrier of the left arm, and on the contrary a pulse wide or slack at the level of the spleen, located in the right arm, always to the barrier.

The normal pulse

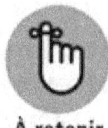

À retenir

The normal pulse, still called Chang Mai, is a pulse that is not floating or hollow. It never is neither too fast nor too slow. Normally, during a respiratory cycle, it must beat 4 to 5 times, which corresponds to 60-80 beats per minute. When the takes, it must have a feeling of softness, power without that it is compelling. After a physical effort, it should return to normal very quickly and must not have large amplitudes.

It is said that the pulse is normal when it obeys to three criteria:

"What is important, when we found this pulse is to see if there is *the energy of the stomach, see if it normally arrives with a good quality of the energy of the stomach. The Chinese then say that "it gives the impression of the footprint of a leg of chicken"*.

"The pulse must have the Shen, the mind, the vitality. We had already seen this in the study of colors. It is very subjective, but it knows when a rose has the Shen, of the vitality or when it is at the end of life.

"Finally, it is said that the PULSE must have a root. This term covers two meanings. First of all, the pulse of the two kidneys, located elbow side of the two forearm, must be present and of good quality. Furthermore, when we support very in depth, it must find a root, one must still feel the pulse.

When these conditions are present, then we know that the five Zang, six Fu, as well as the blood and energy are of good quality.

Le saviez-vous

It is necessary to know that the normal pulse can vary in function of physiological and psychological factors, without that it is for as much pathological. For example, the pulse is to put in relationship with the age, the sex and the physical constitution of an individual:

"Among the child, it will be small and fast.
"Among the Adolescents and Young, it can be smooth, slippery.
"Among the elderly person, it will normally be more hard and tense.
"There may also be a difference of pulse in the Man and the woman adult. In women, it will normally be flexible, soft and End. In humans, moderate and powerful.
In the acts of daily life:
"The pulse may be fast, powerful and slippery after a physical effort. This is not pathological and this must be returned in the order, once the rest found.
"Even after a good meal, it can have these same characteristics of power and speed.
"In case of anxiety, anxiety, it may be tense. It can be erratic in the case of fear.
"The Seasonal factors also have their importance. The pulse can be stretched slightly in the spring, floating slightly in autumn, Slightly hollow and deep in winter.
"It may also vary throughout a day. It may, for example , be floating and powerful during the day and slightly deep, end and slow, during the night.
Finally, there may be specific anatomies at the level of the radial artery. In some cases, it may be on the dorsal side of the wrist. It is then called "Pulse ectopic radial".
So we see that several factors can affect the normal state of a pulse. But as long as the pulse has the three fundamental characteristics that are therefore the Shen, the Qi of the spleen and a root, we can say that we have to deal with the normal pulse.
The 27 kinds of pulse
We will now proceed to the consideration of the pulse that can only be described as abnormal, of pathological. To characterize a pulse, we are going to have to attach to the variation of pace, or to morphology, force and to the form of a pulse. Certainly, there are a lot of subjectivity with regard to the study of these different pulse, but differentiate a superficial pulse of a deep Pulse, a tense pulse of a soft pulse, a pulse with or without root, a pulse regular or arrhythmic, a

slow pulse of a rapid pulse, already gives us a very good indications, provided of course that the conclusions that it draws are in concordance with the other parts of the diagnostic, that this is the study of the language, the observation and examination.

Therefore the pulse of base are very easy to learn, then to the force of experience, to force of years of practice, the practitioner will be able to refine its perception, its sensitivity and will be able to use this tool which is one of the most effective of the diagnosis.

Are therefore studying now the 27 kinds of pulse, derived from the ancient texts and reinterpreted by our master. Professor Leung, at the time of their study, were placed in a particular order. To use, you will see that this order allows us still easily to understand and remember.

Table 8-1 The 27 kinds of pulse.

Floating Pulse Fu	When installing the three fingers on the wrist, as soon as the ignition light, one feels much the artery. If one supports stronger, more deeply, at this time, the pulse gives the impression to be less strong, more low, less flowing. This sign in General Rule of diseases of the external, of Biao. The body has been attacked by external elements.
Soft Pulse Ru	It also evokes a cotton which floats to the surface of the water and disappears under a pressure too high. Although it is soft, it is the place in the category of floating pulse. It is said that it is a pulse inconsistent. It underlines a lack of energy and strength of the patient.
Hollow Pulse Kou	It is floating to the area, and when we supports a little more deeply, it feels a hollow, and when we still supports more deeply, we feel again the pulse. That is why it is said that the middle is hollow. This is a pulse Fu and hollow in the middle. When one observes this

pulse, it is that there is always a lack of blood.

Pulse by drum skin GE	When we touch very slightly to the area, it is very strong, very hard. When one supports a little more strong, it feels that it is hollow, that in the middle it is empty. When supports more deeply, there is a root, but it is very low, it is not the almost smells not. This pulse, in almost all cases, sign a state of weakness important.
Pulse scattered SAN	This is a pulse without root, floating, but not concentrated: it is dispersed. That is to say that from time to time we feel, at other times it is not the feels more of everything. There is intermittent stops and it has not enough force. But its characteristic, it is not to have root. This pulse is also part of what is called a pulse deadly. When the meeting, it may be considered that there is no more hope.
Deep Pulse CHEN	This pulse, when the traces in the area, gives an impression of insufficient; it has not enough force. When supports more deeply, we feel that it is more abundant. He must know that we can find this pulse in the winter and that it is then normal. Indeed, in this season, the water is under the earth and this can be felt at the level of the pulse. When you find this pulse Chen, this means that the disease is entry more in depth. It is in general a disease of internal cause and rarely of external cause.
Weak Pulse RUO	This pulse Ruo is low, sinking and small. Its quality is to be soft. This pulse shows before any weakness of the original energy.
Hidden Pulse FU	This pulse is part of sombrants pulse. When the key slightly, it is not felt. We must strongly support for the obtain. This pulse Fu, hidden, is also called "Pulse buried". This pulse Fu,

141

	hidden, often sign the presence of tan, and in particular of tan stagnant, linked for example to indigestion.
Hard Pulse LAO	This pulse is therefore very strong, but very in depth, it is for this reason that they say that it is almost drive. In all cases, in depth, it is stronger than the pulse fu, is that we are in the presence of a disease Shi.
Delayed Pulse CHI	This pulse Chi depends on the number of heart beats. During an inspiration and expiration of the practitioner, it must feel between four and five beats: the normal pulse. If there is less than four beats, this is called a pulse Chi, delayed. It arrives late. In some cases, there may be that three beats. When the patient has this pulse, this means that in its body there is an accumulation of cold. It is especially disease of Type yin.
Intermittent Pulse DAI	This pulse DAI is of the same category as the pulse delayed, Chi. This is a pulse that comes slowly. Then there is a rupture, a judgment from time to time. We meet especially these cases in the problems of spleen, or if there is cold to the inside of the body.
Rough Pulse SE	This pulse is rough. It is not fluid. One has the impression that there has, from time to time, a time of judgment. But it is only an impression. It is a little as if he could not come. It is end, slow and short. It has often been to make to a patient in lack of Jing Qi and blood.
Relaxd Pulse HUAN	It can be viewed as the pulse of reference. It is a quiet pulse. It is neither too low nor too fast. This is a pulse which shows that there is energy in the stomach, which has the vitality. This pulse is therefore the normal pulse . This

is a pulse which shows that there is no disease. Under the fingers, it is a pulse very nice; it is soft.

Pulse forged JIE	It looks like the pulse Huan, relaxd. But here there is a small stop after a certain number of beats. These judgments are very irregular. There will be for example ten beats and a stop, then thirty beats and a stop and two-three beats and a stop. This pulse shows that there is a stagnation of blood and of energy.
Fast pulse SHU	What characterizes this pulse, it is its speed. If we take as a reference a complete breathing, there are more than five, or even six or seven beats. It is in the presence of an abundance of Yang. Most of the time, this means that we are in the presence of heat, but this pulse may also indicate a extreme cold.
Pulse wide HONG	The pulse Hong" pushes hard, but withdrew weakly," same as when the wave restarts, it is lower than when it arrives. This pulse indicates therefore, before all, an abundance of Yang. If it is summer, it is a normal pulse because of the Yang external.
Precipitate Pulse CU	This is a pulse characterized by its rapidity. There is in fact more than five pulsations by complete breathing. But what makes the difference is that there is a judgment which is not found at fixed frequency. It is foremost a pulse of nature Yang. The potential symptoms related to this pulse are relative to a rise of IQ.
Sliding pulse HUA	The pulse Hua, slippery, gives the impression, when it is key, to be fast. But when we account the beats in function of the respiratory cycle, it is found that its speed is normal it is a pulse of nature Yang, and it appears when there are of

	the Tan.
Empty Pulse Xu	This is a pulse without force, which lack of vitality. It characterizes a state of empty, lack of vitality, of weakness. Eventually, it can be felt great, wide, but it is low, does not present any resistance.
Short Pulse Duan	This is a pulse without force, which lack of vitality. It characterizes a state of empty, lack of vitality, of weakness. Eventually, it can be felt great, wide, but it is low, does not present any resistance.
Small Pulse Xi	It looks like a wire when the traces. Overall, this pulse sign a disease of nature Yin and a lack of energy.
Full Pulse Shi	This pulse is part of the large pulse. It is loud and long. Its shape is wider than normal. This is a pulse which reflects rather a body in good health. However, compared to pulse Huan, relax, it is stronger, more long and its shape is more wide. This is crucial when we found this pulse is to see if there is the energy of the stomach, see if it normally arrives with a good quality of the energy of the stomach. The Chinese then say that it gives the impression of "the footprint of a leg of chicken".
Tight Pulse Jin	When installing the fingers on the artery, we feel an important resistance under the fingers. This resistance is similar to that of a rope tight. When the key, it is very strong, very tense. This pulse means that there is in the presence of a disease of cold type. We know that the characteristic of the cold is to tighten, obstruct the movement and this obstruction very often leads to pain.

Filiform pulse, tense XIAN	The pulse Xian is therefore light, slippery, fluid, with an idea of righteousness and flexibility. It gives the impression to go directly to the PULSE Chi to pulse Cun, of the cubit to the inch. It does not offer, under the fingers, excessive resistance. We can meet frequently in the spring. If this pulse Xian, tense, skinny, lack of flexibility or is too strong, it is then in the presence of a pathology. This means that there is not enough energy of the stomach.
Pulse large DA	When the key, one feels he is full. This is a pulse which is two fingers wider than normal. In effect, if this pulse da is accompanied by a pulse Shi, if it is therefore wide and full, and that in addition the pulse is Suo, fast, we will deduct that there is the internal heat, and that the disease is more and more serious. On the other hand, if the pulse da is accompanied by a pulse Ru, soft, we are in the presence of a state of weakness, of a State Xu.
Pulse stirring, jumping DONG	All pulse have a certain characteristic of power hop. But it looks like a ball and we do not feel it virtually in only one place, namely to the Guan, to the barrier. We can meet after a very great fright. This pulse Dong may also characterize a poor circulation of the energy. The energy can then be blocked at the level of the chest, especially if the person has a tendency to put very often in anger or, on the contrary, if it is easily sad.
Long Pulse CHANG	The pulse Chang, long, is a pulse much larger than normal. It must avoid the fingers for the felt. When you find this type of Pulse, it must not be thought any of following a pathological condition. It sign, in effect, a state of good

Of course, all these pulse can be combined between them, but their description this is beyond the scope of this study.

The study of the language

À retenir

The observation of the language, Wang ze, is an essential point of the diagnosis. This is before any because the language reflects the state of health or illness of the person as well as its Constitution. The practitioner will see if the energy and blood in the body are sufficient or not, if the subject is low or high. Thus, if the language is normally thick and strong enough, it is considered as a general rule that the subject is resistant, in good health. On the contrary, if the language is thin and soft, this indicates a constitution Xu, of weakness.

A red coloration tension of the language is considered normal. On the other hand, if the red is dull and Pale, this also indicates a constitution of weakness and a deficiency of blood and of energy. It may also occur that the language is too dark, that the red coloring of the language is too pronounced. This certainly indicates the existence of a disease.

À retenir

What it is essential to observe on the language, it is the moisture of the oral cavity, i.e. the presence or the absence of Jin Ye, organic liquids. We know that they play an essential role in the organization, particularly for the protection in respect of the diseases come from outside, from external attacks. In effect, the Jin ye to withstand the attack of perverse energies. They also promote the proper functioning of the bodies, either at the level of the digestion, respiration or cardiac contractions. All these bodies have need of Jin Ye, organic liquids for their proper functioning.

Observation technique

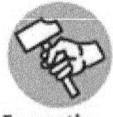

En pratique

The patient is sitting in front of the practitioner. The latter has just to study its pulse. This is the time to ask him to leave his language. For this, it is not necessary that it opens too the mouth. It is

146

necessary that the patient remains relaxd and that its language is well flat. It must not be too pulled or contracted, because if that was the case, we could observe a dark red color by excessive influx of blood.

In practice, therefore, the practitioner asks the patient to show its language without effort. It takes 15 to 20 seconds to properly observe a language. About the staining of the language, if it is located in the presence of an abnormal coloring, it will be necessary to ensure that this staining is not caused by food. For this, it must be to ask him if he does not come to consume the liquorice, chocolate, olives etc. which are foods which may color the language and alter the colors.

As well, we will see that a black language and dull is not an excellent prognosis. Of course, the practitioner must first request to his patient if it has not consumed food dye. When you are drinking red wine to the army, everyone had the language with a black coating: it is the bromide that it contained which gave this result!

The five parts of the language

According to the **Nei Jing, the language can be divided into five parts:**

" The tip and the end of the language represent the Lung and the heart.
" The Center, the spleen and stomach.
" The root of the language, its base, is to be put in relation with the kidney.
" The left side of the language represents the liver.
" The right side, the gallbladder.

147

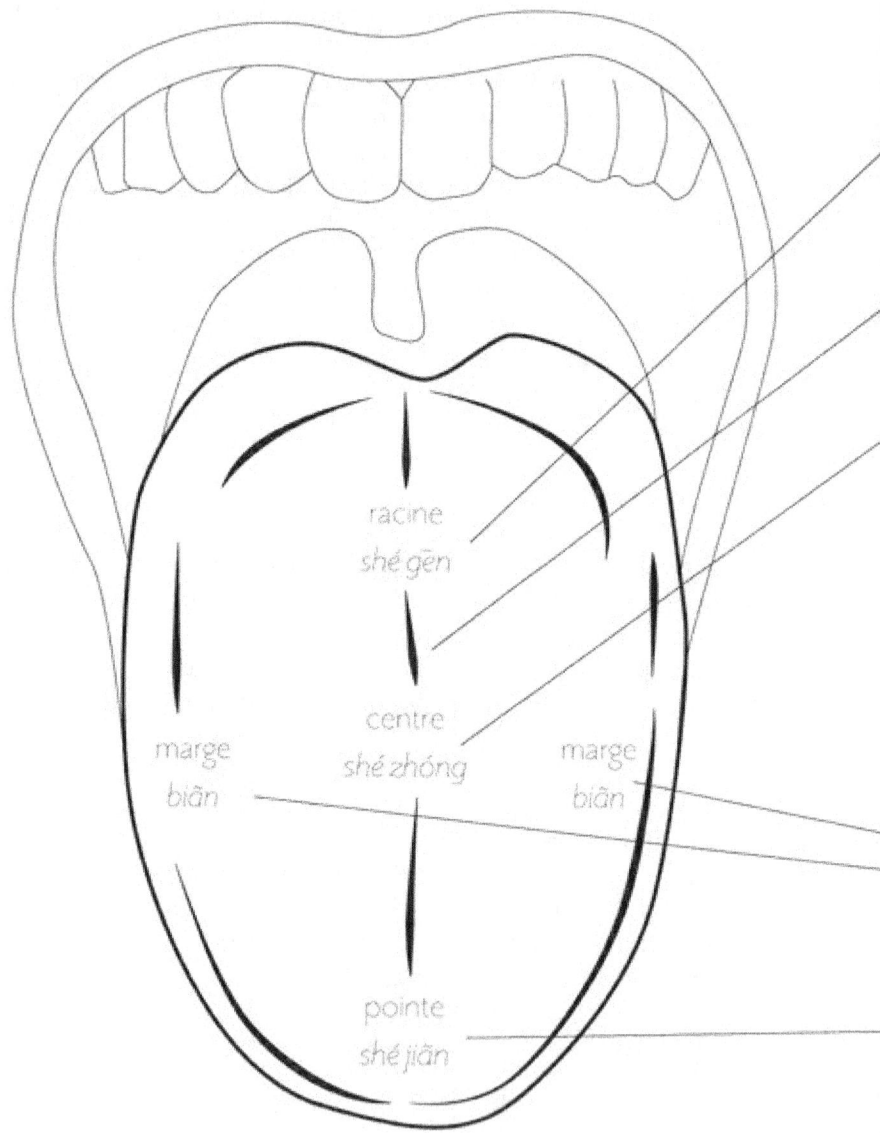

racine
shé gēn

centre
shé zhōng

marge
biān

marge
biān

pointe
shé jiān

Figure 8-2 The five parts of the language.

Observation of the body of the language

This part is directed to all those who want to go further in this exciting study.

Observation of the Shen Qi, the vitality of the language

To determine the vitality of the language, we must see: if the movements of the language are easy and flexible, if it is not numb. It should also be to assess if the color has the brilliance. If the language is mobile and that it has sufficient brightness, then we are saying that "language is prosperous". On the contrary, if it is numb, dull and dried, it is said that the "language is poor."

Table 8-2 morphology of the language.

Swollen Language	- The language is swollen and at the same time white, but that it is sufficiently lubricated, we can then assume that we are before a state of moisture. - If the language is swollen and at the same time pale red, this sign very often a state of moisture and heat. - A language inflated and color bright red, dark, shows that the heat has reached the layer of the blood. - If it is located in front of a language inflated and dark so that it gets almost a purple color greenish, this indicates that the topic is poisoned, intoxicated by either food, either by the alcohol.
Tapered Language	- A language Lean, tapered, of white color lack of energy and blood and at the same time of Yang. - A language Lean, tapered and dark red shows on the contrary that it is in the presence of an insufficiency of Yin, a Yin Xu and fire.
Firm language, Hard, stiff	- A red color dark, and at the same time that lack of mobility; which is stiff indicates that the heat has penetrated in the pericardium. - The Language Soft, without force and

	without force. It is a different type of language with as an example: if it is white in color, this indicates a constitution Xu, of weakness accompanied the impairment of blood and of energy. If on the contrary, it is dark red, this indicates a deficiency of Yin.
Language is pulled to the side	- She sign the penetration of wind perverse in the Jin Luo, the meridians. The penetration of this perverse wind causes the deformation of the language to the side. - If there is no symptom related to the penetration of wind perverse, this indicates that the topic is predisposed to the attack of wind, i.e. to an attack of apoplexy. It must of course distinguish between these two pathological situations of cases where the language is drawn on the side for reasons hereditary or accidental.
Language that aspen	- If it is white, this indicates a deficiency of Yang, a Yang Xu which prevents a normal supply of the muscles. This earthquake in this case a weakness. - If, on the contrary, this earthquake is accompanied by a language dark red, it indicates that there is a Yin deficient, a Yin Xu, who may be at the origin of a wind internal.

Table 8-3 Variation of the surface of the language.

Language with small points	It can often be led to observe of small points to the surface of the language. They can appear on the sides, on the edges of the language. They are often red in color. When precisely they are red in color, they appear in subjects nervous, restless, who do not sleep enough, or who consume too much spicy foods, acids or quills.

Cracked Language	- When the body of the tongue is pale and that it shows cracks, it is a deficiency of blood.
	- If the body of the language is well red, with a yellow coated thick and cracks, this shows a presence of heat abundant in the zang-fu which depletes Jin Ye.
	- If the body of the language is slightly red and it presents shallow cracks that can be covered with plaster and if the patient has no special problems, it is congenital cracks not to be confused with a problem pathological.
Toothless Language	It is a language whose edges are marked or fragmented by the pressure of the teeth. It indicates in general, a disability of the spleen with an abundance of water and the internal humidity.

Staining of the language

We have seen above that a language should have a red color soft and have the Shen, shine, of the Vitality.

Table 8-4 staining of the language.

Pale Language	In general, the white color is to be put in relation with the Yin, the cold or the costs. If the language is white, it is usually a lack of blood.
Language Dark red	There are two degrees in the excess of red: the dark red, and the red very dark which is still more red than the dark red. In all cases, an accentuation of the Red color indicates a state of heat to the inside of the body. But this heat may be due to an excess of Yang; it is then a case Shi. Or a deficiency of Yin and it is then a case Xu.
Language	It indicates a restriction in the flow of blood.

greenish Purple	Therefore, each time that it is in the presence of a language violet, we know that the blood is reached.

The coating of the language

A normal language has a coated thin and light. It normally covers the language. But it must be noted if it is located at the end of the language indicating that the disease is located at the household level higher. If it is in the center, the disease is located at the level of the average household. If this is the root of the language which is covered by a coating, this indicates that the disease has reached the layer in the lower furnace.

Table 8-5 the coating of the language.

Wet coating	We can observe the presence of a large quantity of water and humidity inside the same of the coating, in the layer of the coating itself. It usually indicates the presence of a cold and moisture to the inside of the body, or even the presence of stagnant water.
Dry coating	It does not contain enough fluids. Not only is it dry, but also rough; it looks like a little of the sand. When a language is dry, it is necessary to know if this drought is due to an external heat which by penetrating injured the Jin Ye, or then know if it is not located in the face of a lack of Yin to the inside of the body itself.
Coated rotten" "	It is a coating which is thicker. It is said to be very free, that is to say that it does not have a root. It gives the impression of paste on the language. It presents itself as a layer is very thick and can easily be removed. When one observes this type of coating, we know that the energy of the stomach is troubled by the heat and the moisture. The heat has as a property of the DO evaporate, and it is this

	evaporation that creates this type of coating.
Fatty coating	It gives the impression to be very bold. It is said that it resembles the lard which sticks to the language. This coating fat is often caused by the Tan Yin, phlegm-drink. The TAN is accumulated to the interior, for example at the level of the stomach or in the lungs. And this accumulation of tan is often accompanied by a condition of moisture cold or warm.

Table 8-6 The different meanings of the coatings of the language.

White Coated	- The first case is the attack of a perverse energy to the area of the body. At this time, the coating is white and thin. It is a disease external, superficial, benign. - The second possibility is that the heat has attacked the body, for example of the heat in the lung. Normally in the case of heat, the language should be red. But here as it is an external attack, at the beginning of the attack one often sees appear a white coating that covers the red of the language. This coating white indicates a disease of heat superficial. - The third case possible is an accumulation of cold and humidity. If the coating is white and thick and that one has the impression that it is dirty, rather fat, if there are difficulties in the remove, it is inked, rooted, is that it is located in front of this case of figure. - The fourth case possible is the heat Shi internal. In this case the coating is white with crevasses and, consequently, dry and rough and more at the end of the language, we can observe a white coated in powder form. Under this type of coating, as a general rule, the language is well red.

Yellow coated	- An external disease which has started to turn into heat. The quality of the hue of the yellow is a function of the severity, the degree of penetration of the heat to the inside of the body. This can therefore go of the thin white to yellow thick. - If the yellow is darker, more pronounced, this shows that an external element is entered in the body, but it already existed previously heat to the interior. - A yellow disorder, bold, with or without membrane, is due either to the moisture, to the internal heat, either at the Tan, either to a poor digestion. Then it is an accumulation of food triggering a disease of heat-moisture.
Black coating	- It can be linked to excessive heat which injured the Yin. That is why the coating is colored in black. But this type of black coating drift of the yellow. It has a texture very particular with appearance of black spines and crevices. - Moreover, in case of weakness of Yang, there is the presence of Yin and cold. The black contains white traces. - There may also be a weakness of the water of the kidney. The black is then dull, without the glare; the coating is dry, not smooth. We think of heat if the patient has a thirst for cold drinks. But if it is a Yin Xu, the patient has thirst, but not want to drink. The language is then rather tapering.

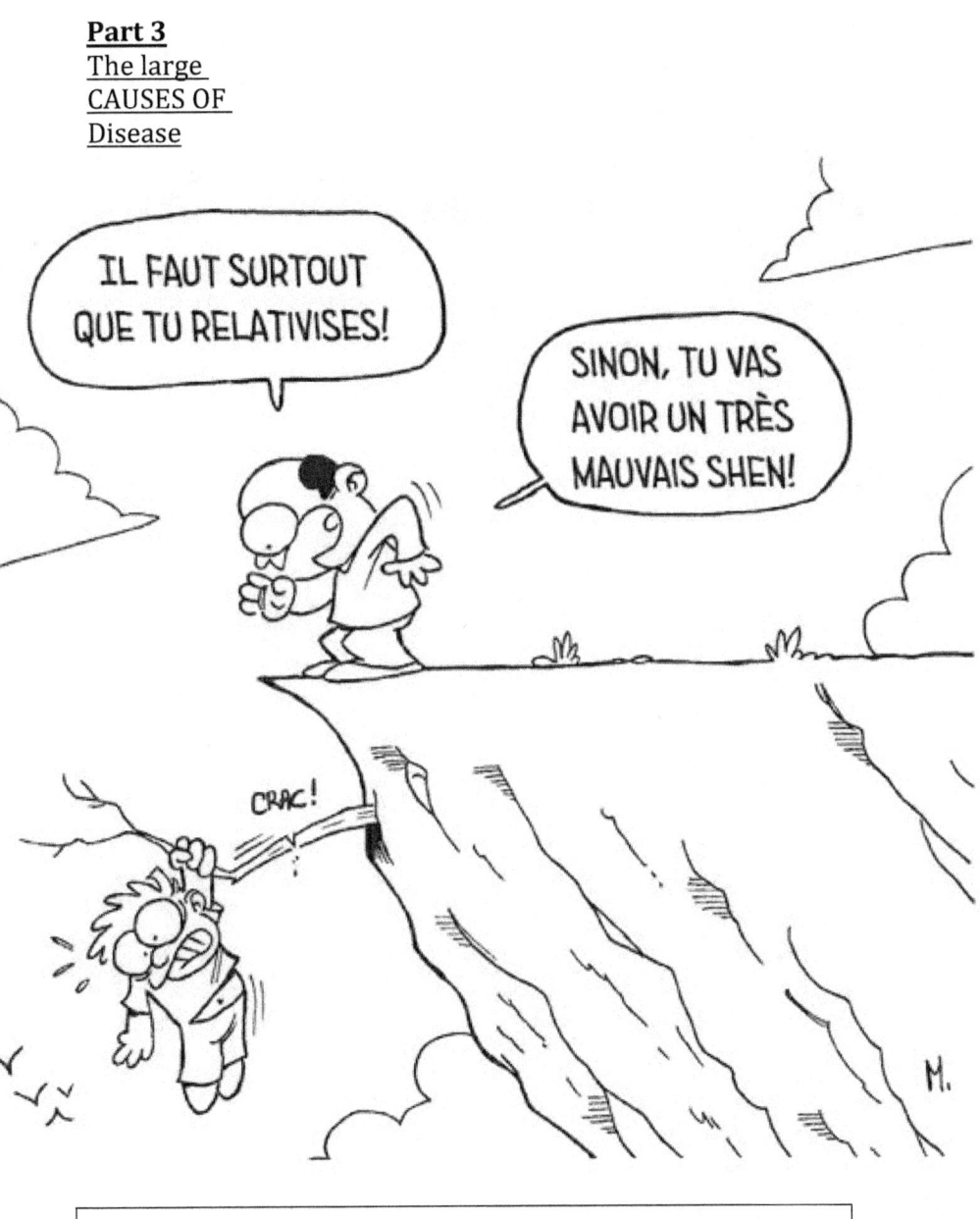

In this part...
A disease, whatever it is, does not appear without reason. In this very important part, you will learn that the different factors of disease, that they are external or internal, could be avoided if we had access to the knowledge.
In addressing all of the major causes of illness, this part will help you, "without fear and without reproach ", to take all necessary precautions.

Chapter 9
Differentiate diseases
Both internal and external
In this chapter:
" The prevention at the heart of the MTC
" Identify the main causes of disease to regain a full health

EN theory, the organization according to the principles of the MTC, has not been designed to fall ill, but to autoguérir continuously. Then why so many people are they carriers of pathologies, for most chronic conditions? It is of course the great question that arises any medicine.

Whose fault is that?

A few responses will be data in this chapter. It may be that the first, so simplistic, but which nevertheless overflows of truth, it is the non-access to knowledge. And this book is there for you open the eyes and help you regain a full health.

A second obstacle that he will have to learn to dissolve. In our current formatting, we remain convinced that if we are sick, it is the fault of the other and that we have for nothing. We are an "effect" in our evils, but not a "cause". The MTC you will learn the reverse. It is through ignorance of the modes of operation of energy in our different software components, taught by this multimillénaire medicine that we not create to not internal diseases, or that we are more permeable to external diseases.

Why some develop-they an allergy and other non?

The Allergies, under a few forms that this either, tend to become a true pandemic rampant, both the number of individuals who suffer increases. Two conceptions of the functioning of the human body, two philosophies of health are facing.

À retenir

Inevitable?

In the West, it considers that an allergy is an excessive reaction of the body to the contact of a regular substance therefore denounced as "Allergen". It is sufficient simply to be in contact with this allergen to develop a defense reaction exaggerated. As well we are going to be able to find in front of hundreds of agents potential allergens. The most well known are the pollen of the flowers. These are not strictly speaking of poisons, but just of irritating substances that the body ends up by no longer bear. Outside of the red eyes, they are at the origin of the allergic rhinitis that can go up to the broncho-pneumonia as the respiratory distress of children, more and more young people to type of bronchiolitis and even of cardio-respiratory diseases. In extreme cases, because of some agents called "highly allergenic " as the egg white, the peanut, the bites of wasps and I happening, it can go up to the anaphylactic shock, state of distress of the body that is potentially very dangerous.

There is a perverse effect in this approach of the allergy in Western medicine, of the "This is not my fault." It is this impression of fatality and fear of the outside. If we are allergic, it is because of the other, of the external, of this poor pollen that yet has not been "manufactured" by Mother Nature to harm the man, but on the contrary to encourage the growth of plants and thus indirectly feed the man.

Then we will detect with devices, we are going to hunt, we are going to protect itself, to confine in homes; wear a mask at the time of peak of the appearance of the said pollen. It is the fear which is distilled and insinuates in our whole being, which is very déséquilibrante. Because fear affects the very basis of the functioning of the Organization, namely, the energy of the kidney. And the life of people allergic to some so wasted can very quickly become hell. Then we will attempt to desensitize. But for us in Chinese medicine, this is that the transfer of the problem to an external layer toward a deeper layer of the Organization. It is the risk of creating in the months or years to come the problems much more difficult to treat as chronic eczema and psoriasis. That is the disease that from external to penetrate more deeply in the body to go up to the layer of the blood. In short, this western vision tends to make us believe that we are a "effect" and not a "cause".

The approach of the MTC

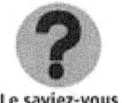

The Chinese medicine, it, will reverse the gives. In effect, its approach is not at all the same. It part of the basic axiom: "An allergic reaction is always the manifestation of a lack of the capacity of adaptation of the organism to its environment. "So it customizes, individualizes the disease. If such was not the case, all the world should suffer of allergy. It is a weakness of the protective energy of the body, that is called Wei Qi, often combined with a weakness of the battery of the kidney, what is called Zhen Qi in MTC, energy right, the healing power of the Organization.

Internal disease or illness External?

The disease is a complex phenomenon. When we find for example before a hypertension or a symptom of headache, it does not stop there, and we must determine the nature as well as the causes of this pathology, this symptom. It is therefore necessary to deepen what is meant by "cause of diseases" IN MTC.

There are generally two: the external causes and internal causes.

External causes

The external causes mean that there is a struggle that opposes an attacker, what is called the perverse energy, Xie, QI and the energy of Defense, the right energy of the body still called Zhen Qi, the force that allows you to resist disease. Zhen Qi is a part of what is called "immune defenses" in modern medicine.

All external energies in excess as the wind, cold, humidity, the drought, the heat, fire, but also the Tan, dietary factors or adverse respiratory, blows and swellings that cause clots, all this constitutes what is called "energy perverse".

It must understand what is meant by external attack in Chinese medicine. It is a real "battlefield". The two fighters are therefore the perverse energy and energy right. The physical evidence of this

159

battle, the objectification of such a fight will be precisely the symptoms that will present the patient.

Internal causes

Independently of external causes, the body itself can generate diseases. In particular, if there is an imbalance in the body.

You know that there are two forces in the body still called Yin-Yang (see chapitre 3). It is one of the essential principles underlying the MTC.

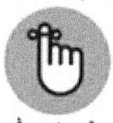

Western medicine has a tendency to consider the disease as a result of an imbalance of the chemical properties of the body. This imbalance will be

À retenir caused by bacteria, viruses and microbes, etc. The Chinese Medicine obviously recognizes the existence of these bacteria, viruses and other, but it considers however such phenomena as the effects and not real causes.

The Oriental designs are based on the concepts of energy and strength. It is the strength of the energy that is at the origin of the physical and chemical transformations. This is why this method is based on the principle of the Yin and the Yang. In some way, energy precedes the matter and any energy imbalance will have an effect on the latter.

The principle of Positive Negative

Yin and Yang are simply an energy or a force which has a negative polarity or positive. These two polarities are necessary to obtain a balance. This bipolar energy flows throughout the body and nourishes each cell. A definition of health in MTC could be: "It is a balance between two opposing forces Yin-Yang, which is never acquired permanently, but should be worked on a daily basis. "

In life, everything seems based on this principle of "Positive Negative". Any thing has its opposite, its opposite which is at the same time complementary. The day is the night, the hot and cold, the male and the female, the Summit and the base, the right and the left, the YES and the No, the speed and the slowness... As we can see the Yin is also important that the Yang and their balance depends on their mutual report.

These two forces coexist in our body and fluctuate alternately. Sometimes it is the Yang which increases, sometimes the Yin. When the Yang increases, the Yin decreases, but when the Yin increases, the Yang decreases. This movement of alternative fluctuation allows the circulation of energy in the body.

À retenir

The balance between these two forces is the real factor which depends on health. If there is a disturbance in this movement of ebb and flow of these two forces, for example if the increase of one of these forces or the reduction of the other is excessive, if the balance between the two is broken, this may then be the cause of a disease, and in this case we will say that the disease is internal. Without that there must be the attack of a perverse energy external. The internal in the body can produce diseases.

But what can also occur commonly, it is that a internal imbalance authorizes, allows the attack of an external agent. In other words, an external agent cannot penetrate in the body and trigger a war that if the prior internal is unbalanced or deficient.

A choice in the order of the study

In the ancient texts, in the Treaties of pharmacopoeia, it was of use to begin by the study of external diseases and then to those generated by the Internal. We are going to do the reverse here. In fact, daily, this are not the epidemics that we bother them, but well the internal diseases with their batch of self-destructive disruptions: rheumatism, cardio-vascular diseases, diabetes, cancer, mental illness and emotional. This being said, a reversal of the situation will take place in a few decades if we continue to weaken our battery. We will then be able to ask the following question: when the great epidemic?

Chapter 10

Internal causes

In this chapter:

The discharge of the battery of the kidney

In a previous chapter, we have extensively explained what was this battery, called Yuan Qi in MTC (see chapitre 3). It is located in the lower furnace, at the level of the kidney. Its means of recharge daily are multiple:

" The restful sleep. We sleep 33 years in 100 years of life: it is the most natural way that we gave Lady nature for us to recharge.

" The practice of mediation, qi gong or of the relaxation which thanks, among other things, in the control of breathing, greatly favor this recharge.

" The energy surplus given by the air that we breathe and the food that we digérons.

It is empty or is charging at the discretion of our emotions. A chronic fear literally drain this battery. On the contrary, the joy, the Interior smile potentiates the uptake of the energy around us.

This battery represents:

Le saviez-vous

"
The immense power of adaptation of the organism. This battery boosted, your body is able to adapt to sudden changes in time, the extreme weather conditions, to the factors Mental and emotional dimensions that can attack you suddenly. But also, adaptation to the changes that occur in the interior of your own body. For example, to a woman, the passage to the menopause.

" *The immense power of self-healing and self-regulation of the body. It is between other what is called in modern medicine, the immune defenses. But the MTC goes well*

162

beyond! It takes place at the level of the imbalances of energy, which precede the imbalances of the material. This battery is fully recharged at daily, you have very little chance of "sick".

However, by lack of awareness of this global vision of the functioning of the human body, and especially by the non-practice of methods of bias that will be studied throughout this book, this battery has a tendency to always be discharged. The progressive loss of the understanding of the meaning of life, the climate of fear and anxiety which becomes our daily food, the multiplication of conflicting theories which do not encourage the passage to the Act, especially in the field of dietetics, are all factors of non-charging this battery. It is for this reason that a whole chapter is going to be spent.

Spiritualité

I remind you that the goal of this education is the return to the uniqueness which has as a corollary the simplicity. Learn to breathe well, well move, eat well, drinking well, well thinking is to the scope of all. It is still necessary that things are explained simply, and do not proceed to theories" abracadabrantesques".

The battery of the Kidney discharged, your body is no longer autocontrôlé, emotions become exacerbated, the desires and the impulses become self-destructive. These are the internal diseases - very often characterized by their chronicity - which appear.

The stagnation of blood and energy

What happens when it stagnates?

It is, after the discharge of the battery of the kidney, the second major cause of internal pathology. If we take a little hindsight regarding the functioning of the Organization, all is that traffic: the blood circulation arterial and venous, the lymphatic circulation, the circulation of the nervous influx in the nerves, the hormonal circulations, intra- and extra-cellular, organic liquids through the different compartments, fluid etc. In MTC, we add the circulation of energy along the meridians, along the three homes, to the surface of the skin... In short, everything must circulate in the body, and this, in

163

perfect freedom. We are going to see that many of the causes will hinder these different circulations, the first being the weakness of this battery, considered in MTC as the engine of all the circulations.

As soon as an obstacle is circulatory product, physical or energetic, either on the surface of the body, at the level articular, or at the internal level, at the level of any organ, appears what we call in the West The Trilogy: "rubor, calor, Dolor", namely redness, heat and pain. It is the inflammatory state which is at the end of the path.

Le saviez-vous

History of the type that decides to plastering his wrist for nothing!!!

While his wrist is completely healthy, flexible and without any particular symptom, our friend has a fad and decides the plastering for three weeks. Around the wrist spend nerves, of the arteries, veins, of lymph circuits, ducts, tendons and six meridians of energy. By blocking his wrist, he comes to hamper all these circulations. To the ablation of the plaster, his wrist is hot, inflated, inflammatory and painful. It will rehabilitate, expose to the light, find the flexibility. And little by little, all resets in place. The blocking of the wrist, who is here an external cause is the origin of all these imbalances. The recovery of its flexibility, the antidote.

The stagnation of Qi, energy

We have previously seen that the Qi, energy originated basically with three "Software bodies" that are the kidney, the spleen and the lung (see chapters 2 and 3).

The Kidney software

It includes a innate energy, the Yuan Qi (the oil lamp) and a energy gained, the Jing Qi, that which comes from the respiration, power supply, and the emotions. The surplus is stored after the Agency has met its immediate needs. It is the Zhen Qi (the battery).

The Yuan Qi, the energy gained, contains within it a fire (the flame of the oil lamp), a nightlight, called "fire of Ming men". This fire has the property to enable the spleen (digestion is

164

38 degrees). It is the driving force of the Vitality. It then becomes " Fire Minister". This fire triggers the growth of the organism. It is the driving force of the Vitality. It is a very soft fire, slow, constant, which radiates continuously. It is in link directly with the liver. It is said that "it is the Yang Qi of the Liver". (The liver is to put in relation with the wood: C is the quiet strength of the sap that rises in a tree and that allows the slow development of leaves.) There is a third fire, very powerful which does not ensure the development of the vitality, but used to rotate the entire machine: it is the " Fire Emperor", emblem of the heart.

But any part of the kidney, the small flame. It is for this reason that it is said that "the most important body for the Qi is the Kidney".

À retenir

The software spleen and lung

The body needs to be powered by the earth to form "the energy of foods", the gu Qi. But this energy is far from being sufficient to itself. It has need of the energy of the air, the Yang Qi that The Lung must assimilate. It is said that "The Lung directs the qi". The two lungs are housed in the upper home. They naturally occupy the highest position in the body and, of this fact, they regulate and control the flow of energy, of the Qi. When the lung is weakened, he is unable to lower the energy and therefore the kidney no longer has the strength to escalate the Qi (see the cycle of five elements: the lung is the mother of the kidney). This will also have an impact on the spleen, which has a dual function, the function to raise and lower. The whole mechanism of the circulation of the Qi is based on the lung. (Where the fundamental importance of conscious breathing.)

The blocking of the QI or Qi Zi

How the stagnation, blockage of the Qi, can happen? As very often, we can incriminate external causes and internal causes.

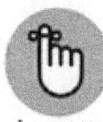

As regards the external causes, some single wickedness can disrupt the process of

À retenir

transformation of the food. For example drink too much during a meal generates an excess of moisture which slows down the digestion. And this stagnation of the circulation of the food bowl can easily lead to a state of rotting the latter. It is one of the causes of production of tan, of waste in the body. The Tan and the moisture that stagnate can easily be transformed into "poison", re of the Chinese, which can clog the circulation of energy in the meridians. A chapter will be devoted to the tan.

Le saviez-vous

Another example. It is said in the MTC that during menstruation, a woman should not touching the water cold. A cold bath risk by example to stagnate the energy at the household level lower. It is a great cause of fibroids and other local pathologies. Similarly, sit long in the wet grass can trigger a lumbago by blocking of the Qi at the level of the kidney.

Among the internal causes, the most frequent case, the great cause of stagnation of Qi in the body, it is the poor management of emotions! We know that the whole of the emotions is under the control of the heart, where fits the Shen, the Spirit. When the Spirit is concerned by conflicting ideas and haunting, emotions are disturbed and affect the heart and spleen. The Qi no longer flows in the body and becomes stagnant.

A grief, a prolonged sadness can literally block the energy at the level of the lung. We said then that the body "increases": the person stands the head lowered.

We can find this case among people who are much too work their mental, or well insist too much on the exercises of introspection, meditation, without practice in consideration of the external exercises such as walking or the qi gong.

Attention

As we have said previously, the worst of the emotions generating the stagnation of the energy is the Internalized anger, which blocks the function of the development of the energy of the liver. When such a blockage occurs, the Yang energy of the liver can no longer fit and can come to attack the spleen. It is a great cause of diabetes and in cases ultimate outcomes of acute pancreatitis or cancer of the pancreas, but also other cancers or mental illness and emotional as the Depression.

It is said in the **Nei Jing** that "the 100 diseases are caused by the interference of the circulation of the Qi". It is for the MTC, one of the first causes of cancer. It is appropriate to any implement, to avoid such a State. We will revisit this in the methods of treatment.

Attention

History of the mother who does not happen to forgive her daughter-in-law!

This is the mother who does not happen to share its filial love with his daughter-in-law. Cases, of course quite exceptional! Everything becomes subject to emotional lock. Little by little is being put in place what is called in MTC a state of "blocking and stagnation at the level of the Liver" (The Internalized anger belonging to the liver). It is a internal lock. The symptoms of departure will be bloating, difficulties in breathing, neck pain, insomnia of three hours of the morning, headache. At the end of the path, when that lasts, the outsourcing of the symptomatology, on the side of the breast, where passes the meridian of the gallbladder: C is the breast cancer. Or even later, it is the organ liver which is reached. And this is more serious. One of the great antidotes, we will come back to in Part psychotherapy, it is "forgiveness", or even the ability to "get out of the scene," no longer be actor, but spectator.

The stagnation of blood, Yu Xue

The stagnation of blood is called Yu Xue Chinese. First of all, it must know that the blood circulates because the Qi, energy the shoot. Therefore a stagnation of Qi is translated as soon as possible by a stagnation of blood. But the reverse may also occur: a poor circulation of blood can foster a stagnation of Qi.

A few reminders on the blood

It is a material substance acquired, composed of a mixture of the essences of the food and the air inspired, produced mainly by the energy of the spleen. The earth produces food for the Man While the spleen product of nutrients to the body. This is the spleen, which transforms the foods in gasoline which will then be mixed with the energy of the sky (respiration).

The **Nei Jing** said that "the spleen is the source of the transformation". But the spleen and the lung are going to be also the source of the production of the energy. We can say that "the Qi is the driving force of the organization while the blood is the nutrient element".

But the second function of the spleen is to circulate the blood throughout the body. It is said: "The Spleen directs the blood".

The heart is the "master of the blood". But he controls the state of the ducts, of the vessels. Regardless of the amount of blood required in any part of the body that it is, the Heart evaluates exactly its needs. It is a mechanism very late. If there is too much blood in a place, it will decrease the pressure. If we get hurt, it sends the blood to form a clot.

The liver stores him the blood product by the spleen. But not only is it the stores, but it the filter, the cleans.

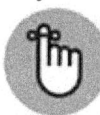 A very important concept: when the man is in the activity, that it moves during the day, the blood circulates to Full in the vessels. It is said that " the physical activity done the blood out of the Liver".

À retenir

The State immobile, at rest, at night when sleeping, the blood reflux at the level of the liver. It is moreover to "the time of the Liver", in the second part of the night, that its metabolism is the most important. If the blood is stagnant too long (Internalized anger), the waste are transformed into poison, also because of a multitude of pathologies. The liver is therefore involved in the regularization of the blood flow and its distribution.

What is it that produces the blood stasis ?

Before all, energy disruptions and functional requirements of the heart, liver and spleen may raise issues of blood stasis.

If the foods are too charged in sugar or grease, this fatigue the spleen, and it is a major cause of waste production, tan or humidity, which will thicken the blood. It is also a major cause of slowdown and blocking of the Movement.

If there is not enough energy in the body, the blood no longer has the strength to move forward.

The internalized emotions can also be at the origin of the slowdown and the stagnation of blood.

The STAGNATIONS of sustainable blood

The stagnations of blood, the Yu Xue which last a certain time generate the production of a toxic substance, of a "poison" called Re The. The body hates it. It is the role of the immune defenses to proceed to its elimination. But if the battery is flat, that is when the problems begin. Remember that the stagnation generates heat: the waste of the blood are transformed into poison. It is a great cause of eczema, psoriasis, but also one of the main causes of cancer.

Conclusion: When there is no of stagnation that this either of blood or of energy, there is no internal pathologies. Circulate. There is nothing more to see!!!

Simultaneous Impairment of blood and energy

Always in these internal causes of diseases, we may be faced with a simultaneous state of impairment of blood and of energy.

A functional disturbance of one of the five bodies software is sufficient to cause a general imbalance. Therefore, the driving force of the qi can weaken with such consequences as to lessen the production of blood or of the slow down. It is this that the MTC calls a state Xu, of weakness.

Very many factors in our life habits can contribute to this state as physical surmenages, a exaggerated loss of organic liquids, Jin Ye (let us not forget that the seminal fluid is an integral part of these Jin ye), a hemorrhage too important (after an injury or childbirth or even of Menstruation too important).

The deficiency of the qi can also come from a disability of the innate.

With regard to the blood, c is the liver which may lose its storage capacity, because the spleen may not produce enough blood. It is a cause of anemia.

When this state appears, the body can no longer withstand these famous poisons which we talked about earlier. It is said in the Nei Jing that "it is a premature aging which is being put in place. The body is fading and weakens easily. "The barriers of defense have a tendency to collapse and suddenly the single wickedness external, whatever they are, can easily penetrate in the body.

The Emotional disruptions

 A bad management of emotions is the iron-of-launches of almost all internal diseases. In the theory of the five elements (see chapitre 4), we

Attention saw that each family of emotion was to put in a relationship with a component software specific. An emotion nourishes in some way the body "target." In contrast, as in all, the excesses of this same emotion imbalance this same body. It is a major cause of internal pathologies. As well each emotion will have a direct impact on the circulation of energy.

" *The joy* is to be put in relation with the heart, the fire. When she is not excessive, it allows you to make energy relaxd. It is like when we light a fire. At the outset, it is just a point of combustion. Then, the flame develops, disperse and spreads harmoniously. Be Happy Time and time is normal, and it is even necessary to stimulate the activity of the Yang, and circulate the blood in the body. But if the joy is excessive, or if it is continual, this can disperse the energy.

" *The anger* belongs to the liver, the wood. It is fit the energy. It is like the wood of the tree which grows toward the top. It is a force Yang that rises easily. An excess of anger may any ravage on its passage. Anger on repetition could be at the origin of hypertensive diseases, cardiac...

" But the anger may be repressed. It fact stagnate then the energy at the level of the liver. This is the "worst" emotions to the origin of very many cancers.

" *The Remembrance* belongs to the spleen, the earth. It is also the reflection. It is an emotion that can regulate the spleen. But in excess, the energy is forged, concentrates, accumulates. It is like the Earth whose nature is to accumulate, of piling, make block. It is then a great cause of depression, but also poor digestion of the food bowl favoring the emergence of moisture and tan in the body, of waste.

" *The fear, the kidney and the water are of the same nature. A good fear allows you to feed the kidney and quickly to take good decisions. In contrast, an excess of fear makes lower the energy toward the bottom. It is a characteristic of the water that descends. A child who has very afraid urine in his pants. It is a major cause of low back disorders, descents of organs, exhaustion of the battery of the kidney.*

" *Sadness and concern* are to be put in relation with the lung. An excess of sadness decreases the energy. But conversely, if the energy is too concentrated in the lung, this creates the sadness. This emotion which literally leaded the energy can be at the origin of very many diseases of self-destruction, lung cancer including.

An emotion, a learned balance between the Yin and the Yang

À retenir

We know that each software component is made up of a part Yang and part of a Yin. Whatever the emotion considered, it is an energy, a force, a pulse whose nature is to install. Inherently, an emotion is therefore of nature Yang, which will excite the part Yang of the body. When the Yang energy is thus energized, energy Yin of this same body is there to calm, inhibit, maintain a balance. The **Nei Jing** said: "Yin is to balance the Yang. If Yang becomes excessive, Yin The tempers. Yin and Yang are constantly in balance. "

The man cannot live without experiencing of emotions. There is no of days without that one has of the emotions. We all spend by phases of sadness, dissatisfaction, concern and even moments of depression. When they occur, these emotions are excitatory and Yin is there to restore the situation and to recover a new balance.

171

The disease can appear if we find ourselves in the presence of either a lack of Yin which prevents the control of the rise of Yang, either to an external factor which contributes to make the Yang too active, and to do so fit too violently.

If the Yin is low and the Yang is hyperactive, then it will be necessary to locate in what body is located the insufficiency of Yin. For example, if you are located in the presence of a Yin deficiency of the liver, the subject will easily in anger, without an external cause is not necessary. The person gets angry without reason, it is irritable, it quickly loses patience. Similarly, if the Yin of the heart is low, the Yang will be too active; the person will laugh for a nothing, without reason and even in circumstances which do not lend to laugh.

The innate characters

Spiritualité

Eh yes! The MTC explains to you that you are not all equal to the birth. Not only do you inherit the nonsense made by your ancestors (one goes back to the three previous generations: lawyers are going to rub the hands!), but come take place, in their remains to your birth, of energies very subtle, the Hun and the Po, the sides Yin and Yang of the soul with all their baggage, what the Chinese call very poetically the "previous sky". Call it the subconscious the deeper, or any other thing, we are all born with predisposition. As well, as soon as the birth, some people will be carriers of a character, a innate temperament. In MTC, it considers three types of profiles and we are going to see their main characteristics.

The Nervous temperament

"It always wants to prove that he is the best in everything.
"It hate to lose (in the game, for example).
"He likes the glory, honors, good places social.
"It is always ready to fight both within the family, that in professional relationships.
"He is proud, vain.
"It is a "upstart" which not only supports to get across its path.

172

" If it is braked in its impulses, or that something is not achieved, it becomes very tense and nervous.
" If it encounters of the competition, it can very quickly become malicious.
" It can be without mercy to his enemies.
" It is often a perfectionist. It is concerned about very quickly and becomes tight as soon as something is not perfect.
" It is difficult to supported by his entourage.

The diseases that threaten these people are numerous. Include cardio-vascular diseases, hypertension, stroke. The end of their life will often under the mode ON-OFF. They can die brutally after for example a big crisis of anger, a stroke or a heart attack.

The pessimistic temperament

" It is very introverted, does not expressing that very little.
" It keeps the problems for him.
" It does not even want to talk about the evil that other have done.
" It is inhabited by a feeling of inferiority.
" It has not enough confidence in him and becomes easily neurasthénique.
" His dominant emotion is the anxiety.
" You have beautiful speak with him, try to make him see the good sides of life, the positive aspect of things, even if it follows your reasoning, it found very quickly its old habits of pessimistic.
" It Sees without stops the negative aspect, negative tests of life.
" It stare constantly for his problem.
" Even if it has no problem, it will think about the problems that it would be likely to have.

It is a profile where the Shen, the mind is constantly tense, wince, in blocking situation. These psychological attitudes lead very frequently to the Depression, to pathologies by stagnation and especially to cancers.

173

The Optimistic temperament

"In the face of serious events, disturbing, attristants, it reacts very properly.
"It is confident, imperturbable.
"He loves the life.
"He smiles very often.
"It all positive.

The optimists are of the people in the shelter of mental illness and emotional. And if they are sick, they are very easy to treat. But if their daily habits (feeding, sexuality...) are misadjusted, this will not prevent them for as much to create a pathology.

À retenir

A Council of Practitioner to practitioner

Fortunately, these innate behavior are not If sliced. Let me add a note of optimism. By having access to the knowledge as you made in reading this book, and practicing daily to recharge your battery in the kidney, all these predispositions will only remain that scars at the inside of itself. On the other hand - and here I address to the practitioner, you can leave your Health to tire you to try to treat people pessimistic of nature. In all ways, they will try to demolish everything that you will try to make positive for their health.

The imbalance of desires

It is another important cause of emergence of internal pathologies. The desires, the passions are inherent to life. They are necessary to maintain the vitality. However, the wishes of the men are very complex. While generally, those of other living beings are summarized to the satisfaction of their hunger and the need to reproduce, in humans, the ego, the affects, the feelings interfere with the natural desires.

Le saviez-vous

At the beginning, a desire is that a feeling, a need that is felt in the conscience. When it is decided to satisfy, the desire appears. I hunger (a sensation), I will lift up to open the Tablet of chocolate (desire). But if this desire is not controlled by the energy of

174

the kidney and by the Shen, the mental housed in the heart, it can be devastating (I eat the whole tablet!).

In effect, when the desires are met, it is happy. In the contrary case, it is either in anger, or sad, or even shot or desperate. This is called in MTC: "The Fall of Shen, spirit, its bursting. "As well the desires lead-they always emotions in their wake.

When you leave a desire we invade and become excessive, it occurs sooner or later a sense of disappointment that ends by disrupting the flow of Qi. And we have seen that this interference was the cause of almost all the internal diseases, cancer including.

In MTC, it is considered that there are six major types of desires.

The desire hardware

It is a desire found in all living beings and that it is vital to meet. Find to eat, where to sleep, where to stay his family...

But it can become excessive. Although we have obtained the object of our desire, we always want more. It is like this that works our modern society.

The spirit of this person is still tense. It is said that the Yang of the heart to ignite. Very many pathologies may appear, especially if its desires are not satisfied. These include certain types of insomnia rebels, of hypertensive pathologies or cardiac disease.

The desire of glory

These are people who have always need to feel superior to other, more strong.

They are looking for various exploits to be covered of praise. They need to believe that they are famous. They want the best social place possible.

These people often generate a fire of the heart, with a propensity to high blood pressure and cardiovascular diseases.

The desire of possession

The person sees something that she likes and wants everything to suite the possess.

It is normal to admiring a flower and, possibly, the pick for the bring home to us. When it is a desire casual, nothing abnormal. But let us take a desire uncontrolled, the collector of antiques. It wants to accumulate all what it finds in relation with the period in which they are interested. It can fill in a house and why not buy another for the also fill.

The "collectionnite" can become a true obsessive compulsive disorder (OCD). As well, some people accumulate fortunes, that an entire life would not suffice to spend. The accumulation of wealth becomes an end in itself.

This type of desire can bring people up to the madness. They are no longer constrained by the conscience. We are in full in the self-destruction.

The indiscriminate desire

It is a desire that comes from the subconscious the more profound. It is innate. He escapes to the education gained. It is the dark side of the force, the Po, the body soul that attracts you toward the earth. It vehicle sometimes much of violence.

The person has the desire to injure his entourage without reason, destroy, and in a manner that is free of charge.

It is a desire which leads to a lot of social disruption within a family, a village or a society. It is a desire dangerous.

This desire is obviously generator of mental illness and emotional functioning up to the madness.

The sexual desire

The sexual desire, libido, is a natural need, an innate human need for the dissemination of the Yuan Qi, of the original energy in the goal of a future reproduction.

But what differentiates us from the animal, is that it can become act of full consciousness with all affects which ensued.

In MTC, it is considered that any report excessive, with emission in humans of seed to rehearsal before the total maturation of the sexual organs (21 years for women and 24 years in man), is quite damaging for the result of events! This desire quenched in excess eventually deplete the Yin of kidney and generate a excessive Yang at the level of the liver (low back disorders, prostatites, hypertension, bone fragilisations, loss of teeth and hair, etc.). What made you

176

want to of this finding purely physiological and find a track of the middle!

Sex or not sex!

The intercourse which are the expression of our unconscious are healthy. Those who are the fruit of our conscience can be detrimental to the health, in the same way as to continue to eat when there is no more hunger. Excessive behavior related to a permanent excitation generated by the images, films or other, eventually create a false libido.

The schema is simple. The emission of seed to repetition exhausts the Yin of the kidney. The latter no longer in control of the liver. The Yang of the Liver increases. The liver is the place of the development of the projects, but also of the Toc and states of dependency. And the more the act is repetitive in the same week, if this is in the same day, the greater the energy of the Kidney weakens. At the end of the path, a early aging and all internal diseases that ensued. The MTC is far from being puritanical. It has put in place many exercises of seminal containments in order, why not, to have daily reports that will regenerate the body. It is said in the texts: "The sex can kill as allow you to make immortal! "

The illusory desires

This are the desires close to the alienation.

You can find them among the **serial killer** who always give good conscience with regard to the practice of their impulses. This is for example the individual who killed systematically the young girls of 13-14 years. Without any remorse, he considered it their made service and that it allowed them to arrive Virgin at the paradise. It is an extreme case, I agree.

But is that the destruction of mass in the purpose of clean up a race were not what the MTC called "illusory desire"?

Attention to all these impulses which, under the guise of altruism, can give to fanaticism in certain cases.

The food imbalances

The dietetics is a subject of such importance in MTC that any part is going to be devoted in this book. In the West, it is mainly based on physical designs biochemical or of the human body. It follows that the food will be analyzed, dissected, quantified, weighed, past to the magnifying glass. And the conclusions as to its therapeutic role may move away from the reality.

The chocolate, so good for the Health?

Le saviez-vous

Let us take the example of the spasmophilie which is the signature in MTC a stagnation of blood and energy at the level of the liver. In the West, it is said that the magnesium is good for treating this type of state. However, the chocolate contains a lot of magnesium. Therefore the chocolate is good for treating spasmophilie. Except that the chocolate, consumed in excess, it is four poisons in MTC: A tablet contains the equivalent of two tablespoons of saturated fats that are gradually coming to plug all the filters of the body. It is the equivalent of 10 pieces of fast sugars which distort the software spleen. It is an excess of bitter flavor which turns against the organization by generating a internal cold, a fluid retention and therefore a weight gain (the chocolate to the origin is consumed in countries very hot and dry). Finally, the seed of grilled Cocoa contains substances assimilable to a drug which, in exciting the liver, put very often the person in a state of dependence.

The dietetics of the middle

The Chinese dietetics takes account of concepts much more subtle, such as the concept of energy of food through their colors, odours, flavors, natures. But also the notion of symbiosis between man and the Universe. We shall see later the fundamental rules, adaptable to everyone who will allow you to become the leader of the orchestra of your own food of the season and region.

A poor diet is one of the sources of almost all internal pathologies generated by the Organization: cardio-vascular diseases, rheumatism, diabetes, cancers, etc.

Le saviez-vous

We will also see that one of the major sections of the dietetics, namely the hydration of the body, is virtually never addressed in the West. And, too often when we talk about it, there is a tendency to move away completely from the physiological reality. In the West, we do not know drink, we drink too much, we do not know split the quantity of beverage. And by that we are depleting progressively the Yin of the kidney and bring too much moisture at the level of the spleen, with all of the implications on the health that may have. This topic, of a major importance, will also be developed at length in this book.

Therefore learn to opt for a dietetics of the middle, without any Radicalism, too often generator of fear. Do not forget, the fear literally drain your battery of the kidney. Not become extremist, and do not isolate yourself in a straitjacket which could you make life impossible.

Attention

The BIO has good back!!

It is obvious that it is very important to "eat Own, "as close as possible to the nature and therefore to turn to the food "bio". But I remember, at the detour of some lounges bio to which I was invited, have seen regularly before me the same people. Sometimes they consumed a ice bio, and then of the Chocolate Bio, a glass of rosé wine bio, sausage bio, cheese from cow bio, an orange juice Bio, and this, in the same day. And I said to myself: "This person can only shorten its life expectancy, but it will have the satisfaction of die early bio! "

The overwork and fatigue

Here too, it should be to learn to spare its mount. Another constant in our society is to be a huge generator of fatigue, of overwork and burnout. The consecutive fatigue to a overwork affects in the first place, after the MTC, the software spleen-pancreas.

Le saviez-vous

In other words, a overwork which causes fatigue both physical and mental wounds the spleen. The spleen then loses its ability to provide energy to the body.

We know that the spleen is the conductor of the digestion of food bowl. It produces the blood and energy. The energy goes to the lung and the blood goes to the liver. But it is also said that globally" the kidneys are the residence of the postnatal energy," in some way the battery of the Organization. Therefore, the overwork will disrupt in fact directly this energy postnatal.

It is a very great cause of outbreaks of disease internal.

179

The irregularities of the Sleep

Le saviez-vous

Let us ask ourselves the following question: why is sleeping? If we intend to 7-8 hours of sleep per 24 hours, in 100 years of life, we sleep 33 years! It is the most natural way that has given us Dame Nature to recharge our battery of the kidney, to boost our faculties of adaptation and our immune defenses. But everything is done in our civilizations for the less hectic to do harm to this daily act so important.

Some people lack of consistently sleep. They are perhaps too inactive, or the opposite is surmènent due to excessive work, or they do not have enough time to sleep. The normality for the sleep time is between 6 hours and 8 hours, no more, no less. This lack of sleep will generate an imbalance between the Yin and the Yang. In effect, the SLEEP Allows the yin to reconstitute themselves to accommodate the period Yang, activity of the day.

Other people sleeping enough, but in an irregular manner. They do not have a regular schedule of sunset and sunrise and the number of hours is not fixed.

It is obvious that this number of hours can vary according to the seasons. A little more in winter where it must store of Yin and a little less in the spring and summer.

Among other people, the schedule for the period of sleep is not regularly set. They sleep a little, and then they work, and then redorment and so on, and this according to irregular cycles.

Normally, it must be awakened the day and sleep the night. Some do not live as well and Sleep intermittently. Some have periods of work alternatives, the day and then the night.

All these situations, even if they are difficult to preventable in the modern context of work, are quite harmful to health. It is then creates an imbalance between the Yin and the Yang at the inside of the body and it is one of the major predisposing factors for mental illness and emotional, to arterial hypertension and many other pathologies internal.

Chapter 11
External causes
The six climates
Among the external causes of illness, it is essential to take into account climatological factors. According to the **Nei Jing, it is only when the man is low - the inside of the body is unbalanced - that the external elements can attack. It is therefore this internal disability which has allowed the external attack.**
How these external elements can they cause disease?
The six perverse energies
According to the **Nei Jing, there are six external elements which attack the human body. These are what are called the "six perverse energies". As well, the sky has six climates, this are the six normal climates.**
There is:
" The Wind, Feng;
" The cold weather, Han;
" The heat, Re;
" The humidity, Shi;
" The drought, Zao;
" The Fire, Huo.
For example in the spring, the time is warm, the been him is hot. Between the end of the summer and the beginning of the fall, the time is rather wet. The fall is a season rather dry. The winter is obviously cold.
We have the five single wickedness corresponding to the five climates. The sixth, the fire is not fundamentally considered as a climate. This fire is produced in the human body after the attacks of one of the five other perverse energies.
What is meant by a climate which would not be normal? That means a time abnormal?
It is when he arrives too early, or that it does not arrive on time. For example in the summer, it should be warm. If it is

181

too hot, the heat is excessive. Or if in summer, even after the solstice, it does not still hot, the heat is called insufficient.

There is also the case of the time which does not correspond to the season. For example in the summer, he would have had to make hot, but it has snowed. Or then, it is a time to fall in the summer. The climate in these cases, is not appropriate, does not correspond to the season.

Attention

Climate Change are not always where we think!

With current means of transport, it can be a few hours change abruptly in climate and, for example, find themselves in the heat of the desert while it is winter where one lives. Another case of the figure, is to have a temperature of 30 degrees to the outside and that there are brutally to 18 degrees, thanks or rather because of the air conditioning. If we are resistant and in good health, if our Yuan Qi, our energy of the kidney is recharged, the body can then adapt. But if the body has not force, if it does not happen to adapt, then he is attacked by the Climate abnormal and the disease appears.

These external elements which attack the body are then called Xie Qi, the perverse energies. This are the external causes of disease. The Chinese Medicine therefore spoke of six Xie Qi that we will now review.

The wind, Feng

When we speak of wind, Feng in MTC, it is as well of the wind of the climate, but also everything that is mediated by the wind, Germs, viruses, pollen, toxic agents, "fine particulate matter", etc.

The **Nei Jing** said: "The wind is the cause of the Hundred Diseases". It is of course here of the wind harmful, still called "perverse wind". It is a wind which, attacking the body, has triggered a number of pathologies. It must be under-hear here "The energy of the wind".

À retenir

This wind is not harmful in itself. It becomes such only if the body is weakened, weakened and that it leaves the penetrate to the interior.

This Xie Qi, this energy perverse, this harmful wind can cause a multitude of diseases, and even cause diseases that are not clean.

182

The wind, Feng, is to be put in relation with the liver which, you know, corresponds to the spring and to the element wood.

When the wind rises in the spring, it is said that it helps to growth, that it wakes up any thing, that he gives life to all things. But if this wind is abnormal, it can also harm, Destroy. This same wind therefore has the power to generate and destroy at the same time.

If the person is weakened, if it is not strong enough, balanced enough to cause for example of a addition of fatigue, the irregularity in its mode of life, in its Schedules to sunrise and sunset, in the decision of its meals, in the nature of the absorbed food, if it is under the control of emotions, if it does not know how to manage her sexuality, this person is no longer able to adapt to its environment and when a wind is too strong appears in the spring, it falls ill.

The diseases that are more basic than we all know, related to this attack of Feng, wind, are colds and the flu. Initially, the symptoms are more benign. It may have onset of cough, headaches, blocked nose, sneezing. That is what is called in Chinese medicine a disease simple. It is just a penetration of the perversity in the body which remains on the surface. We cannot strictly speaking a real lack of the resistance of the body.

But often the wind does not attack only the body. It may be the vector of other single wickedness as the cold, Han, humidity, Shi, drought, Zao, heat, Re.

" For example when the wind combines with the cold, this is called an attack of wind-cold, Feng Han. The symptoms will then be of Diffuse pain in the whole body, in all joints.

" If the wind combines with moisture, Shi, it is Feng-Shi. The humidity is an element which descends. We will therefore often symptoms related to lower home. For example the heavy legs, without forces.

" In the fall, the wind can be combined with the drought, Zao, and summer with the heat, Re. You know that the heat is in the nature of An Yang and has a tendency to fit in the body. That is why these attacks of wind-drought and wind-heat will cause a history that will often be localized at the throat or to the head. One can find sore throat, eye pain, bleeding from the nose, cough.

" All these diseases of the wind, that they be combined to cold, heat, drought, moisture, when they last too long, can transform into fire, Huo. We will talk then of wind-fire, Feng Huo. This will obviously be a disease that is warmer than the Feng re, wind-heat.

If the one is led to make a differential diagnosis on the pain, one could say that the diseases due to the wind are often localized to the joints. In the Feng Han, the wind-cold, the pain are fixed, strong and acute. In the Feng re, wind-heat or the Feng-Shi, wind-humidity, Feng Huo, wind-fire pains are more Deaf and more diffuse. One feels without force.

When the pain is due to the wind only, in Feng, pain circulating, they are not fixed. It is said that they are erratic.

Le saviez-vous

Doctor, what is a chronic rheumatism?

Diseases due to the wind are often related to rheumatism that the Chinese call Feng Shi. There is a particular case. If the attack is due to a penetration of the wind and the cold and that then adds an attack of moisture, the Chinese call this PEI Jing. It is a disease feature, called in the West a chronic rheumatism. So, at the start, it will have taken an attack of wind-cold. These single wickedness, these two energies will not have had the strength to be expelled and will be remained several days, even several weeks, or more, to the inside of the body. Then, another attack perverse, the humidity, will wake these single wickedness previously hidden and trigger this rheumatic disease chronic. Several cases of possible figure:

" **The first category of chronic rheumatism will be one where the participation of the wind is the strongest. It will be called then Feng PEI. There will be triggering of rheumatic pain who have particularity as to be erratic, to circulate, as the nature of the wind.**

"In a second category, this will be the cold, the Han which will be dominant. This will be Han PEI. The pain here do not circulate. They are fixed, very localized. At the same time, they can be very acute.

"In the third category, there will be a preponderance of moisture, Shi. It is called Shi PEI. It is said that the pain will focus, it will be located. And often, in this place, there will be a swelling, because the nature of the moisture is to inflate. This pain is not circulating because the wind is not very important, and it is not very badly, because the cold does not dominate.

"When one of these energies perverse or a combination between these three stagnating energies too long in the body, either Feng, Feng Shi or Feng Han, he will be able to have the presence of heat. The Yang will then become too important. Do not lose sight of that as soon as there is stagnation, there has appearance of pain and heat. These different types of rheumatism will then become chronic with acute phases inflammatory. This is called " rheumatism to dominant warm ", because the place where the patient has evil is very hot. It then calls this rheumatism Feng Re.

These four types of rheumatism are very common. When they are present in the body for a very long time, the pain that result may affect the tendons, bones, vessels, the muscles, skin. In effect, there is talk in MTC rheumatism of skin, rheumatism of OS. The people complained about actually of pain more or less chronic in the OS. Each rheumatism will then bear the name of the affected area. If the time still passes, the pain can then directly affect the organs. We will talk about at the time of rheumatism bodies such as rheumatism of the heart, liver, spleen, lung, kidney! It must then examine the symptoms to be able to attach to such or such a body.

The cold, Han

The cold of the six single wickedness is the perverse Cold, Cold external.

It is a normal climate, an energy that can enter the human body when it is in a state of weakness and cause a disease.

Most of the time for that the cold can penetrate in the body, it must be accompanied by wind.

It sometimes happens that the cold can penetrate all alone in the body. There will be as symptoms:

˝The fear of the cold ;

˝Of the fever;

˝Headache;

˝Poorly in the OS.

If it is accompanied by wind, this is called Feng Han, the wind-cold.

If it is accompanied by moisture, it is Han Shi; of drought, it is Han Zao. Often, when we think of the drought, we the assimilates to the heat. However, it is necessary to know that the drought may also be of cold nature. In the fall, the time may indeed be dry, but also cold, and these two single wickedness together can penetrate in the body.

It may be in some cases to attend a gradual transformation of cold in the heat, then in fire. In effect, when the cold penetrates the body, it is likely to undergo an evolution.

According to the state of the digestion, the resistance of the body of the time, of the emotional state, it may evolve toward a disease lukewarm. And if the temperature increases, it can evolve into heat.

If this perversity is still longer in the body, and if the temperature is even more strong, this cold can then become the fire.

 The main symptom linked to the illness of the cold, Han Bing (Bing, meaning disease in Chinese), is the pain in the joints.

À retenir The **Nei Jing** explains that "The cold has as a characteristic of acquiring the energy in the body."

But the cold also enters into the skin, it promotes a slowdown of the circulation of the blood. The combination of contraction and slowing of the blood circulation fact that there is a lack of blood to the periphery.

Slowdowns, stagnations, or even blockages, that is how we explains the genesis of these pain. The pain will occur where the stagnation will predominate.

The heat, Re

The **Nei Jing** says that "in the sky there is the heat and on earth there is the fire". In the sky, we will find the heat of the climate. We have to do then to a hot climate. When this heat penetrates the body, it is called a disease Shu of the summer.

These hot diseases appear after the summer solstice. The **Nei Jing** said: "before the summer solstice This are diseases tepid, Wen Bing, who appear, and after the summer solstice of warm diseases, Shu Bing. ". These two diseases, warm and hot, have the same hot characteristic according to the BA gang. They only appear at different times.

Outside of the time of onset, another difference between these two diseases, c is the temperature that presents the patient. In the lukewarm disease, Wen Bing, the heat will be less strong than in the disease of the heat.

At the level of symptoms, we will find:

" An evil of constant head;

" Fever. It is then a high temperature;

" A sensation of thirst, whereas in diseases due to wind and cold, there is not this sensation of thirst.

" These warm diseases have as a feature to enter very quickly in the body, and "disturbing the Heart", as it is said in Chinese. The person will then be agitated.

" We will also find of the sweating, since the disease Shu is a perversity hot.

" The Pulse In this case are very sharp and rapid.

This disease may be hot, as the other combine with other elements perverse. We have already seen when we talked about the wind, the combination wind-heat that could attack the body.

The heat can also combine with the drought, Zao. The drought is the most often in the fall, while the heat is found in the summer.

In another case, the heat will be able to combine with the moisture. When these two single wickedness penetrate together in the body, it is called heat-moisture. This type of disease often appears at the end of the summer. It is still hot, but the external moisture can easily be present and therefore penetrate together in the body.

The Touareg in the desert hot drink in small quantities split.

He must know that the heat and moisture can not penetrate together in the body. It can be found in front of the case of following figure. In the summer it is very hot, and there is a tendency to drink too much. When we had too much to drink, the intestines and stomach no longer arrive to eliminate the excess of liquid. If, at that time, the heat penetrates the body, this can cause a difficult digestion, indigestion. The water that has stagnated at the inside of the body is transformed in moisture and form, with the heat, the "illness of heat-Moisture" with a good indigestion to the key. We will therefore have, the penetration of a external heat on a problem of internal humidity.

Another case is the one where the heat of the summer is not eliminated by the body, and that the humidity is already emerged: one is then in the presence of a genuine disease of heat-moisture. There is therefore, attack of external moisture on a pre-existing heat in the body.

The diseases "delayed"!

There is another disease of heat that is called Fu Shu, Fu meaning risen, and Shu, summer, heat of the summer. The perversity heat has entered the body in the summer, remained somewhat hidden, and it reveals itself later in the fall. It should be noted at the level of symptoms that this heat at the moment of entering the body is often accompanied by moisture. This disease has between other as symptoms a high temperature and a whole history of moisture, swelling at the level of the throat, gastro-enteritis. It is for this reason that the Chinese have the habit of consuming for example of the melon yellow in the end of the summer which has precisely the property to eliminate this heat accumulated during the summer.

The moisture, Shi

It is the moisture of the climate which appears at the end of the summer and early fall. Often for the Western calendar, this corresponds a little to the change of the season which is put in place after the 15 August. At this time, the time may suddenly change and become very wet.

 Having taken the habit during the summer of very little cover themselves, and not to bear that very little clothing, when appears this change in time, especially if it was taken the habit of going out in the evening and go to sleep late, or to get up early,

Attention

the ambient humidity risk of penetrate then in the body.

This moisture is often found in nature in the form of a mist or dew.

When this moisture enters the body, taking advantage of a weakening of the latter, it then becomes " Humidity perverse".

Other situations can encourage this penetration of humidity. For example, when one is led to work in the water, in the rice paddies for Asians, in swimming pool for the Western.

It can also be tired by a long walk and be surprised by the rain, and find themselves the wet clothes.

For some, the fact to search the freshness, lie in the grass can predispose them to this penetration of humidity. And many other situations...

What are the symptoms that may appear during the penetration of such a perversity:

" The body can be very heavy, tired.

" There will a sensation of pain in the bones, and stiffness in the Lombes.

" All the joints we do evil. When there is joint pain, they have as a characteristic to concentrate in a same place.

" The digestion becomes difficult and diarrhea may appear.

" Urine may become rare, which is a factor of a worsening of the disease.

As in the other cases, this perverse moisture can combine with other single wickedness to enter in the body. It can, for example be accompanied of wind. This is called an attack of wind-humidity, Feng Shi. It can also be combined with the

189

cold. It is then a attack of cold-humidity, Shi Han. If it is with the heat, this will be Shi re, heat-moisture.

There is a case where the humidity remained too long in the body eventually transform into fire. This fire will dry the organic liquids. It is only in this case that we will be able to say that the humidity is transformed into drought.

If this moisture external Shi combines with the internal humidity already present in the body (excess of drink, saturated fat, dairy products, sugars, fast) and that it persists for too long, it can transform into perversity fire. One of the classic symptoms of moisture and fire is the abdominal pain violent.

This moisture can also become what is called, in MTC for the tan, including a translation closest would be "the phlegm". This term is very important, we will talk about it at length by the suite. Already, remember that the TAN is produced by the spleen.

If the humidity is too intense, too important in the stomach and intestines, if it cannot be eliminated, it is said that "she remains in the spleen".

If it meets the fire of the lung or the fire of the other organs, or if the fire in the kidney is too strong, these different types of fire evaporate moisture which then becomes the phlegm, of the Tan. He should know that this tan can circulate throughout the body and a very great cause of internal pathologies including very many cancers.

The drought, Zao

It is in the fall as a priority that the dry weather appears. This season is intrinsically a dry season. If this drought of the fall attack the body at that time, taking advantage of a weakening of the latter, we will call this a "disease of perverse drought in the fall".

The drought "dries "Often the internal liquid, which can cause symptoms such as:

"A reddening of the eyes,
"A sensation of thirst,
"The nose and lips dry,
"Dry cough without phlegm,
"Pain costales,

" Of the constipation.

As the other single wickedness, there may be combinations of different single wickedness at the time of the attack.

" If the Drought combines with the wind, this is called a disease of wind-drought.

" If it is combined to the cold, this gives a disease of cold and drought. In addition to the Symptoms specific to the drought, there will be wrong everywhere in the OS.

" With the heat, this gives a disease of drought and heat. We may have sore throat, or then bleeding of the nose in addition to the symptoms mentioned above.

The Fire, Huo

Let us look now at the last of the six single wickedness, fire, Huo.

We can understand that the wind, heat, humidity, cold, drought can each belong to one of the five seasons, to one of the five elements. But to what season can we attach the fire?

According to the **Nei Jing, it is said that "in the sky there is the heat, and on the earth there is the fire". We must understand, that when we talk about climate, we are talking about of heat. This represents what is hot. On the Earth, we are talking about of fire which has also of course, a characteristic hot.**

According to the Pr Leung, this fire should not enter into the category of climates. This would be according to him, an error of transcription of the copyists. Normally, therefore, in the series of six single wickedness, instead of the fire, it should instead have the lukewarm.

If one puts aside the problem of error and the need to talk about Tepidity in the climate, the fire is the resultant, the product of a transformation.

After that the five single wickedness, wind, cold, heat, moisture and drought have attacked the body and y are entered, when they remain there too long, they become the fire. Therefore, when we talk of the external fire, that means the fire produces by the other five single wickedness. The fire is therefore not an attack directly on the body.

In a disease of fire, is found mainly of symptoms to Yang characteristic.

191

Since the fire is nature very Yang, the first thing that is affected in the body, this are the Jin ye, the organic liquids. The symptoms are then:

" A high fever.
" There is what is called "an agitation of the Heart" with as a symptom of the agitation, of the concern.
" There may be of the thirst.
" Sore throat.
" The face and eyes are red.
" The pulse are swift, strong, and Floating.

We have said that this fire could be produced by any perversity. However, the more often it is the incoming heat in the body which is transformed into fire. At the beginning of the transformation in fire, we still speak of disease Huo. But as soon as the heat becomes the "true fire", we then speak of disease Huo SOS, or Yang Huo.

If it is the moisture that between in the body and which transforms into fire, we then speak of pathologies Shi Re. If the temperature is not high, there is talk of moisture-hot. On the other hand, if it is very strong, it is of the moisture-fire.

When it is the drought that penetrates the body, you know that this perversity already has in it a character hot, it is for this reason that the drought can very easily be accompanied by fire.

Environmental Factors

By the time that run, it is undeniably one of the major causes of the emergence of internal pathologies. And what are the problems of air pollution which will be the more serious.

Pollution

There may exist a pollution of the air "natural." For example, in wetlands, forests are difficult to access, in some caves, near the lakes, swamps where the water stagnates, there is what the Chinese call "miasmas", of harmful energies in the air. Often the atmosphere there is wet, heavy, loaded. If the man is exposed for long periods of time, this may be the origin of many internal diseases of type stagnation and heat.

The dust in suspension, such as in quarries or areas of work, can penetrate into the lungs and y result in obstruction of the respiratory tract. Those who work the plaster, cement, who

192

were manipulating the asbestos, but also many other substances while also irritating, are very exposed.

Our modern cities with their cortege of polluting factories, of pots of exhaust of cars are of the champions of the pollution. In MTC, it is said that "the gases emitted by the cars are a dead air". All of these odours, these fumes are particularly heavy and contain many toxic substances. We are talking about in our modern language of "fine particulate matter".

It goes without saying that it is important to live in places, without air stagnant and without smoke perverse, cigarette smoke understood.

À retenir

Do not forget that the skin is to put in relationship with the lung. The skin is an organ breathing: 30% of the respiration of our organization is ensured through the skin. The toxins in the air can penetrate through the skin.

In addition, the wounds of the skin will facilitate the penetration of these substances. Stop you to gnaw the skins around the nails. It is an incredible track of penetration of toxic substances, directly in the layer of the blood.

It should be particularly wary of this problem among the professionals at which the hands are frequently injured, especially if these cuts occur repeatedly in the same places.

Radioactivity

The radioactivity, the effect of the radiation are as many external factors likely to trigger internal pathologies. We all know the harmful effects of solar radiation when it is exposed to the sun for too long, without protection. There is talk in MTC of "Poison-fire", Huo-Du may in some cases cause for example a cancer of the skin.

There is a natural radioactivity, as in the marble quarries, which in the long run can become harmful to the workers.

But it is the artificial radioactivity which is going to be very worrying in the next few decades. The first are the X-rays, thus the action is cumulative. However, as these rays are invisible, the man gets used to the danger and the fails. The dentists for example can easily develop a brain tumor. And that also say of radiation atomic""!

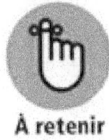

À retenir

193

A small note of hope in this table rather alarmist... If your battery of the kidney is perfectly recharged, it is capable of adapting to conditions themselves the most extreme. As well, in Hiroshima, the "practitioners", those who knew the methods of prevention, preservation of health were statistically much less achieved that the common mortals. The body is then able to reject in large part the "poisons external".

?
Le saviez-vous

The Cigarette: A danger can hide another one!

In modern medicine, we focus the dangers of cigarette smoking on the toxins, poisons that it contains: tars, and dozens of other harmful particles that the smoke vehicle. The vision of the MTC is a little different. It highlights the fact that the smoke of the cigarettes has a desiccant power significantly higher than some other smoke. If in a closed room, two or three people smoke throughout the day, the relative humidity will increase from 50% in the morning to 20-25% in the evening. However, the cigarette is at the same time regarded as a food (swallow the smoke which goes into the digestive tract), but also as a stale air that it inspires and which goes into the lungs. We are therefore going to attend a progressive drying organic liquids with as a consequence, a drying up of liquids of the lungs (chronic cough, sputum...), a dewatering and premature aging of the skin (skin = lung), with appearance of wrinkles, wilting, a drying up of liquids of the stomach and digestive tract (heartburn, constipation...). But outside of this early aging, the big problem is that the drying of organic liquids will foster the emergence of stagnations of blood and energy in the organization. These are the stagnations which are very dangerous as we have developed previously. It is only at this time that the poisons conveyed by the smoke will potentiate the danger of the cigarette. All traditional societies had been aware of these dangers. It is for this reason that they were moving the smoke through the water. This are the famous narghiles, water pipes and other which decreased very strongly to the harmfulness of the cigarette. Smoking then becomes a true act of meditation.

The Tan, waste
What is the tan?

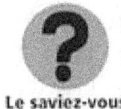

The Tan IN MTC is a concept to mid-way between the external causes and internal causes. As the fire, it is also the result of a transformation internal under the effect of a stagnation of organic liquids. But it can also be directly imported into the body through our diet.

It is a generic term which, with a connotation of concentration, qualifies of substances that the body would normally have had to eliminate, among others by the stool and urine, but it has not had the force. Where because of the battery of the kidney is too low, or that this Tan is too important in quantity. The fats that are circulating in the blood stream, atherosclerotic plaques, the bad cholesterol, free radicals, the balls of fat, adenomas, cysts, the nodules...: all this is of the Tan.

We will also see that stagnation of blood, energy and tan are very good household. An excess of tan promotes the stagnations and the stagnation "factory" of the Tan.

À retenir

For the very "zero", sinking the nail

How to differentiate between, the organic liquids, moisture and the tan? When you eat out of the water is a liquid also clear that tears, saliva, lymphatic fluid. This is in comparison what we call the Organic liquids that bathe all our bodies. We are constituted 80 per cent of these liquids. When you eat a yoghurt, a compote, a thick soup, a part of liquids "clear" has evaporated. The product is then more concentrated. It is of the moisture. In the body, it is for example of the thick pituite which flows out of the nose, the grease that accumulates under the skin by retention, stagnation of fluids. When you eat of the butter, cheese, it is of the Tan. It is a substance that is very concentrated, which will require a lot of effort to the body to be evacuated. In the body, this Are lipomas, cysts, calculations, of nodules... Everything is therefore a question of concentration.

The concept of disease of the "water-drinking", Jue Yin
The **Nei Jing** said: "The Tan, is produced by the spleen and retained by the lung. But it can also circulate throughout the body, in the four members". Let us look at this more closely. To better understand the Tan, are trying to see how to develop the liquids in the body and the different processes of the digestion.

The **Nei Jing** said that "the kidney controls the process of the elimination of urine and excrement". Therefore, when we absorbs too much water, to eliminate this excess, there will be a need for our energy of the kidney. As there is a relationship internal-external of kidney with the bladder, before to be eliminated, this water will be retained by the bladder.

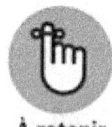

À retenir

We must therefore know that in the first place, when there is an excess of water in the body, it is that the energy of the kidney has not had enough force to eliminate this too-full.

But a second component may be involved in this fluid retention, c is the heart. In the cycle of the five elements, we know that the heart is in internal relationship-external with the small intestine. According to the Chinese doctors, when the food have been digested by the stomach, everything that is not digested between in the intestines. Then the waste are disposed of by the stool. After the assimilation of the water by the small intestine, excess water begins to accumulate, and then is then eliminated through the urine. It is said that "the excess water overflows from the small intestine". As the small intestine is controlled by the Heart, it includes there that this body is responsible for the metabolism of the water.

When the water remains in the body, this is particularly evident at the level of the members, of hands, feet, skin, muscles. It can also have edema of the face. The hands may be swollen. As the water has a tendency to go to the bottom of the body, there is a high probability that the feet are also swollen.

All that we have just see a as a generic term: "disease of the stagnant water". The water to the inside of the body and the water of the beverage to be quite comparable, it is for this reason that the This is called together: " water-drinking" or Jue Yin.

While the "diseases of the water" are often of diseases of the heart and kidney, the diseases of the drinks are often due to the spleen and stomach.

If the water comes in the spleen and the lung and is not eliminated, it is kept at the level of the average household. If there is too much fluid in the average household, it can easily fit in the home superior. If the water stagnates in the average home and in the home higher, it is because of the spleen and stomach. It gives them then the disease name Yin, drink.

This liquid is no longer really as of the water. It is already more concentrated. It becomes of the moisture that can also call Jue Yin.

This concentration fact that this Jue Yin flows more difficult and therefore can easily stagnate. In this disease Jue Yin, we note that:

" The person can easily coughing.
" She may have difficulty in the heart and it is said that "the lower part of the Heart" hardens.
" Water is concentrated in the flanks.
" The breathing becomes difficult.
" Another characteristic symptom is a noise of water in the intestines.
" This type of disease can drift toward what is called in the West: the acute edema of the lung, the PAO.
" This water can circulate everywhere in the body. The person feels then his body very heavy. There is a swelling of the flanks.
" In another case, only the thorax is swollen at the top, and bottom occurs a swelling up to the hips.

To treat these different diseases of jue Yin, it is necessary to use of the theory of the meridians and regularize the energy movement (see chapitre 2).

Overall to the inverse of the Tan, these diseases of the water-drinking are characteristic to Yin, and therefore their treatment is different from the treatment of the Tan, strictly speaking that is of such a nature Yang.

197

Difference between the diseases " water-drinking" and the tan

You begin to glimpse that the origin is the same. It is the same root cause. It is always of the water which is stagnating. When the body is unable to remove this excess water, if the water stagnates in the stomach and intestines, if it meets the fire, that is to say of the Yang energy, this fire evaporates the water which is then mixes with the other substances in excess.

More fire is large, the more the Tan, is concentrated. If the fire is not strong, the Tan, is more liquid. The concentration of tan, shows the intensity of the fire.

The key thing to understand about the Tan, is that it is produced by the Rate-Estomac.

If the energy of the kidney has not the strength to eliminate these liquids, it can then occur of the phenomena of stagnation. But if at this moment, there is a fire in the stomach and intestines, if there is an excess of Yang, there is going to be a phenomenon of evaporation of this water that will start to thicken. Gradually, this can become the tan. This Tan, Monte and will then be retained in the lung.

Another body may be concerned in the production of tan. It is the liver. We know that the liver belongs to the wood. If the energy of the liver does not circulate freely, if there is stagnation, then there may be production of fire. It is a State that is called " fire of the Liver". When this state persists, there may be an assault of the spleen. If the Yang of the kidney is not sufficient and that the water stagnates, the fire which attacks the spleen fact evaporate this water and at this time, the Tan, appears, and as previously, Monte in the lung.

Two cases may arise then:

" If the lung is low, the TAN remains in the lung and triggers the history that we have a view over the top.

" On the other hand, if the diaphragm is resistant, tan, don't stay there. It is said that the diaphragm pushes this tan in the rest of the body. At that time, it can be found in any part of the body.

At the time this Tan flows, it is called the Tan re, i.e. " fire of the tan".

This Tan, product therefore by the liver may, for example, go in the tendons, muscles, the meridians, vessels, etc.

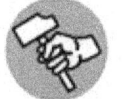

There may be:
" Dizziness.
" Headache.
" Pain in the ribs, etc.

" Then that if the tan remains in the lung, there will be cough, gasps.

The Tan can therefore circulate everywhere. It can also enter in the heart. It then affects the barrier of the heart, namely the pericardium. Chinese doctors then speak of "Tan which obstructs the hole of the heart". It is an acute illness produced by the entry of the Tan, in the meridian of the pericardium. The patient reached can then fall into a coma. It is the crisis of the heart.

But the pathology can enter in the chronicity and be less violent. We said then that the Tan, affects the emotions of the Heart and causes palpitations, insomnia, disorders of the heart as the concern, dreams excessive.

To treat diseases related to tan, it never discusses a body alone, or a single meridian. It is very important not to forget that the TAN is produced by the spleen, but it should also examine the Yang energy of the kidney. If the symptoms show a relationship with the diaphragm, it must also deal with them.

If the tan is not in the lung, but that it is caused after the fire of the liver, it must in this case, deal with the liver.

The diseases related to tan are not simple diseases. There is of course not of mono-processing. The diagnosis is fundamental then to come to the end of such imbalances. And of course, if one applies the rules of dietetics that we will see later, but also, if we learn to manage our emotions that are iron-of-launches of the production of stagnation, therefore to tan, we will immune to such pathologies.

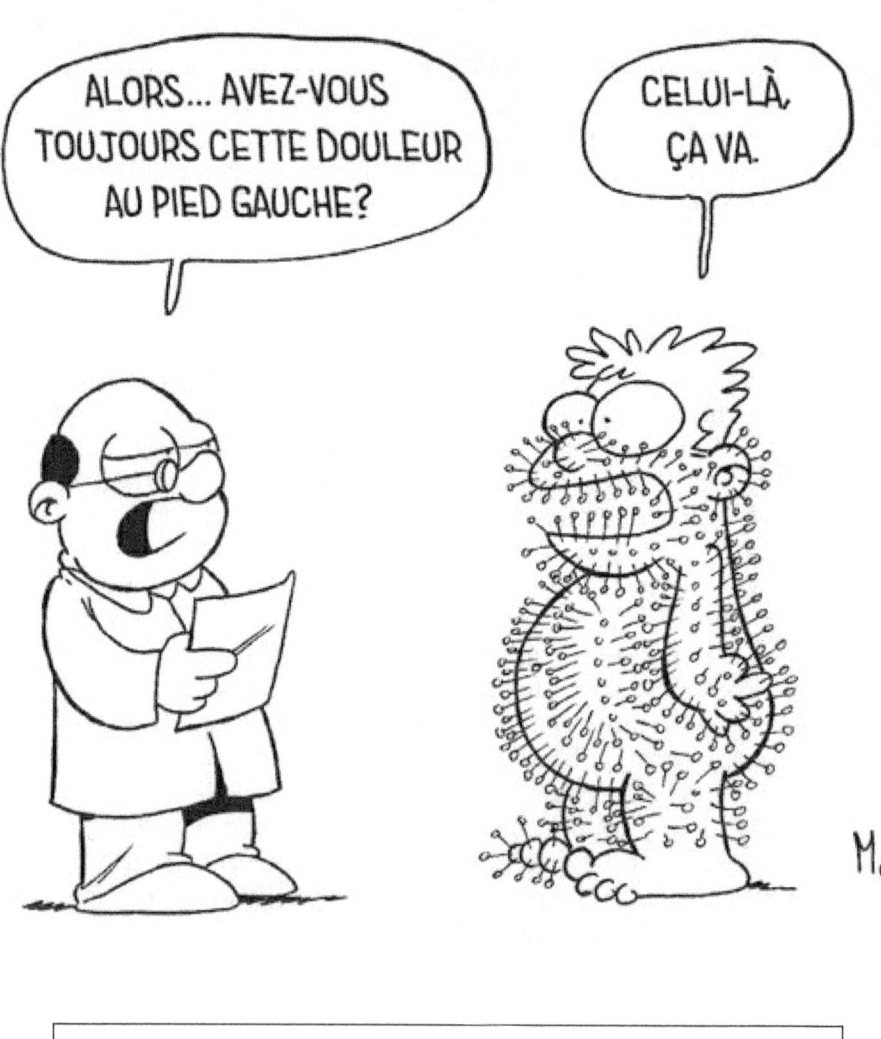

In this part...

This part covers a very wide range of therapeutic techniques and preventive measures taught by the MTC, of the acupuncture in the traditional pharmacopoeia of the practitioner. But this part is directed mainly to all "null" that we are: How to really deal with his health, "without fear and without reproach ", avoiding any radicalism and any excess? You will learn in effect to breathe, to sleep, to relax, to you automasser, to move your body, to meditate. A broad place will be given to the ancestral technique of digitoponcture, with a few large formulas of passable points by everyone. As a bonus, you will find a very simple method to learn in a few minutes the localization and the journey global of 12 meridians of energy.

Chapter 12

The major principles

In this chapter:

" The four disciplines of the MTC

" The big question: should we deal with first the Crown or the root of a disease?

" The three major types of treatment

UN practitioner in MTC must be a multicard professional. In effect, when it is in the presence of a patient, once the role of detective completed (see chapitre 3**), when all indices have been met, when the weapons of the crime have been found, when a Diagnosis melded well will have been installed, it will have to decide of treatment methods to implement. Thus after the end" of the implementation review", it should rebalance its patient.**

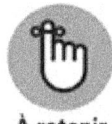

À retenir

If you have well understood the basic principles which underlie the MTC, a practitioner has never healed a patient! He has made that giving back to the body of the patient, by different rebalancing, the ability to autoguérir.

For this, this same practitioner will be at the same time acupuncturist, digitopuncteur, masseur, dietician, chiropractor, psychotherapist, sophrologue, herbalist, sports educator. Of well-conducted studies of MTC are that a good practitioner must be broken to all these techniques. And according to the patient that he has in front of him, he will choose such or such of these methods. Once more, the MTC is not summarized that of acupuncture! Let us look at this more closely.

The Disciplines

The four major disciplines

The MTC includes four major disciplines as to the methods of treatment.

" **Acupuncture, digitoponcture and moxibustion** *which will be widely developed in these pages.*

" *The use of medicinal plants:* the Chinese pharmacopoeia is one of the most developed and older than we knew. The drugs are compounds of mineral products, sometimes animals and especially plants. As we will see, each plant is chosen according to its color, its form, its smell, its flavor and often it is necessary to use several simultaneously. If a mixture of plants is not sufficient, for the minimal part remaining, there will be a need in some cases to use of mineral substances, or even animals. (Sensitive soul refrain! Eat a scorpion is not in the scope of all!) but it is before all a medicine by the herbs.

" *The exercises and the massage.* exercises such as the Qi Gong that are of type either internal or external.

" *The method Dao Yin, DAO meaning "guide", instruct the patient. This are all the advice that the practitioner must give to his patient to the outcome of the treatment. In this method, the psychotherapeutic treatment held a central place in view of the multiplication of the internal diseases. However, we have already seen that the disruptions was mental and emotional the starter and the profound cause of almost all major pathologies generated by our western way of life.*

The complementary methods

The practitioner may also have other methods such as:

" Methods to rectify the posture of the body. There are similarities with the western osteopathy. These techniques are called "readjustments," when the skeleton is not right, or when the OS has been broken, disconnected, the articulation luxée.

" There is also a whole science of poultices. These are methods of application of drugs on the skin, known in China for thousands of years. It was thus able to count thousands of forms to use very varied.

But all this would be incomplete if the practitioner was not able to learn to his patient the methods of preservation of life, or Yang Sheng FA. This is a whole series of methods intended to keep the body in good health. It must learn to his patient how to:

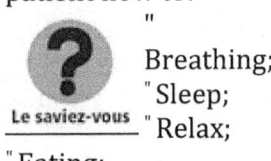

" Breathing;
" Sleep;
" Relax;
" Eating;

"Do the love;
"Move his body;
"If automasser;
"Manage its emotions.

In sum, once the patient is rebalanced, he must learn to do more "falling" ill by daily practices of charging the battery of the kidney.

Should we deal with first the Crown or the root of a disease?

At first glance, the answer should be obvious. The practitioner must deal with the root causes of the disease and not any of following obscure the symptoms. That is what differentiates TCM and Western medicine. Medicine so-called "modern" is very efficient to treat acute symptoms, emergency. But it very often lost foot when it comes to chronic pathologies, lack of treatment of the cause deep.

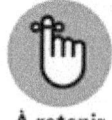 I remind you that a symptom is that the objectification of a battle that occurs between an aggressor (that he either external or internal) and "energy right", the defense of the body. If this is

À retenir

done disappear immediately, the disease risk of progress at low noise, for a single blow, go toward a state of self-destruction of the body. Therefore pay attention not to take painkillers to Tower of arm, as soon as the emergence of a simple headache.

In MTC, it objectively these notions of root causes and superficial causes of a pathology by the terms Biao and Ben.

"The Biao, "the surface", relates to the demonstration of the imbalances and therefore, here, to the symptoms presented by a patient.

"The BEN relates to the deep root. This is the cause, the factor causing the affection.

You have just to catch cold: Ben of the disease, it is the penetration of the perversity wind-cold to the inside of the body that it is going to have to hunt. The headache, vomiting, pain in the joints are the Biao, the objectification of this penetration.

In nature, the Ben corresponds to the root of the tree, while the branches, the trunk, leaves represent the Biao.

That must treat first?

We are going to see that everything is a question of logic with respect to the appreciation of the table presented by the patient.

In the case of benign, there will be able to treat simultaneously the Ben and the Biao. If the practitioner is sure of gentleness of the disease, that the syndrome is not serious, it will at the same time act on the two factors. For example, in cases of flu, there has a fever and headache. It will at the same time enable the Agency to reject the perversity, but also use of the means to bring down the fever and calm the pain.

But when the disease is more severe, the practitioner in the light of the table symptomatologique that presents the patient decide to begin or by the Ben or by the Biao.

If for example the person manifest, during the course of his illness, a state of weakness very important, it will be necessary to select the plants, treatments by powerful needles to reconstitute rapidly its forces. Once the Zhen Qi (Energy right) restored, we will then be able to deal with the symptoms.

In another case, if there are symptoms of blocking of faeces and urine (the Biao), before treating the cause (Ben), it will be immediately release these symptoms of blocking and stagnation.

 If a pain, whatever it is, is not very serious, that the patient is likely to accommodate, it is by the Ben that it must begin. In the opposite case, if the pain is intolerable, it will be necessary to treat the symptom.

À retenir

Another example. It is said, in MTC, that the energy of spleen allows to keep the blood in the vessels. When one is in the presence of a weakness of the energy of the spleen and kidney, the person can very easily bleed. It will be necessary to treat the root of the imbalance. But if the person has a bleeding very important, for example at the level of the nose, it will take a very quickly if attach to treat this symptom. In such a case, you may also consider to deal at the same time the symptom and the cause.

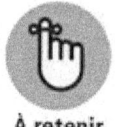

Everything is a matter of appreciation and "profound vision"!

When the disease is acute and presents a character of emergency, it is appropriate first to treat the Biao, the symptom, the surface of the disease. In contrast, when the pathology is of chronic type, slow evolution, it is fundamental to treat the Ben, the deep imbalance of one or several of the five software bodies. It must then be that the practitioner is able to find the root cause of the affection, and then to deal with priority. It is the history of this patient who goes to see his doctor for pain in the eyes. The latter does not have the "profound vision" of the MTC, will prescribe any painkillers to treat the symptom. The Practitioner "Chinese" having pushed the examination until the end just going to say to his patient to remove the small spoon it retains in its glass and which injures him permanently his eye when he drinks!

Three major types of treatment

The same formula for several disorders

This principle of treatment is called Tong Zhi: "a same treatment that applies to several different conditions." It exists in MTC formulas of Pharmacopoeias types, as well as series of points of acupuncture for treating such or such a type of disruption.

Let us take the example of a formula that treats the heat that has been able to penetrate the layer Yin. It allows to remove the fire. We will be able to use for example the same formula when the heat is present in the three homes. But also, when a stagnation-moisture is present in the stomach, generating of fire (gastro-enteritis). It is a common treatment for some types of pathology which are not acute.

Different treatments for a same pathology

This type of processing is called yi Zhi: "It is applied different types of treatment, then that it is a single disease, in the same patient. "It means that it will have to adapt to the state of the patient, but also that the same disease can have, according to the ground, several different treatments. The treatment will also be able to be adapted on the day according to the evolution.

Type "support and eliminate"

A third type of treatment is fu Zheng Qi Xie: "support and eliminate". In this case, it must support the right energy, Zheng Qi, which has need to assist, to be assisted, reconstituted in order to be able once again to fight effectively against the perversity, the Xith Qi.

"When the attacker is not very powerful, if it effectively supports the right energy, defense, it can then arrive any only to eliminate it.

"However, if the attacker, the 11th qi, is powerful, it must be not only support Zheng Qi which is damaged by the attacker, but also implement techniques to eliminate directly the Xie Qi. As the symptom is acute, it also deals with the Biao.

Attention

But attention not to tone up to the hilt. In effect, if the practitioner is not the correct diagnosis, it risk. At the same time toning the right energy, but also the agent perverse, the attacker. And suddenly all the pathology flames.

Therefore, if the state of weakness is very serious, it is necessary to deal with any of following by plants or points to type toning. In contrast, if the state of weakness is not very serious, it must be careful and choose tonics in function of the state of weakness found. As well, it is necessary to see if it is a state Xu, of weakness of blood, the Qi, the Yang or the Yin, as well as the stage of development of the pathology.

Chapter 13
The true
Acupuncture
Traditional
<u>In this chapter:</u>
" <u>The eight therapeutic methods</u>
" <u>The nine needles according to the **Nei Jing**</u>
" <u>The method "fair" according to the **Nei Jing**</u>
" <u>The Route of the meridians for Dummies</u>
" <u>The acupuncture points</u>

SI we refer to what has been said in the first part, rather than getting lost in the maze of "10 000 techniques" of our own civilization, where the explosion of the Yang outweighs the interiorization of the Yin, this course on acupuncture is going to be some kind of a return to the Uniqueness. Certainly, this can be disturbing for some who have followed some types of curriculum. But I prefer to trust the Pr Leung Kok Yuen which has been considered as one of the best acupuncturists by his peers of our time" "modern" (see chapitre 1**).**

Acupuncture is therefore a therapeutic system which goes back to the night of the time and which consists in the stimulation of specific areas of the body, yet appointed "point of Acupuncture". These points are most often found on journeys of meridians well defined.

The eight therapeutic methods

We will see in the study of the pharmacopoeia (see chapitre 16) that there are "Eight therapeutic methods", the Ba FA that are:

"Sweating or perspiration, Han Fa;
"The vomiting, Thou Fa;
"The purgation, XIA Fa;
"The harmonization, he Fa;
"The warming or the calorification, Wen Fa;
"The clarification or refresh, Qing Fa;
"Dispersal or reduction, Xiao Fa;
"And toning, Bu FA.

Among these eight therapeutic effects, acupuncture allows to obtain four to know Heat, regularize, toning and disperse.

Things are simple:
" Heat is implemented in the affections of cold type.
" Regulate is used in the case of illness of nature hot.
" The toning is used in the case of weakness, Xu, lack.
" The sedation, in the case of fullness, Shi.
We know that when one is in front of an imbalance, a disease, we must identify it we used Ba gang, of the eight classifications (see chapitre 3). This is very important for understanding the function of the points.
We will see as well that some points are in direct relationship with the bodies, Zang-Fu, while others concern the meridians, the Jing Luo. Obviously," the five solid organs (FU) and the six hollow organs (Zang)" being housed in the depth within the same body, they fall under the heading of internal, then that the meridians more at the periphery of the body are the responsibility of the external field.

The Technique

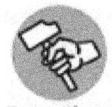

To achieve a treatment by acupuncture, it is therefore necessary to:
" First, whether the disease is internal or external.

En pratique " Secondly, to choose points rather in relation with the internal or external and the Yin and the Yang.
" Thirdly, according that the disease is hot or cold, we will implement one of four methods. If the disease is of cold nature, it will heat, if it is of a nature warm, we will regularise.
It is then necessary to see if a disease is Xu or Shi, in weakness or in fullness. We will use the toning for a State Xu and sedation for a State Shi.
It is considered that, by acupuncture, toning has a heating effect. When the tones, it stimulates, it increases the strength of the body. To this title, it is considered that the toning and the warming are two methods close to one another. It is mainly implements thus in cases Xu, of weakness.
Similarly, for sedation and regularisation. The sedation applies to the case Shi, fullness, and the regularisation in the case hot. The two cases, Shi and hot, fall under the heading of Yang.

In acupuncture, heat requires the implementation of the moxibustion (see chapitre 15), whereas the regularization is obtained strictly with the needles.

Therefore, we repeat, the actions of tone or heat are equivalent. The same that disperse or regularize. That is why the methods implemented in acupuncture can bring, in the interests of simplification, in a first approach, to the toning and the dispersion.

Our Master s is before all concerned in its course to teach simple methods and which ensure a maximum of security. We will therefore see the standard method of base. It is direct from the teachings given by the Nei Jing.

À retenir

When a problem is difficult and that we must return to the knowledge the oldest, what are the methods that will be exposed later who will offer the most guarantees. And if they are familiar with the basic theories of elders, the applications will be easy and it will be seen that acupuncture is not so complicated that this.

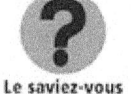

Le saviez-vous

Do not get lost in the maze of "10 000 techniques" Some are served, to discern the methods of toning and of sedation, the direction of the movement of the energy flow in the Jing Luo, the meridians. Other have concentrated on the speed of inserting a needle. Others, on the way we are going to rotate. You can insert the needle slowly or well the remove quickly, or give him the flicks, the oscillate, the rotate in one direction or the other. You can also rotate as to widen a hole. It may involve the respiration. For example, coordinate the insertion and withdrawal with the inspires and the expires. You can also insert the needle in three steps or the insert directly in depth. Similarly, the effect may vary, if we withdraw this needle in three stages. You can also use the rhythms that one puts in relationship with the Yin and the Yang. A rate based on the Figure 9 is rather Yang, while a different pace based on a cycle of six is rather Yin. For example, if it is done by rotating the needle nine times, it has an effect Yang, six times, an effect Yin.

Therefore, already in ancient times, we had a plethora of techniques of poncture. And, of course, these techniques have only to complicate to our so-called modern era. Some thought that the right side and the left reverse its effects depending on whether it is a man or a woman. The problem is complicated then it immensely. Therefore, the more one looks in the study of the texts, even old, dealing with the acupuncture, more the concepts that will be found will be complex. To such a point that the problem could become insoluble. And if someone really wants to attach to summarize all beliefs, all studies of former time to develop a practical method standard, this would prove to be an impossible task. The return to the Uniqueness is required.

The nine needles according to the Nei Jing

In the **Nei Jing, it is considered that there are nine types of needles. Each of them has a particular use. Each needle, depending on its form, allows you to get some specific effects.**

Needle No. 1, needle Chan

Its length of after the Nei Jing is of 1.6 inch. His head is swollen while the end is sharp. The tip to the end is very short.

In these nine needles, the Digit 1 is in relationship with the sky which is therefore itself attached to the Yuan Yang, in the Yang originel, to what we call in MTC "the sky previous". The highest position of the organs is the lung that corresponds to the sky. The skin belongs to the Lung software. The area of the skin is also the most external part. The external is yang. That is why it is called "the needle no. 1".

 This needle must in no case be inserted deeply. It allows you to disperse the Yang, obtain a sedation of the Biao, of the external.

À retenir As this needle can be used only under the skin, of our days and by extension, it qualifies this type of needle and needle of "sub-skin". These needles can have different forms and can be left in place.

It is from this needle No. 1 that the Japanese have designed the "hammer to flowers of plum tree". It is a long handle accompanied by a variable number of needles. Here also, the needles are designed not to enter deeply into the skin. If there is penetration, it may not be only superficial.

There are mainly two kinds. Either with a central needle and four other needles around, or then a central needle and six other around. It is then called in this case "hammer to seven stars." It taps the skin with this hammer, or on specific points, or well on the path of a meridian. All needles penetrate simultaneously, but in a very superficial manner.

The difference between the needle **Chan** and the hammer to flowers of plum is that the first does not penetrate that in a single point while the flower of plum several key points in a same area in only once.

Needle No. 2, needle Yuan

He must know that the figure 2 was to put in relationship with the earth. The earth corresponds to the spleen, which control in the body, the muscles.

This needle has a rounded shape. It is thick. The shape of the needle is quite similar to an egg.

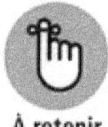

The important thing to remember is that its sole aim is the sedation.

With this needle, it rubs the surface of the skin. Unlike the previous needle, there is here no skin insertion. In rubbing, causes a relaxation between the valleys of muscle. We can thus raise tensions.

À retenir

It is from this needle that was created the "scraper", or even "knife to scrape". It comes from a stone which was worn against another stone to eliminate the small irregularities. It uses to "scrape" the meridians of the bladder in the back. We can also use the installment of a coin.

This type of massage is particularly effective in people who have a nature too hot, among which muscles are very tense, painful. It is an excellent means of sedation of energy between the muscles.

Needle No. 3, needle Ti

According to the **Nei Jing, the form of this needle, as well as its end are rounded. It is therefore not pointed as in some representations. It presents almost the same diameter on the entire length. It therefore cannot cross the skin.**

It is used when the disease affects the blood vessels, the Xue May. It uses, among others, when the person has a low energy which must be it toned.

It therefore makes it possible to exercise pressure on the points or to support on the surface of the skin. Therefore, you can either rub, either press, either exercise a pressure. It is a form of treatment are very effective.

We can compare this process to what today is called "digitoponcture", or acupressure. In ancient times, it was not using the fingers to exercise these pressures.

Needle No. 4, needle Feng

The needle Feng or triangular needle has the shape of a small sabre. The form of this needle has evolved according to the times, up to reach a certain grandeur. However, it is necessary to ensure that the insertion depth is nevertheless limited.

The figure 4 refers to the seasons that are the spring, summer, autumn and winter. Because of these seasons, the individual is exposed to the Xith Qi, to single wickedness which assault the meridians, blood vessels. Then they are achieved and can be retighten, to contract, causing an obstruction, a stagnation. The blood circulation and energy is then disrupted. In this case, it uses this needle for Obtain a sedation thanks to the bleeding. The 11th Qi stagnant in the vessels are eliminated, especially if this stagnation lasts for a long time. The blood and energy will then go back to circulate harmoniously.

Needle No. 5, needle Pi

It is similar to a knife. As a scalpel, it serves to cut, to rend the surface of the skin.

This needle allows therefore to incise the abscesses when there is training of pus. It inserts the needle in the abscess to allow him to be empty.

Needle No. 6, needle Yuan Li

It is a needle that is thick enough and its end is relatively sharp.

It therefore makes it possible to harmonize, to intervene on the six pairs of meridians, in order to treat, adjust.

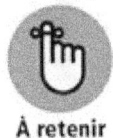

À retenir

213

Therefore the needle No. 6, among the 9 needles, is the one that allows you to rebalance the Yin and the Yang through the 12 Jing Luo, 12 meridians circulating in the human body.

Its main action is to obtain a sedation. In particular when there is a penetration of Xie Qi important, linked, among others to the penetration of perverse energies of one of the four seasons.

It allows you to restore the balance Yin and Yang and, by the same token, to evacuate the Xie Qi, the perverse energy.

Needle No. 7, needle Hao

The word Hao means End, end as a hair. The figure 7, him, is to put in relationship with the stars.

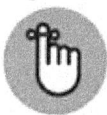

In current acupuncture, this needle no. 7 is, in the eyes of the Pr Leung, the most important of the needles.

À retenir In the sky, there are 7 groups of constellations which are to be put in relation with the 7 holes that are: the eyes, nostrils, mouth, the two ears. It is said "that there are 7 groups of constellations in the sky and 7 holes on the Earth".

We know that when a perverse energy between in the Jing Luo, in the meridians, a conflict is declared. If a Xie Qi stays too long, it can cause pain and numbness. From there, the ancient Chinese created a needle very pointed, very thin and sharp, relatively short, comparable to the sting of a mosquito. This needle must be particularly sharp and ready to be able to penetrate very easily the barrier of the skin. It allows to maintain and nurture the Zheng Qi, energy right, one that protects us and, unlike most of the other needles, it allows to root out only the Xie Qi, the agents "vicious", preserving the integrity of the zheng Qi and even in the tonic.

Needle No. 8, needle Chang

It is a needle that is longer than the previous one. It looks like the Nos. 6 and 7. Generally, these needles are between 1 and 1.5 cun (Le Cun = 35.8 mm).

The long needles are between 3 and 4 cun long. Some may even reach 7 Cun. It is very rare today to use such lengths.

Symbolically, This needle is linked to 8 winds. Then one can be in the presence of arthritis at the level of the joints when the perversity penetrates very in depth. These needles allow to reach great depths, penetrate even in the joints.

They allow to prick points such as the 30VB at the level of the buttock to achieve the articulation coxal-femoral.

Today, we mainly use of needles Long, short, thick or thin. The thickness of the needle may vary. Generally, we find the needles which vary from 26 to 36, 26 being the thicker, and 36 the most thin.

Not even wrong!

Le saviez-vous

Formerly, we used needles properly larger. There is an explanation for it. Formerly, living much more in the open air, there was exposed steadily to the weather, that this is the wind, cold, heat, sun, rain, etc. the skin to adapt was much thicker and possessed a layer of protection is much better. At the present time, of the fact of our new mode of life, it is quite otherwise. Living much more to the interior, being more and more sedentary, wearing clothes more and more masking fluid, the skin is much more fragile. If we used the same needles than in the former time, the fact of this embrittlement of the skin, there would have persistence of scars and holes to elsewhere would surely have of evil to heal. And the assurances of the practitioners would increase in arrow! As well more the resistance of people decreased, the more it became necessary to use needles increasingly thin. Our Master, in his cabinet, had not used exclusively that of the needles of 36. Of our days, it considers that the needles 28, 30, 32, being thick enough, can be considered as the needles No. 6. The Needles 34, 36, they are to be regarded as the needles No. 7.

Needle No. 9, needle da

This needle is larger and thicker than the needle No. 6.

After insertion, it creates a port by which liquids may elapse. Thus, when there is accumulation of liquids, for example in the case of moisture perverse, with such needles, we will be able to allow these liquids to drain and the situation can then to improve more rapidly. The needle thus allows a kind of drainage.

In ancient times, were also used of warm needles. According to the **Nei Jing, it heats the needle before the insert. This**

215

technique was used in cases of infringement of cold perverse. It was then to proceed to an insertion very fast. Similarly, the withdrawal must be also very fast. If we used then a needle too thin, it would have bent or broken.

The method "fair" according to the **Nei Jing**

According to Chinese tradition, the living being, and here more particularly the man, is an organization resulting from the combination of matter (the body material or physical) of nature Yin, and energy (which animates matter) of nature Yang. The harmonious balance between these two components determines the state of health. The disruption of this balance are responsible for the disease. Any disturbance of nature to break this balance first assigns preferentially energy.

For example, an excess of Yang will generate a sudden pain, inflammation, spasms, a headache or an increase in the voltage. An excess of Yin can translate by Diffuse pain, a sensation of cold, the retention of water or a large fatigue.

The energy, the Qi is movement and any disturbance will impede this movement: the blocking in is the consequence. The energy stuck in a region of the body material accumulates upstream of the blocking, while areas downstream of the blockage will find in energy deficit.

In the presence of a state of pathology as well described, the acupuncturist will establish his diagnosis by searching for the levels at which the energy is blocked, and that it is the reason of the blockage. It will then apply its treatment by lifting the lock and correcting, if it can, the reason for this blocking. The needle, among other things, will enable him to direct the course of energies.

The **Nei Jing** quote four fundamental points with regard to the Act of puncture.

First point: the correct patient position

After you have properly determined the points that we will prick, it will be necessary to install the patient as a function of this choice, and this, in the most comfortable position possible.

In practice, some points require more a sitting position for their puncture, others a recumbent position. But, in all cases, it will be appropriate to prefer the extended position. In effect, in the sitting position, the patient will eventually move.

He must know that the muscular relaxation is an indispensable condition for the proper conduct of a meeting. If the release is not sufficient, if the four members or the trunk are not in a natural position of relaxation, this uncomfortable situation will disrupt the work of the practitioner, the manipulation of the needle.

À retenir

The second point: the good attitude of the practitioner

The practitioner at the time of his gesture must be very careful. It must take a lot of precautions in order to avoid any error.

The needle must be maintained with masters, otherwise it could him escape of hands or, at least, it could make a handling error. At the same time, the other hand deals with the location of the point. It is used to perform massages or pressures. The two hands are thus put to contribution.

The practitioner must, of course, think only of his patient and must not be disturbed or distracted by something else. When he place a needle, there is more than this that account. It must look to the right or to the left, and he must not be that breathing. The spirit is fully involved, concentrated on the action that is in progress.

It must also be held right, with dignity and even a certain solemnity and especially do not leave the eyes the patient. The Eyes, we now know, are the part of the body where best manifests itself The Shen, the Spirit. By monitoring the eyes of the patient, it also captures his attention.

The concentration of the practitioner calls in some way that of the patient. It is only in these conditions that will quickly the Qi, energy at the end of the needle.

Third point: the insertion of the needle

The insertion of the needle will be done in three steps.

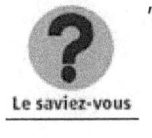

"

The first step is superficial. This first step is used to eliminate the perverse energy, Xie, qi, in order to allow the blood and to the energy, Xue and the Qi, to reoccupy as well the space, to leave the place to the blood and the Yuan Qi who can then assemble under the skin.

"*The second step* is to insert more deeply the needle in order to dislodge, disperse the perverse energy which has been able to penetrate more deeply in the part Yin. It must therefore be to dislodge go more in depth, under the skin, in the region Yin.

"*Finally, in the third step, it pushes the needle more deeply, up to reach the level of the real energy of the organism, the Zhen Qi. I remind you that Zhen Qi is a substance that is very subtle which is produced from Zhong Qi that represents the whole of the functions of the average home and by EIF Qi, the energy of the lung. Zhen Qi is the subtle substance that circulates in all meridians and which, with the blood, contributes to the substantial contribution necessary to the whole of the functional dynamic which is under the emblem of the "Five Zang, six Fu", of the five software bodies.*

It is therefore defined three stages and the needle is not pressed a single blow up to the normal depth. It is therefore necessary to move by a superficial step, then average, before joining the depth that we must normally achieve at this point. And it is only at this level that we reached the real energy of the body. As soon as we reached this area, it is necessary to stop the progression. It must not be push more the needle. This insertion can not be made of a single blow up to the proper depth and this good depth varies in function of the point that we spades.

Fourth point: the obtaining of the Qi

Obtain the Qi wants to say that the energy comes to the meeting of the tip of the needle. The tip of the needle really affects the energy of the body and it is the indispensable condition for that the processing has an effect.

The effect of treatment by acupuncture, c is the disappearance of the disease exactly as the Hunting wind the clouds in the sky and leaves behind him a clear sky. The brightening of the sky under the effect of the wind is observed in a way immediate and very distinct. It is the same here for the treatment by acupuncture.

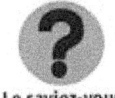
If you do not get the Qi, the treatment produces no result. On the contrary, if the Qi was obtained, the patient feel the effect immediately, he finds it immediately a state of relief and relaxation.

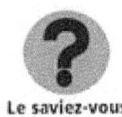
Le saviez-vous

219

The obtaining of the QI or the passage of the "rude" to the "subtle"

He should know that this concept has been completely distorted, even distorted in our contemporary world. When a practitioner acts on a point, it search before everything to reach the Qi, the energy which circulates along the meridian. It should not be forgotten that this energy is the outcome of a mixture very subtle between the quintessence of the energy of the air and the quintessence of the digestion of food bowl. And that this energy goes well beyond any materiality. Our master insisted on the following fact: "This energy can never be quantified, measured and no device will not be able to view it." This can only be a feeling on the part of the practitioner. And this felt will be, not with our cognitive faculties, our Shen, as one feels a point hot or cold. This felt will proceed in what is called the "intuition", the intuition of the point. And that is what differentiates us totally of acupuncture and the modern digitoponcture. This is not the patient who must feel a sensation, or if little. It is the practitioner who through a transmitter, here the needle must "feel" that the Qi is there, present. The Pr Leung compared it to the fishery. A fisherman warned, once its line jetty in the current of a river and which takes a expert hand his fishing rod, will be able to distinguish, to feel what is happening at the end of his line. In effect, the shaking that it will feel may be due to a fish by train to eat the bait without touching the hook. It will have a felt different if its line is pushed by the direction of the current and even more important if the hook is clinging to the bottom of the river. At a time, eyes closed, he may even "see", feel, having the intuition, the profound vision of the fish in the process of the bait. It is the same when the practitioner pushes a needle in the energy flow of a meridian, or when we support with the pulp of our thumb on a point of acupuncture. It is a sensation that must be proven by the practitioner and not by the patient. And it is this same practitioner who must be capable of controlling this flow of energy during the whole duration of the stimulation. However, the modern treatments do not contain any more this notion very subtle, that the ancient texts called him "the obtaining of the Qi". They do not retain more than the sensation of tingling which must at that time be felt by the

221

patient. "The tingling is a Sensation own to the patient, while obtaining the Qi is own to the doctor. "

Regardless of the number of inserts in a same meeting, or the number of treatments performed, or the time that lasts the establishment of the needle, you can get results that if you arrive to obtain the Qi in the tip of the needle.

If you have not reached the Qi, it is necessary to repeat the treatment or lengthen the duration.

As soon as the Qi is obtained, it is necessary to remove the needle. It should be especially not the press more.

The obtaining of the Qi is more rapid in some subjects, a little slower in others. Everything depends on the preponderance of the Yin and the Yang in the body.

If the method is fair, there will be no side effects to the acupuncture.

The five faults and the four infringements of the practitioner according to the Nei Jing

The five faults

" *The first default* : Do not search for the causes, the origin of the disease. The doubt and uncertainty can be install in the mind of the practitioner and, if it begins the treatment in this state of mind, passing in addition to a further investigation, which aims to remove this uncertainty, the result of the treatment may not be as poor.

" *The second fault* : do not take into account what may reveal the mode of life, the hygiene of life of the patient and, from there, perform a treatment to misuse.

" *The third default* : to determine the nature of the disease by the single palpation of the pulse. In reality, the palpation of the pulse rate should be confronted to other comments, she must be relativized. Outside of the problems related to climatic variations, so the external causes, it must be well know the physiology of internal organs. Indeed, some organs can contain a lot of Qi and a lot of blood, or few of QI or little blood. Therefore, before

222

deciding on the character Xu or Shi a affection, he must know what is the body which is reached, and what are its proportions of Qi and Xue, energy and blood.

" *The fourth fault* is to put in relationship with the attitude of the Practitioner vis-a-vis the patient. In fact, in some cases, the patient has need of precise instructions and strict that it will have to implement on the opinion of its practitioner.
"

À retenir

If the practitioner does not feel safe enough of him, that he has not enough confidence in him, the patient will lose in its turn confidence in his doctor and this will affect the treatment of the disease. If there is a lack of firmness, for example if it has a tendency to assign when a patient does not like the treatment, that it prefers to follow the inclinations of the patient, it will not be able to defeat the disease.

" *The Fifth Default* : not to recognize the first cause of the disease. He must know that some diseases are before any psychological in origin and non-somatic. The emotional stress can affect the body physically and it can appear of pathological signs observable. Indeed, we know that the psychological disorders greatly disturb the balance Yin-Yang in the body. We can thus find themselves in front of stagnations of Qi, Yang who can foster the emergence on the surface of the body of abscess, and even of tumors, benign or malignant. The fifth error is therefore to ignore the cause first and to poncturer for the sole purpose of restoring the balance Yin-Yang at the level of the symptom.

The four infringements

" *The first breach:* do not discern the variations in relative of the Yin and the Yang. We may know on the theoretical plan the theory of Yin and Yang without being able to assess their relative variation. There is indeed a stream of evolution, a mutual variation between the Yin and

Yang, this flow can be in the direction of the current, in the right direction or then against the current. If the relative balance of the Yin and the Yang of the man follows the nature, which must be the normal state, it is then in the presence of a stream that goes in the direction of the current. If, on the contrary, the flow, the variation of the Yin and the Yang in the man are not adapted to those of the environment, it is in this case in a flow against the current. An example: in autumn, the pulse is superficial. Autumn is the season that corresponds to the metal in the human body. The metal element is the lung. The Lung corresponds to the descent. This descent extends to the element water which corresponds to the winter and to pulse deep. Indeed, we know, through the cycle of five elements, that the Yang begins to descend from the lung. This are of seasonal variations of the pulse which are in agreement with the ebb and flow of the Yin-Yang. However, if it is observed that the pulse is deep in the summer, that is to say that if the pulse of the winter is manifested in the summer, it is a pulse pathological. It indicates the presence of a disease. Similarly, if the superficial pulse occurs in winter, it is also a pulse pathological. In these cases, the normal dynamics of the Yin and the Yang is upset and there is talk of against the current. Therefore, a same pulse may be interpreted differently in function of the Yin and the Yang of the universe. Ignore these phenomena by insufficiency of learning is the first error.

"*The second breach:* stop her studies before having completed its learning of Chinese medicine. If, for example, it is not confined to the acupuncture, that it decides to stop learning and that it is merely to learn of the formulas of points indicated for certain disorders or some symptoms for example the headache: by lack of study, it does not seek to know if it is a state Xu or Shi, which would have been able to guide our treatment toward a toning or sedation. If it is simply a few elements of the medical theory and that are considered to have learned everything already, this attitude leads to the second error described here by the Nei Jing.

" *The third infringement* : Do not take into account the mode of life of the patient and particularly of its place in the social scale, its level of life. For example, the most disadvantaged persons are generally not turbocharged as are the people most fortunate. They have in general a power supply more abundant, rich in meat and lack of exercises. Conversely, the poorer people tend to be more physically active, overworked, whereas their power has a tendency to be rather inadequate, or at least not varied enough. For this third error, it is also mentioned that the practitioner may not make enough Differences, distinctions in the analysis of the signs. He may miss nuances, interpret one way the signs he observes instead to refine its analysis. The same sign may in fact lead to different conclusions. Do not qualify her interpretation, not the weighed, lead to install false diagnostics.

" *The fourth breach* : Do not query in sufficient depth to the patient, to find the true cause of the disease. It is necessary that the field of investigation as broad as possible. It is therefore appropriate to inquire on the psychological state, emotional, of our patient, but also see some morbid habits such as smoking, alcohol, the irregularities, the Food aberrations, the irregularities affecting the mode of life, or at its own pace. See if there is no possible causes of poisoning.

The journey of the meridians for Dummies

Before studying more before the acupuncture points on which the acupuncturist must act, assume that you have no concept of the journey of the 14 main meridians. In the paragraphs that will follow, I will give you a mnemonic unstoppable, so that you can not only locate these meridians on your body, but also that you have very quickly the possibility of locating the points in space.

For example, with this method, if in a formula, you spoke of Item No. 3 on the meridian of the liver, you will know that he can only be at the level of the foot, which is more, on the column of the big toe and close to the end.

225

I remind you of what has been said in part 1:

"At the level of each of the members, you have six meridians, three Yin meridians which are to be put in relation with the vital organs, "full" and three meridians Yang, to put in relationship with the organs "hollow", receptacles, which have among other things such as action to protect the vital organs.

"

The meridians Yin begin at the level of the foot, because they capture the energy of the earth. Conversely the meridians Yang ending at the level of this same foot. In contrast, at the level of the hand, it is the contrary. The meridians Yin ending at the level of the hand. Indeed, thanks to the hand, it gives its energy through the meridians of the Heart and the pericardium. And therefore the meridians Yang begin at the level of the hand.

"The meridians and therefore returning at the level of the foot will contain many points, because they are far from the vital organs (for example 64 points for the meridian of the bladder). In contrast, the meridians of the hand will contain a few points, because they are close to the vital organs (for example, 9 points for the meridians of the pericardium and the heart).

"The meridians Yin will be on the faces Yin of upper and lower limbs (skin side "white"). The reverse for the meridians Yang. I remind you of the position to the four legs for zones Yin and Yang of the body.

Method of visualization of the six meridians of the foot

And to start this mental visualization of the meridians, serve us of one of our men current policies which is Mr Raffarin! It is that when you take your foot in your hands, at the level of the column of the big toe, under the arch, in a hollow near the metatarsal of the big toe begins the meridian of the kidney, the 1RN. Then, when you look at your big toe, on the side of the internal nail, we find the 1RT, the first point of the meridian of the spleen. And Nail side external, on this same toe, starts the 1F, the first point of the Meridian Yin of the

226

liver. Spleen, liver, kidney, this gives us ra (spleen) FFA (liver) Rin (kidney), Raffarin.

If you remember these three meridians, by deduction, you will find the path of the other nine meridians. Indeed, if one refers to the different couples of organs contained in each software component.

" The Meridian Yang corresponding to the kidney is the bladder. The latter will be located, and will end on the side of the external more of the foot.

" The Meridian Yang corresponding to the liver is that of the gallbladder. It will be located and will end on the external side of the fourth toe.

" The Meridian Yang corresponding to the spleen is that of the stomach. It will be located and will end at the level of the external side of the second toe. It browses therefore the center of the foot, such as the stomach which is at the center of the average household.

Just remember that the third toe has not of meridians which the travel.

Symbolic of the provision of the six meridians of the foot

Le saviez-vous

It must be based on the basic principle in MTC which is: "The Yang protects the Yin. "This is not the fruit of chance if the three meridians Yin of the foot are located on the internal side, big toe. On the contrary, the three meridians Yang are on the external side, that of the bladder and the gallbladder being the most external. In martial art, a kick is worn with the external side of the foot. If an experienced practicing happens to you take the internal, and if the strike is very powerful, this can become a deadly blow.

Method of visualization of the six meridians of the hand

If you know the three Yin meridians of the feet, by deduction, you will find the three Yin meridians of the hand. This are:

" The Yin meridian of the lung that is located on the external side of the thumb and ends on its nail angle external.

" The meridian of the Pericardium which goes through the center of the palmar face of the hand to finish" at the end of the end" of the major.

227

"The meridian of the heart which ends on the angle external nail of the atrial, annular side.

Symbolic of the provision of the six meridians of the hand

Le saviez-vous

It is a little different from the previous one.

Let us start by the clamp thumb-index, where are located the two meridians of the same software component, Poumon-Gros intestine. In India, it is the mudra Jnana. The Inch (the lung, the sky, the pure Yang, the i) covers the index (the large intestine, the cloaca, waste, the ME, the ego). The ego must be put in removing vis-a-vis the spiritual. In MTC, this software component is to put in relationship with the metal. The metal is driver. When the pulp of the thumb and the index are met, this forms a ring conductor of energy of the two bodies!

Then, if we refer to the point 9C. It is located at the level of nail the atrial, annular side. It is the point of Croque-death. In ancient times, there croquait this point to see if the heart could leave. In MTC, it is a great point of resuscitation. However, the meridian of the heart, which is the Emperor of all bodies, must be super protected (the heart stops beating, you die!). Two meridians Yang will load on the hand: the meridian of the small intestine which is the most internal (palms of the hands in the face of itself) on the same finger and that of the three homes on the external side of the finger. When, in martial art, it is a blow with the edge of the hand, C is the Meridian Yang who strikes, the Meridian Yin is protected.

Finally, in the center of the hand, we have the point 8cc, lao gong, a minor chakra you will learn how to open later. It ends at the end of the major. It is by this meridian and this point that we give our energy (massage, imposition of hands...). This meridian ends at the level of the pulp of the major, "at the end of the end," as a stream of energy which would leave of the hand.

It does not remain more than three Yang meridians corresponding to the three Yin meridians of the hand. This are:

" The Meridian Yang corresponding to the lung that is the one of the large intestine. It begins on the angle external nail of the index and runs along the side of this finger dorsal side.

" The Meridian Yang corresponding to the pericardium which is that of the three homes. It begins on the nail angle internal to the annular, atrial side. It runs along this finger, dorsal side of the hand.

" The Meridian Yang corresponding to the heart, which is that of the small intestine. It begins on the angle internal nail of the atrial, and runs along the inner side (hand facing you) of this finger, side Yang, dorsal of the hand.

The two previous meridians and post

In our view, we still have two fundamental meridians to see. You stand, legs spread apart and arms raised, themselves excluded: the man of Vitruvius.

On each side, 12 meridians which circulate continuously, thus 24 meridians. In the median axis, two meridians, a anterior and the other posterior which form a loop. These two meridians put in relation the meridians of the two sides of the body and have a direct relationship with the 12 internal organs.

" *A previous Meridian, the vessel "design", or REN May, which begins at the level of the perineum to fit on the anterior and median of the abdomen and chest. It ends under the lower lip. Ren wanting to say "take charge", it controls all the meridians Yin, and by There has an action on all the organs Yin internal. He has 24 points.*

" *A posterior Meridian, the "governor vessel", or of May, which also begins at the level of the perineum. It goes back on the median line of the back, along the spinous processus, to finish at the level of the upper lip. It is said that this vessel "governing" all the meridians Yang (the back is yang), and therefore all the viscera "hollow,", Yang of the body. He has 28 points.*

To make it short, under the control of the energy of the kidney, these meridians absorb the energy of the main meridians and their return when they need it, in the manner of an expansion bottle. They circulate the protective energy in the chest, abdomen and back.

The acupuncture points

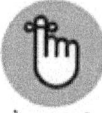

À retenir

A point of acupuncture is a point which is located along the route of a meridian. Next to a Meridian Energy, which, I would remind you, is a pipe located in depth," between the OS and the muscle," we have on the surface, hollow, differences of textures in the skin, small depressions where are usually these famous points.

The palpation of a point allows us to know what is happening in the energy flow the underlying, a little like a look on a water pipe. And when it is on the point, it acts on this flow. We can thus circulate, open a valve when there is an excess or add of energy when there is not enough.

Traditionally, there were 360 on the 14 main meridians. Are then appeared to the Use the points out meridians. There are more than 2 000 at the present time!

Le saviez-vous

In the pages that follow, you will see that in reality very few points, about 60, are sufficient to prevent or treat the pathologies. For the rest, it is local points which can be used on some stagnations, pain or swelling. We will return there.

It is necessary before any Learn the journey of the meridians, and then the points. Indeed, in many classic works, among others in the Nei Jing, only the name of the meridians was indicated, without reference to the points, when it was to treat and regulate certain problems. In other words, it must first choose the meridians before choosing the points.

Traditionally the Chinese doctors say: "It is better to be wrong on the points, but not on the meridians. "

About bodily measures of reference

To locate a point of acupuncture, three methods are at our disposal:

"The Cun, or "measure of proportional unit". It is a method which is to subdivide the parts of the body to know head, trunk, members in equal parts between them. Each unit is called Cun, thumb.

" The cun can also be measured as a function of the fingers of the patient. For example, the distance between the two flexion folds of the medius is equivalent to 1 Cun, a distance. The width of the thumb is equivalent to 1 Cun. The width between index and middle finger tight to 1.5 Cun. The width between the phalanges of the last four fingers outstretched equals 3 Cun, 3 distances.

" Finally, we can choose lairs natural, such as Landforms anatomical, the bony prominences, etc. This can be the line of implantation of the hair, the apple of Adam, the thorny articular process of a vertebra, the umbilicus, etc.

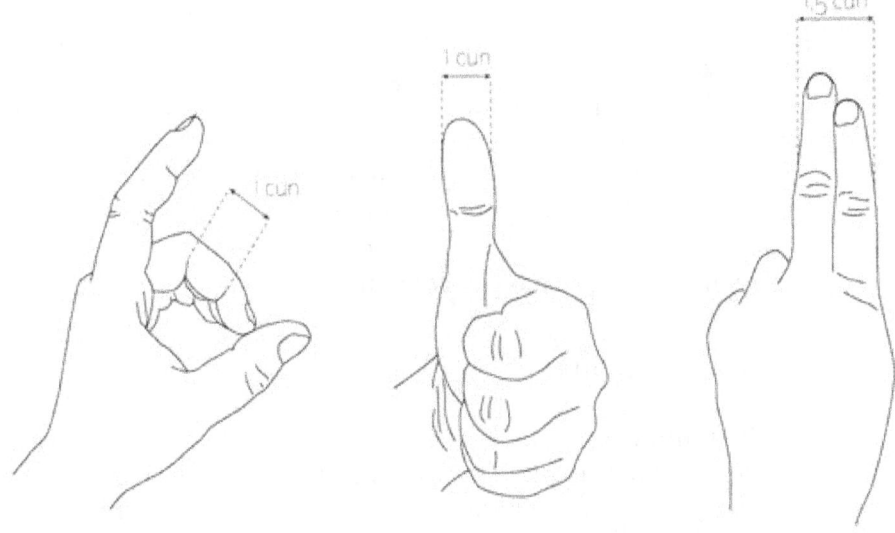

Figure 13-1 methods of locating a point of acupuncture.

In practice, it uses simultaneously the three methods. It uses the anatomical reliefs to locate the area of the point, and then search for the item by dividing the area in commensurate units or in cash with the measures taken from the fingers of the patient.

À retenir

He must know that these measures are necessary for the departure for the layman, to learn how to locate the point. But little by little, the practitioner will know very quickly where the point is located. It will be somewhat "the intuition

231

of the point". Moreover, according to the seasons, or other factors, the point may in a same individual vary from a few millimeters. Do not forget: what counts is to be on the good meridian. If there is a wrong a little upstream or downstream, it has not too much importance.

The different categories of points

The principles of prescription of points, or how to develop a formula are going to appeal to several categorizations of points. In the first place, we are going to differentiate between points called relatives, remote, and median. Then we will see the specific points.

Search the error!
A special feature: Let us take five Masters in MTC in the face of a same patient. Of course they will make a same diagnosis. But they will surely be brought to develop five forms of different points according to their felt. And all five will get the healing of the patient.

Le saviez-vous

This categorization of the points is derived directly from the lessons of the Pr Leung Kok Yuen.

The main points

The points near

Points which are located on the home of the affection or nearby. We will see that in this choice, it takes into account the effects of proximal points, that is to say:

"Eliminate locally the single wickedness;
"Unclog the meridians and vessels, the Jing May of the headquarters of the affection;
"Dispel the stasis of blood;
"Stop the pain.

The choice of these points near is done between other in case of acute or chronic well localized, affecting a specific structure, that this is a body, a meridian, a vessel, a tendino-muscle, a member or an articulation. The points near tonifican and circulate.

232

The distal points

As their name indicates, they are distant points of the home of the affection and chosen according to the pathophysiology of bodies, viscera and meridians. These points are located primarily at the level of the feet and hands. It is also said that they are most often below the elbow or the knee. These points have a local action as any point of acupuncture. But in addition, they can treat to distance the conditions which are located on the route of the meridian. But some of these points can also address the General symptoms such as fever, sweating, etc.

If we take the example of He Gu, the 4GI located at the level of the hand, this point deals not only the disorders of the upper limb, but also those of the neck, the mouth, the head. In addition, it may treat the fever caused by violations external.

As distal points, these points have as the action of:
" Unclog the energy and the blood of the meridians;
" Regularize the operation of the zang-fu;
" Rebalance the Yin and the Yang.

The median points

Most, as we will see, are located along the column side Yang on the back, but also above the elbows and knees. They have a role of harmonization within a formula.

The specific points

They include:
" The SHU points called "ancient points", Wu Shu Xue;
" The Yuan points called "points-sources", Yuan Xue;
" The Points Luo, liaison Luo Xue;
" The SHU points of the back, EIB Shu Xue;
" The Mu points of the anterior, or mu Xue;
" The eight points of confluence, BA may Jiao Hui (BA Xue);
" The eight points of meeting strategic or or Ba Xue today;
" The points of crack, or point of emergency, Xi Xue;
" The Points Xia He, or Liu Fu Xia He Xue.

The 60 points Shu, antiques

This are the five specific points that are found on each of the 12 main meridians, distributed between the elbow or the knee and the end of the members. These five points are called, Jing, Yong, Shu, Jing, Il.

The ancient doctors compared the movement of meridians in the course of natural water. They claimed as well as the circulation of energy in the meridians was comparable to the movements of water. At the outset, water courses are narrow and shallow. They will then to be widening and becoming more and more profound, as they are progressing. In other words, we can say that the depth of the meridians varies along their routes, and their different points have of this fact specific properties.

We are going to have *60 points antiques, five times 12 meridians.*

" *The Jing points:* They are therefore located at the distal ends of the members, fingers and toes, near the nails. The energy is very superficial and very mobile. They are considered as the points of emergence of energy, comparable to a source, Jing meaning well. The action of these points is very powerful, which in fact a category of points called points of emergency or resuscitation. They are very useful to hunt the perverse energy, Xie, qi, in acute phase, or attempt to restore the balance Yin-Yang in extreme cases such as the high fevers, convulsions, hemorrhage, the States of shock, or the loss of knowledge.

" *The Points Rong (or Yong, or Ying) :* after the point of emergence of the energy, the first place where passes the energy looks like the beginning of a course of water where the flow is still low. Who said "points of burst" said points where the energy of the meridian is very powerful, where its potential is ready to manifest and develop, as the water of a torrent which streams. These are points of very effective and powerful to quickly change the state of the patient when he fight against a perverse energy, be it internal or external, especially when there is heat.

234

" *The SHU points:* This are those where the energy pours as the water in which the course becomes more profound, Shu meaning "dump", "carry". Placed either at the level of the joints of the fingers to the hand and toes for the feet, or still in the articulation of the wrist for the meridians Yin, the SHU points are very powerful. It is said that the energy defensive if gathers together there. The points Shu-transport therefore deal in priority the affections of the spleen. They are used in the event of a syndrome of painful obstruction (BI), especially when it is linked to the moisture. This applies more to meridians Yang that the meridians Yin. The Shu points of the meridians Yin are of a nature earth, therefore harmonizing and those of the meridians Yang are of a nature wood, enabling therefore.

" *The Jing points:* these are the points where the energy of the meridians flows quickly as the water in a river. From this point, the Meridian has all its force. If unfortunately the perverse energy stagnates in this place, if it has made its bed, it is in a position to earn the tissues more profound, tendons, bones, joints. The points Jing meridians Yin are of a nature metal. The points Jing meridians Yang are of nature fire.

" *The points he:* these are the points where the energy of the meridians converges and is sinking. They are comparable to the rivers which are all going to be throwing in the sea. The term he meaning also "collect". The journey becomes deeper and it is possible to act on the viscera in depth. The points he deal primarily with the disorders of the kidney. They treat the rise against the current of energy, what is called "The Rebel Qi" and the phenomena of leakage of IQ. The points he of the meridians Yin are water nature and meridians Yang of nature earth.

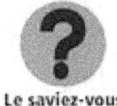
Le saviez-vous

The energy action points on this part of the meridians is much more dynamic than that of other points and it is this which explains that they are very frequently used in clinical practice.

235

Table 13-1 The points shu antiques.

LUNG	11p, Shao SHANG	10p, Hu Ji	9P, Tai Yuan	8P, Jing that	5P, Chi Ze
Pericardium	9CC, Zhong CHONG	8CC, Lao GONG	7CC, Da Ling	5CC, Jian Shi	3CC, that Ze
Heart	9C, Shao Chong	8C, Shao Fu	7C, Shen MEN	4C, Ling Dao	3C, Shai Hai
RATE	1RT, Yin Bai	2RT, Da of the	3RT, Tai Bai	5RT, Shang Qiu	9RT, Ying Ling Quan
LIVER	1F, Da Dun	2F, Xing Jian	3F, Tai Chong	4F, Zhong FENG	8F, that Quan
KIDNEY	1RN, Yong QUAN	2RN, Ran Gu	3RN, Tai xi	7RN, Fu Liu	10RN, Yin Gu
Large intestine	1GI, Shang YANG	2GI, Er Jian	2GI, San Jian	5GI, Yang xi	11GI, that Chi
Three households	1TF, Guan CHONG	2TF, Ye men	3TF, Zhong ZHU	6TF, Zhi Gou	10TF, Tian Jing
Small intestine	1IG, Shao Ze	2IG, Qian Gu	3IG, Hou Xi	5IG, Yang Gu	8IG, Xiao Hai
STOMACH	45E, Li	44E,	43E,	41E, Jie	36E, zu

236

	DUI	Nis Ting	Xiang Gu	Xie	San Li
Gall BLADDER YIN	44VB, zu Qiao	43VB, XIA xi	41VB, zu Lin Qi	38VB, Yang Fu	34VB, Yang Ling QUAN
BLADDER	67V, Zhi Yin	66V, Tong Gu	65V, Shu Gu	60V, Kun Lun	54V, Wei Zhong

The 12 points Yuan, or "points-sources"

The Yuan points are located in the vicinity of the joints of the wrist and ankle.

There is a similarity between the term Yuan and the Yuan Qi. The energy Yuan also called "Authentic energy", "true energy", Zhen qi, is the fundamental energy of the body.

In the upper part of the body, these points are pushing the Heart and Lung to circulate the qi and blood. In the central part, they stimulate the spleen and stomach to digest the food. In the lower part, they encourage the liver and the kidney to drain liquids.

The theory on the San Jiao, the three homes, therefore serves as a reference in the application of the points Yuan. These points can:

" Regularize and toning the Yuan Qi;

"To support the correct energy, the Zheng Qi;

" Assist in the elimination of Xie Qi, the single wickedness.

In addition, these points Yuan have a direct relationship with the viscera Yin. It is said that "if we are familiar with the correspondence between the points Yuan and the viscera which are associated with them, you can diagnose a pathology of viscera Yin".

This are:

Table 13-2 12 points Yuan.

Side Yang of the hand	4TF, Yang Qi
	4IG, Wan Gu

	4GI, He Gu
Side Yin of the hand	7C, Shen Men 7CC, Da Ling 9P, Tai Yuan
Side Yang of the Foot	40VB, Qiu Xu 42E, Chong Yang 64V, Jing Gu
Side Yin of the Foot	3RT, Tai Bai 3F, Tai Chong 3RN, Tai xi

The 15 points Luo, or points of communication

These are the starting points from which the vessels Luo leave their meridian of origin. As the meridians Luo and their ramifications are most superficial that the main meridians, it often uses the Luo points for the problems superficial of meridians rather than the internal problems.

Table 13-3 The 15 points Luo.

LUNG	7P, binds that
Large intestine	6IG, Pian Li
STOMACH	40E, Fen Long
RATE	4RT, Gong Sun
Heart	5C, Tong Li
Small intestine	7IG, Zhi Zheng
BLADDER	58V, EIF Yang
KIDNEY	4RN, Da Zhong
Pericardium	6CC, Nis Guan
Three households	5TF, Wai Guan
Gallbladder	37VB, Guang Ming

LIVER	5F, Li Gou
The May	1 DM, Chang Qiang
Ren May	15RM, JIU Wei
Large Luo of the spleen	21RT, Da Bao

Each meridian Luo joined the meridian that is associated with it in an internal relationship-external. The point Luo may deal not only with the pathology of the Meridian on which it is located, but also the meridian that is associated with it.

Furthermore, the use of a point Yuan can be joint to that of a point Luo, meridian which is associated with it in the internal relationship-external. We are talking about host point and point guest. Example: In the case of empty of the lung, you can take the 9P Tai Yuan, point Yuan and strengthen its action with the 6GI, Pian Li.

Table 13-4 Association Luo point-point Yuan.

Host	Yu AN	9 P	4 GI	42 E	3R T	7 C	4I G	7c C	4T F	40 VB	3F	3R N	64 V
Invited	Lu o	6 GI	7 P	4R T	40 E	7I G	5 C	5T F	6c C	5F	37 VB	58 V	4R N

The 13 points Shu back, or points of communication

The Shu points are points located on the back. It is the place where the energy of the organs and viscera is "dumps". This are therefore points in direct relationship with the zang-fu.

Shu means carry: These points carry the Qi, the energy in the lung.

These points are fundamental to know, in particular in the treatment of chronic diseases.

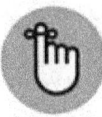

In reality, it is necessary, for the locate, of course take into account the location standardised, but mainly refer to the sensitivity to the pressure of

À retenir

the point. The Pr Leung insisted on the fact that it should not necessarily focus on the measures in distances to locate the point. In reality, it is fundamental, thanks to the palpation, to learn to "touch" this point which will always be in a hollow.

The point Shu takes the name of the component to which it belongs, which facilitates the memory. And the order of disposition of these points corresponds to that of the viscera.

To the origin, these points were not bitten, but only heated at the Moxa for a case Xu or "ventousés" for diseases Shi.

In a general way, the points Shu of DOS are of a nature Yang and is mainly used for toning the Yang. Despite this, we can use in the event of Yin Xu.

In addition, we can use these points for Act on the body of the direction corresponding to the viscera concerned.

When a patient is very tired, exhausted or depressed, the points of the Shu dos are much more effective than the points previous MU.

These points Shu can become a very important element of diagnosis. In effect, they can become very sensitive to the pressure, even painful outside of any pressure when the corresponding viscère is assigned. For example, when the 23V is painful to pressure, it helps to confirm the diagnosis of diseases of the genital organs and the urinary system.

Table 13-5 The 13 points Shu of the back.

13V, EIF SHU	Lung	D3
14V, Jue Yin SHU	Pericardium	D4
15V, Xin Shu	Heart	D5
17V, Ge SHU	Diaphragm	D7
18V, Gan SHU	Liver	D9
19V, Dan SHU	Gallbladder	D10
20V, Pi SHU	Rate	D11

21V, Wei SHU	STOMACH	D12
22V, San Jiao SHU	Three households	THE1
23V, shen shu	KIDNEY	THE2
25V, Da Shang SHU	Large Instestin	L4
27V, XIA Chang Shu	Small intestine	S1
28V, Pang Guang SHU	BLADDER	S2

The 12 points previous MU, or points of gathering
The points MU are previous points, located on the chest or abdomen in relationship with the organs and bowels.
Mu means "gather, collect". What are the points where the Qi of the organs gathers and focuses to the anterior face of the body.
These points are located according to the anatomical location of the viscère, most often on a meridian other than that of the viscère. In effect, there is that the point MU of the lung, Zhong Fu, 1P, the one of the Liver 14F, shi men, and that of the vb, 24VB, Ri Yue, which correspond to their respective meridian.
When the points MU are located on the REN May, they are median and unique. When the points MU are on the meridians of the hands and feet, they are bilateral and double.
In the literature, these points are also known under the name of "points heralds". These points are used to both the treatment and diagnosis.
We have seen that the points dorsal Shu were used mainly to treat conditions of type Yin, while here, the points abdominal MU are primarily used to treat conditions of type Yang. However it is necessary to know that the points abdominal Mu located below the navel can also treat disorders of disability type, Type yin.

241

These points are used most often in acute pathologies. However they can also be used in the chronic pathologies.

When one combines the points previous MU and points Shu of Dos, it reinforces the effects of the treatment. This association is very effective and produces effects more sustainable. In practice, therefore, you can use either the point dorsal Shu or point MU to treat the disorders of the corresponding viscère, but they can also be combined. This is called a "combination before-Rear".

Table 13-6 12 points previous MU.

1P, Zhong Fu	Mu point of the lung
14RM, Ju that	Point MU of the Heart
17RM, Dan Zhong	Mu point of the Pericardium
13F, Zhang Men	Mu point of the spleen
25VB, Jing Men	Mu point of the kidney
14F, Qi Men	Mu point of the Liver
25E, Tian SHU	Mu point of the large intestine
4WD, Guan Yuan	Mu point of the small intestine
5WD, shi men	Point MU of the three households
12RM, Zhong WAN	Mu point of the stomach
3WD, Zhong Ji	Mu Point Of The Bladder
24VB, Ri Yue	Mu point of the gallbladder

The 8 points of confluence of 8 marvelous vessels
It is of eight specific points located below the elbows and knees.

What are the points of communication between the eight extraordinary vessels and the 12 meridians.

Although the eight vessels individuals do not spend all by the four members, they intersect nevertheless certain main meridians.

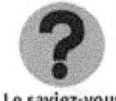

The elders had the habit of comparing the eight extraordinary vessels to lakes and the meridians to rivers. The first serve to regulate the flow of energy and blood in the meridians.

In these eight points, only Shen May, 62V, and Zao Hai, 6RN, are in direct relationship with Yang Qiao May and Yin Qiao May, two meridians curious, because they are located on the route of the latter. The other points are in indirect relationship with the other extraordinary vessels, because their respective meridians to join these at the level of the head and trunk of the body.

You need to know before all that by their liaison with the 12 meridians and the eight vessels wonderful, these points allow to act very effectively on the 12 main meridians, the REN May and the of the May.

Of our days, their use is very widespread. They are also well employees in the internal diseases, external, gynecological, pediatric, trauma, in cases of emergency, etc.

It is said: "The bulk of 365 points of the body is in the 66 points (sub-heard the whole of the 5 points Shu of 12 meridians and the 6 points Yuan of the meridians Yang). And the bulk of the 66 points is located in the 8 points. "

The 8 points of confluence can be employed only (e.g.: 7P Lieque key point of the REN May), by torque according to the method Shang (top) / Xia (bottom) (e.g.: 7P Lieque + 6RN Zhaohai).

Table 13-7 The 8 points of confluence.

4RT, Sun	Gong	Chong May	Heart, chest, stomach
6CC, Guan	Nis	Yin Wei May	Heart, chest, stomach

3IG, Hou Xi	The May	Corner of the eye, ear, shoulder
62V Shen May	Yang Qiao May	Corner of the eye, ear, shoulder
41VB, zu Lin Qi	Da May	Corner of the eye, behind ear, plays, neck, shoulder
5TF, Wai Guan	Yang Wei May	Corner of the eye, behind ear, plays, neck, shoulder
7P, binds that	Ren May	Lung, throat, chest
6RN, Zhao Hai	Yin Jia May	Lung, throat, chest

The 8 points of the meeting

We know that the figure 8, in Chinese Thought is linked to the movement of the wood, therefore the liver/VB. But it is also a figure that allows the regulation and the balance of the Yin-Yang.

There are eight marvelous vessels to ensure the regulation of the meridians. There are eight points to regulate the organs, the substances and the tissues.

Table 13-8 The 8 points of meeting.

Poi nt	Deals
1 3 F, Z h	The me etin g poi	- The blocking of the liver that leads between other a sensation of distension and discomfort in the chest and abdomen.

a n g M e n	nt of the org ans	
	Zan g Tod ay	- The impairment of the spleen and stomach with, among others, symptoms of abdominal distension, diarrhea, of edema. - The impairment of the Kidney resulting in pain dorsolumbar, edema of the diarrhea. - The disability of the heart and spleen. - The accumulation of tan in the lung.
1 2 R M , Z h o n g W A N	The me etin g poi nt of the Fu (or gan s "ho llo w")	- Acute conditions or in the states of re fu, heat of the bowels.
	Fu tod ay	- The Abdominal distension intense. - Gastric pain blazing that may result in a loss of knowledge.

- The vomiting with severe diarrhea.

17V, GeSHU	Meeting point of the blood		- Bleeding from the nose.
			- Vomiting of blood.
		Xue Today	- The haematuria.
			- The rectorragies.
			- The breakthrough bleeding important.
			- All kinds of blood loss or abnormal benign, but incessant.
17RM, Dan Zhong	Meeting point of energy		- Regulates the energy of the lung, heart, liver and stomach.
		Today qi	- Activates the blood circulation.
			- Supports the energy to unclog the vessels.
39VB, Xuan Zhong	The meeting		In practice, since this point can reconstitute the kidney by fortifying the brain, it is often used in: the attacks of wind, the strokes, the stroke.

246

		point of the marrow 	Not only is it the trafficking, but it also allows you to avoid relapse.
		9P, Tai Yuan	Meeting point of Vessels	Regulates the energy, activates the blood.

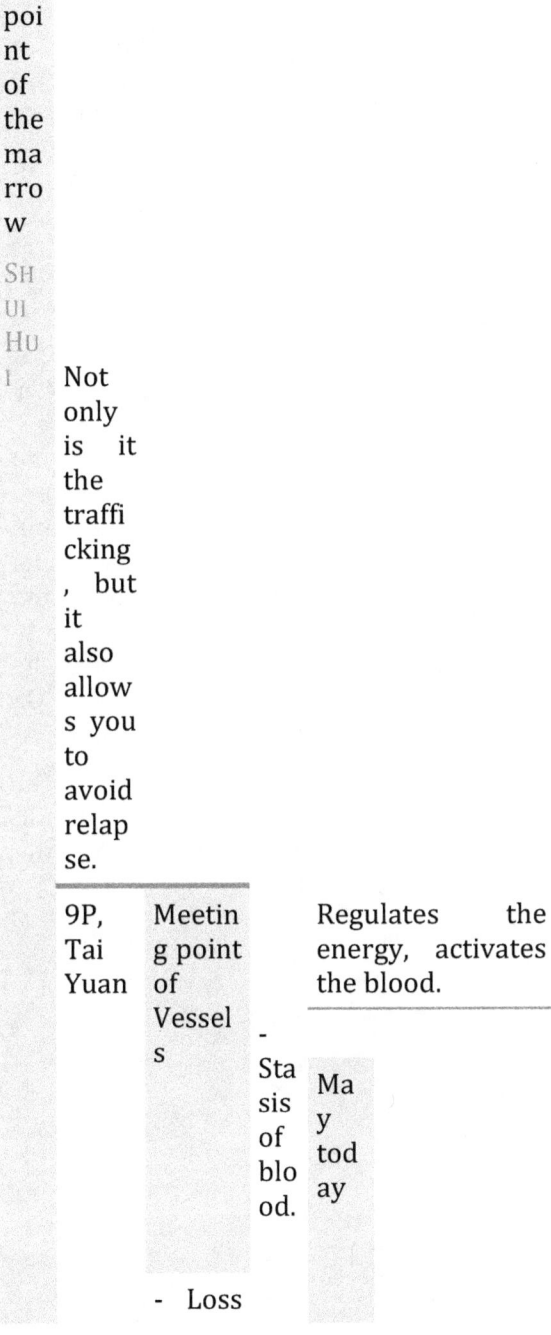

- Stasis of blood. May today

- Loss

	of blood (haemoptysis, Haematemesis).	
		- Weakness of the pulse.
11V, Da Zhu	The meeting point of the OS	Treats the bone disorders such as:
	Gu Shui	- The stiff neck and neck.
		- The pain of the lumbar vertebrae.
		- The stiffness of the knee.
		Strengthens tendons and bones.
		This point can refresh

		the heat and disperse the wind as in the case of infringement external with fever, headache and cough.
34VB, Yang Ling QUAN	The meeting point of the tendons Jin To day	- The disorders of the tendons and muscles, that this be problems of Hypotonia of lower limbs, lumbar pain, contractures , etc. - Unlocks the joints. - Refreshes the liver and

the gallbladder. It can therefore be used in the case of stiffness of the knee, pain in the hypochondres, if there is bitterness in the mouth and vomiting.

Regulates the energy, activates

the
blood.

The 16 points Xi, unblocking

In the term Xi, there is the idea of "hollow," slot. Indeed, the points XI are located in the deep hollow between the bones and tendons, where energy and blood congregate.

They are all located between the fingers and elbows, or between the toes and knees, with the exception of Liang Qiu, E34.

The 12 meridians and the 4 curious meridians Yin and Yang Wei and Yin and Yang Qiao each have their point xi, or 16 points. They are mainly used in acute pathologies, especially when they are accompanied by pain.

He must know that these points can also be very useful at the level of diagnosis. Indeed, in very many diseases, the points XI are very sensitive to palpation.

Table 13-9 The 16 points xi.

	Points	
LUNG	6P, Kong Zhui	Of cough with sputum of blood, swelling, very important to the throat, in the crises of acute asthma, the cough incessant.
Pericardium	4CC, Xi Men	Angina pectoris, vomiting of blood and bleeding from the nose.
Heart	6C, Yin xi	Angina pectoris, vomiting of blood, or transpiration, sweat very important, of bleeding from the nose.
Large intestine	7GI, Wen Liu	Headache very important, and swelling of the plays, swelling and pain of the language, of pain in the throat and anthrax, boils, neck very

		painful, of pain of the arm, elbow and forearm, odontalgies, borborygmes with abdominal pain.
Three households	7TF, Hui Zhong	Pain and numbness in the hand and forearm, of pain in the hypocondres, muscle pain and skin.
Small intestine	6IG, Yang Lao	Of acute pain of the Shoulder comparable to a fracture and back pain, swelling and pain of the hand and forearm, decrease of the visual acuity.
RATE	8RT, Di Ji	Of pain with distension at the abdominal and hypochondriac, urinary blockage and rectorragies. Very useful in case of dysmenorrhea.
LIVER	6F, Zhong of	Of metrorrhagia, pain and swelling of the testicles or vivid pain in the lower abdomen. Very useful in case of acute cystitis, important breakthrough bleeding or benign incessant, of the stasis of blood in the uterus.
KIDNEY	5RN, Shui Quan	Pain and feeling of discomfort at the level of the chest, and pain or swelling at the heel. But also in the event of amenorrhea followed by rules causing considerable pain.
STOMACH	34E, Liang Qiu	Of Acute gastralgie, pain or swelling of the breast especially after a big fear, pain or swelling of the knee, rheumatic pain the tibia, lumbar pain with numbness and cold sensation.
BLADDER	63V, Jing	Of headache rebels and recurrent, abdominal pain Vives, syncope, acute

	Men	cystitis.
Gallbladder	36VB, Wai Qiu	Of headache with pain and stiffness of the neck, with aversion to the cold and the wind, of pain and sensation of distension at the level of the chest and hypochondriac, biliary colic.
Yin Qiao May	8RN, Jiao Xin	Of Rules irregular, metrorrhagia mingled with White mucus, prolapse of the uterus, swelling and testicular pain, contracture of sex.
Yang Qiao May	59V, Fu Yang	Heaviness of head, headache, backache with inability to stand for long periods or to recover after be long remained seated, of swelling and redness of the outer malleolus. But also of pain in the root of the nose.
Yin Wei May	9RN, zu Bin	Of manic-depressive psychosis, swelling and pain, testicular or vomiting of drool. But also in the case of absence of milk in women, with significant pain of breasts.
Yang Wei May	35VB, Yang Jiao	A sensation of discomfort and distension at the level of the chest and hypochondriac, pain in the knees or hypotonia, rheumatism cold type or type heat with inability to move the thigh and the leg.

The 6 points lower He
It also called on these points, the "points of correspondence", Xia He.

What are the points where accumulates the energy of the Fu, of the bowels, where the meaning of the term he, who wants to say accumulation or meeting.

The special feature of the Fu, of hollow organs, is that they are only transmit the food gasoline without the keep. And it is the evacuation to the bottom which determines their proper functioning. As soon as there is a disruption of this function, we have the appearance of a pathology of type fullness.

The points he below are particularly effective in the case of figure, because they allow to identify and to lower the energy of the FU.

Table 13-10 6 points he lower.

Body	Point	
STOMACH	36E, zu San Li	Bloating gastric, of regurgitations acids. It treats the Abdominal pain of the "zone of the stomach".
Large intestine	37E, Shang Ju Xu	Dysentery, intestinal abscess as acute appendicitis, borborygmes, diarrhea. It treats the abdominal pain in the area of the large intestine.
Small intestine	39E, XIA Ju Xu	Of dysuries or oliguries with dark urine. It treats the Abdominal pain of the area of the small intestine.
Three households	39V, Wei Yang	Very useful in the case of urinary retention.
BLADDER	40V, Wei Zhong	Is used in the case of retention of urine. It treats the Abdominal pain of the area of the bladder.
Gallbladder	34VB, Yang	Vomiting, pain cholédociennes or gallbladder. It therefore deals with

254

Ling QUAN	the abdominal pain of the "zone of the gallbladder."

The 12 stars of my Dan Yang

My Dan Yang is a Taoist very famous. He was born around the year 1123 in the Province of Shan Dong, under the dynasty of the Jing. Author of very important books on the Taoism, he has left a legacy of a selection of 11 points called "celestial stars".
These points were considered as the most important points of the body.
Later, Xu Feng, Doctor of the Ming Dynasty, published this list in the classic of the **Jade Dragon** by adding a twelfth star, Tai Chong, the 3F.
These 12 stars are:
" 36Th, zu San Li;
" 44E, Nis Ting;
" 11GI, that Chi;
" 4GI, He Gu;
" 40V, Tong Li;
" 57V, Chen Shan;
" 3F, Tai Chong;
" 60V, Kun Lun;
" 30VB, Huan Tiao;
" 34VB, Yang Ling Quan;
"7P, binds that;

" 5C, Tong Li.

The 13 points ghosts of Sun If Miao

The "13 points of the Daemon" are the main points that the elders used to treat mental illness and emotional.
They are must among other things to Sun If Miao who has integrated in the chapitre 14 of his book "important formulas worth a thousand pieces of gold", the **Qian Jin Yao Fang.**

Normally, these points must all be stung in the order below and without leaving the needles in place.

"The 26DM must be piqué according to the method of the "pecking house sparrow" or of the "shaking up to a depth of 1 cm". This method is to hold the needles of the right hand and to make the coming and going, Ti Cha, of small amplitude and at a speed fast enough.

"The 11P, 0.5 cm in depth.

"The 1RT to 0.7 cm.

"The 7CC to 1 cm.

"The 62V to poncturer with a needle heated.

"The 16DM to 0.7 cm.

"The 6E to 0.7 cm with a needle at the moxa.

"The 24RM to 1 cm.

"The 5CC to 2 cm.

"The 23DM to 0.7 cm.

"The 1RM to 0.7 cm.

"Hai Quan, brake of the language, in bleeding with a triangular needle.

According to the principles of Chinese medicine, mental illnesses are caused by a disturbance of the normal movement of the Qi and functions of 5 Zang 6 Fu, 5 bodies and 6 viscera. They include diseases such as:

"The manic-depressive psychosis, Dian Kuan;

"The syndromes emotional lock, or depression, Yu Zheng;

"Insomnia, Shi mian;

"The Memory deficient, Jian Wang.

The points of the daemon can regulate the Yin and the Yang of the whole body. They can also regulate the blood and energy, Xue and IQ.

Chapter 14
The digitoponcture
For all
<u>In this chapter:</u>
" A technique plurimillénaire!
" <u>Learn How to you create a true "hand of massager "</u>
" <u>Discover the real traditional technique</u>

QEu we called digitoponcture, acupressing, shiatsu, these techniques dating back to the night of the time. Some Egyptian hieroglyphics already represented scenes of punctual massage on certain areas of the body using the use of fingers.

Who has never used his hands or fingers to relieve themselves of a pain? In the event of a migraine for example, which has never worn spontaneously its fingers on the temples to relieve themselves? The MTC, in its methods Dao Yin, has systematized the use for millennia.

Although related to massage, this technique goes much further. We will see that it is a method as well preventive and curative.

We can say from the outset that the digitoponcture is a method much more soft that acupuncture and can therefore be practiced by all the world.

À retenir   A short definition: "It is the activation of certain points, mainly on the meridians, in the aim of toning, circulate or to calm down the flow of energy underlying. "However, we know that the surface of the body through the route of the 14 meridians is directly in relation with the "5 software organs". By the digitoponcture, we can act directly on the imbalances of one or several internal organs.

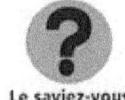

And what is more, this technique can be applied on itself. Indeed, some therapists do not hesitate to show some points to their patient for that they

Le saviez-vous

continue to energetically rebalance their organization between two sessions. The digitoponcture applies the same principles as the acupuncture, but these are the fingers, and in particular the pulp of the thumb, which will replace the needle.

257

During our previous study on the meridians, we saw that there were three layers of energy at the surface of the body:

"The meridians itself, which are located between the OS and the muscle, very in depth, and which are only accessible by means of a needle, the more fine possible, to enter the energy. This point has been extensively developed previously.

"A superficial layer, "on the skin", represented by the capillaries energy. Remember, surface of skin, we do not have a meridians strictly speaking, but zones Yin and Yang, representative of the energy mesh of the three meridians Yin and three meridians Yang present on each member. This "energy layer" is directly accessible by the different massage techniques.

"Finally, a middle layer, located as the say the texts" between the flesh and the muscle". It is this layer that we will achieve in the different practices of digitoponcture.

To create a "hand of massager "

Before addressing the technique itself, we are going to have to learn how to we create a "real hand of massager". It is not only a hand that can become hot and dry very quickly, but also a hand "energy".

Need to open the Lao point gong, at the center of the hand

To make our energy hand, we must attach to act on a very precise point, located virtually in the center of the hand: it is the point lao gong, the eighth point of the meridian of the pericardium.

Gong means "palace" Lao and "work", where a translations of this point: "The Palace of the Labor".

We know that in the software The heart is located housed the Shen, the Spirit. It is also said that the heart is "the master of the five Shen", of the five emotions. It is the heart emperor, the Yang in the Yang, the summer, the red color...

The pericardium, the concept of which goes well beyond the matter, is the protective envelope of the Heart on the energy plan. It was said that the "pericardium should ensure laboriously to the comfort of the palace," where his name: "Palace of the Labor".

In the popular language, it is said of this type of person that she has "a hair in the hand". This makes reference to this point and the fact to do nothing of his ten fingers.

This point is therefore located in the center of the hand, between the second and the third metacarpal, closest to the third, of the thenar eminence. In closing the fist, the end of the annular indicates exactly the location.

For more precision in the acupuncture, it must find a depression next to the back of the hand and hold it between the thumb and the index the two points.

Outside of its therapeutic virtues specific, such as that of draining very strongly the " fire of the Heart", in all traditions, it has a very strong symbolic load.

In India, for example, it is considered a minor chakra. In the traditional iconography, one often sees the representation of a Outgoing radius of the center of the hand. This is what we call the "output of the healing energy".

This is the opening of this point that will give a magnetic power to the hand.

Without entering into the details, remember that this point is in direct relationship with the point Dan Tian, located at two through finger under the navel. This will be a capital importance when we will discuss further the "true traditional technique of digitoponcture".

We are going to see an exercise very simple that will allow you to "work this point". You will be able to practice in a sitting position, elongated, relaxation, or in a position of meditation. All the action that will follow will happen very quickly.

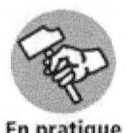

En pratique

"You open your left hand, target the center of the Palm and, with the end of the right index finger, you make a flick powerful enough on the Lao point Gong. Then, very quickly, you go to the other hand and repeat the same operation. Once this double bump performed, if you turn to think of something else, if your mind wanders you go very quickly forget the sensation of the point. On the other hand, and this is an excellent exercise of meditation, if you mentally visualize this point, eyes closed or open, you will fully the feel. In a state of relaxation or meditation, the sensation of this point may be even be amplified.

This felt may take the form of a ad hoc heat which will irradiate progressively in all the palm of the hand. This point may even become transfixiant and the feeling of the side Yang, namely the back of the hand. "

All this work of visualization may last between 10-15 minutes, or even more. And you will be amazed to see that, far to mitigate or disappear, only by concentration of mind, the sensation of this point will increase. You are in train" to open the Lao point Gong". To force of repetition, you will actually bring energy to the center of the hand and be able to provide to good use.

Energizing his hand and eliminate deadlocks

But this is not all. Your hand has need of force.

In the Diagnosis by the observation, great attention is paid to the tonicity of the thenar eminence, when we look at the hand of the patient (see chapitre 6). It is a mass of muscle located at the base of the thumb. It is important that it be well" "mushroom and meaty. If the muscles of the hand are released, this indicates that the energy of the Rate-Estomac is low. Conversely, if the muscles are farms, this indicates that the stomach and intestines digest well, assimilate well the food bowl and by that same produce enough energy the body needs to function. Let us remember that the " muscles and the flesh" are to be put in relation with this software component.

It should also be to examine at the level of the thenar eminence the presence or not of small venules or capillary color of blue or red. It is necessary to see if the color of the vessels has shine, a dull aspect or lively, in order to determine whether the quantity of blood in the Xue May, vessels, is sufficient. Normally, when a person is in good health, we must not see virtually no capillary.

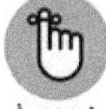

It is therefore very important to regularly work his hand to the tone. There are exercises of Qi Gong specific to act in this sense, to know how to act not only on energy, but also on the tonicity of the muscles of the hand.

À retenir

Use of " balls of meditation"

A method quite traditional, it is the use of Baoding Ball's. This are metal balls, in partitioned, stone, of different sizes, still called " balls of meditation".

These balls are to use a very old. It finds traces during the Ming dynasty, the middle-age of the Chinese, in the vicinity of the years 1400.

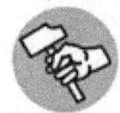

The exercise is to maintain a pair of these balls in the palm of the hand, by rotating them, while the now in constant contact. Little by little, we will be able to increase the speed of rotation. And later, they will be able to turn in one direction or the other, without that they are touching. The entire surface of the hand will thus be massaged. The action of muscle toning is then very powerful.

En pratique

Qi Gong of release of hands

I would like to take the opportunity here to give you a Qi gong is very important to implement, especially when we find ourselves faced with patients who develop a symptomatologique table that we call in MTC "stagnation of blood and energy at the level of the Liver".

To make it short, when we are continuously subjected to situations which are realized by an internalization of the anger, we run the risk of hindering the free movement of energy and blood at the level of the software liver. However, we know that this software component, which is to be put in relation with the element of wood of the nature, must have the movement of its SAP (energy and blood) free of any obstruction.

When we are faced with situations of stress, anger which internalized persist, the blood and energy are stagnating at the level of this software. There is À retenir not enough blood to the ends. The brain is a sponge to blood. If the blood does not happen to the feed, this can be a major cause of fatigue. Moreover, the blood has need energy to circulate until the ends.

If the energy of the liver is blocked, there will be very easily cold hands and feet. At the beginning, this is only a simple symptom alarm signal. But, if we do not take care, little by little, these micro-stagnations of ends can give birth to real pathologies and, among other things, to an autoimmune disease. We will talk about then in this extreme case of "Raynaud Disease".

Obviously, following the basic principles of the MTC, we will be brought to treat the cause of this pathology, namely here unlock the energy of the liver. But here, it will be convenient to make proof of pragmatism. It will at the same time make a symptomatic treatment, especially if our hands are always cold, which not only is unpleasant for the patient, but also signed an inability to create a hand energy.

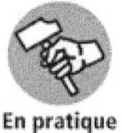

En pratique

A Qi Gong very interesting is therefore to "shake up his hands", as if we were to eliminate droplets of water that would be on the skin. You put your two hands in front of you, elbows bent to 90 degrees, wrists fully released. Then you start to shake them up very quickly before you. Little by little, there is no more mental effort to produce. The movement is self-maintained by the release of the wrist and the force of inertia that is put in place. Your breathing is calm throughout the duration of the exercise, namely 2 minutes. Have fun, without changing anything in the practice of the Movement, to focus your mind on the annular, the atrial, the thumb. In acting thus, you start to feel the power of the mental energy on the physical.

At the end of these 2 minutes of practice, you suddenly stop this movement which has become almost automatic. Feel the impression then of tingling, your fingers being as in cotton. This is the energy which circulates, and small distal capillaries which are in the process of regaining their permeability. Test this exercise twice a day for nine days of suite. The results will be surprising as to the warming of the hand. You will begin to feel what is called "a free movement of blood and energy". We could call this exercise "technical of shaking of hands".

In martial art, there are many other techniques to create powerful hands and energy, as do work in a tray of sand, gloved or, in a tray to mercury. But this exceeds here the framework of our remarks.

The real traditional technique

How to prepare for a session

It is appropriate to have a maximum of concentration before starting a session. Here is an excellent exercise in preparation which will very quickly allow us to make our hand operational.

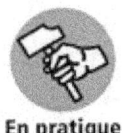

En pratique

263

Start by vigorously scrub your two hands in front of the area of the heart. Then you return before you and made a "washing of hands" for about ten seconds. An operation that you should repeat very often: Once the fingers nested one inside the other, return the palms of the hands toward the front, as far as possible before you in a way that maximum flexibility Fingers and wrists. Then, stretch each of your fingers. If you release them well, you can hear from time to time a "creaking" beneficial. Then massage each finger on any length. Take each end of the fingers, pinch and rotate as if you wanted to carve a pencil. This is called in MTC "the ten statements". Finally joined hands in front of the heart, made a short concentration during a dozen seconds.

Do not get lost in the maze of the 10 000 techniques

Spiritualité

One of the characteristics of our modern world is what we could call "the explosion of the yang." We had spoken at length on this point at the beginning of Part One. The more we are moving in the time, the more we find ourselves in front of a plurality of theories of more and more complex and even the most scholars end up losing their Latin.

In the case that interests us here, the digitoponcture, it will be necessary for example massage in the direction of the current to make a toning and the reverse for sedation. And in other texts, it is even completely the reverse which is explained. But this is not all. To obtain a toning, it is appropriate to make a rotation in a certain direction with his thumb or fingers, and the opposite for sedation. And this change again if it is a man or a woman. As well as according to the sex, it will have to start rather to the left than to the right or the reverse. Some theories are even enter the hourly cycles in practice, which would oblige the practitioner to act on some points to 3 hours of the morning.

We will see that the technique "paramount" of digitoponcture, if we can talk of technical, will be much more simple. This is the theory of the Shaver of Occam which considers that a simple explanation of a fact has a greater chance to be true that a complicated explanation.

Yes, but this simplicity is only apparent, because it goes under-HEAR A total change of point of view and behavior of a practitioner. In effect, the practitioner will be fully invest, but also to give itself the means of this investment for not itself be unbalanced on its cable of life. In the trilogy sky-man-land, it will little by little become a mediator, and at the same time a transmitter and regulator of energy to treat his patient.

To return to our remarks on the digitoponcture, that said the tradition as to the fair technique of the practice? In the **Nei Jing** is a passage which deals of the "Nine needles". Each type of needle has a particular form and each of them, depending on its form, allows to obtain a certain effect. As regards the digitoponcture, c is the needle No. 3, the needle called Ti, which was used to make this type of intervention. It is a round needle that was used to exert pressure on the points of the meridians or to "rub "The journey of the latter. It is only later that if is imposed the massage by the intermediary of the fingers and the thumb. I remind you that the figure 3, C is the action of the man between heaven and earth.

How to create its own formula?

In digitoponcture, as acupuncture, it is the choice of the points which will allow us to know in what direction we want to go with regard to the treatment that we must apply.

The three categories of points

À retenir

"**The *distal points, and which are located in the four ends, the hands and the beginning of the forearms and the feet and the beginning of the legs. And to a lesser extent, at the level of the head.***

"**The *median   points* located   along   the   column   and especially   between   the   elbows   and   shoulders,   and between the knees and hips.**

"**Finally   the *points   near* located,   them,   on   the   trunk, anterior face and for some on the posterior.**

It has been done a fair diagnosis using the four methods that are the interrogation, the visual examination involving the study of the language and its coated, the taking of pulse and palpation. From there, you will give a direction to your treatment. For example, if there is a weakness, a lack, it will

265

have to tone. If on the contrary there has an excess, it should be calm, make a sedation. If you are located in the presence of blockages, stagnations, it would then be appropriate to use of formulas to circulatory referred.

À retenir From these findings, you will develop a formula. If it contains more points of ends that points near, it is that you want to somehow "drain" the excess energy, make a sedation for calm the game of the symptoms of excess. If on the contrary you take more points close is that you turn to a toning. Those are the points that we will be elsewhere very often brought to heat through the technique of moxibustion.

And very often to harmonize a formula, we will be able to use of the midpoints as the 36th or the 11IM.

Attention Therefore, it is not just question here to massage in one direction or the other, but a choice of points.

It is to be noted, moreover, that if there is located in the presence of three practitioners confirmed in the face of a same patient, they will be led all three to make a same diagnosis, but will be able to propose three different forms according to their own logic and intuition. And they will get all the same result, certainly more or less quickly, namely the healing of the patient.

A central point: the concept of intention

Outside of the choice of points, what is fundamentally account in the act of the Caregiver? It is before all the intention.

Spiritualité A classic definition of the intention is: "a deliberate plan to accomplish an action, which will lead to the desired result." This is annoying in this definition, it is the concept of planning. In effect, each part of a plan generates as much of fears and counter-energies which can hinder the success of the treatment. I prefer by far this definition which arises between other the latest research on the Quantum Physics: "The intention is a projection of the conscience, deliberate and effective fashion, with a view to achieve a goal or a given result. "

However, the intention is a central concept, when it comes to treating a patient, which stems directly from the Teachings Taoists. I refer you to the chapter devoted to the Hun and the Po, the spiritual souls and bodily.

In fact, in our societies that we could qualify" of exponential change "at all levels, our Shen (sub-heard our spirit, our mental, our cognitive faculties, our feelings and emotions) is before any fed by our five senses. The excess of information to which it is subjected ends by the put in overheating, all the more that most of the time, this fire of the heart is not calmed down by the water of the kidney. And it is the burn-out, the " TILT " of the body which is often at the end of the path.

Loser foot with the nature, being more and more distant from the uniqueness, we have built a genuine carapace which prevents us from access to our subconscious the more profound, which prevents us from listening to our soul.

The three levels of practitioner

Le saviez-vous

"*The practitioner of level 1* is a practitioner who has not "opened his heart", that is to say that he has not learned to issue its healing energy. He merely that of revenue, he knows of the lists of points corresponding to some of the symptoms and obviously does not know manipulate the energy. He will have an action that we could qualify of hardware, superficial on the point. It will necessarily be a result, but the cursor on a scale of 1 to 10 will remain at 1, and pathology will not long to reappear. It will have that obscure a symptom alarm signal.

"*The practitioner of Level 2* knows the real traditional techniques. He knows how to manipulate the energy. He knows how to listen to his soul, its intuitions. He knows how to tap into its energy, in its battery. Through its hands, its inches, it will act directly on the energy of the patient. There is a corollary to this: this practitioner is then held, in a same day, to charge as much as it has given, under penalty of be quickly depleted and early aging. This profile of practitioner will do fit the cursor to 5 on a scale of 1 to 10, which corresponds to the effectiveness of the treatment.

"*The practitioner of level 3,* him, is located then on a Any other vibration. It is a practicing of long date. He has learned to "open up his heart" through its practices. It becomes a kind of intermediate, an intercessor between heaven and earth. It is a medium in the true etymological sense, namely a "medium-term" between the two polarities Yin-Yang, between sky and earth. It captures the Yang energy of the sky, the Yin energy of the Earth and thanks to the potential of regulation of the Zhi, the energy of the kidney, it occurs an alchemy at the level of the heart, a transmutation very subtle which allows him then to issue the pure "energy of healing" through its hands. Some possess this donation, say to flower of skin very early in their lives. They arrive to heal only by imposition of hands. Other possess buried under layers, carapaces of ego, a little like a hidden gem in its gangue. To force practices, Qi Gong for example or letting go through meditation, this gift can be traced back to the surface. It is at this time that the aphorism that "a point is sufficient to cure a patient" takes on its full value. Of course, this profile of practitioner will climb to 10 the cursor of the healing. It will be necessary, for the vast majority of us" of entire lives" to arrive at this level. But do fit the cursor to 7-8 is to the scope of the whole world, provided of course to give themselves the means.

What we call "return to the Uniqueness" in the tradition is to divest itself of this shell of the ego, remove layer after layer residues of the excess of our thoughts, our emotions, our affects: se to bare in some way for our spiritual soul, our Hun can finally express themselves freely.

This vision will allow us to draw the following conclusion. As we will see, the digitoponcture is a pure intuitive act, where the power of the issuance of the Thought, the emission of "the energy of healing," which is nothing other than the energy of love, the intention in the Act are not under the direction of our Shen, of our ego, of our mental, of our cognitive faculties, but of our Hun, of our spiritual energy.

And to be listening to our Hun, he should know, as it is said in some initiatory societies, "remove its Metals", let the outside the armor of our ego. And this is working.

Our master insisted very often on this which should be a clear: "Any practitioner, or any person who wants to help the other must put in place a **À retenir** policy of so-called "selfishness salvateur" and take care of his own home for the soul to want to stay there and can be express. "

A practitioner of Chinese medicine or any other person having the ardent desire to deal with the other and who does not practice the exercises on a daily basis, such as the Qi Gong, meditation or other techniques, will come to resemble what was called at the time of the Cultural Revolution, "a doctor at the foot nu", that is to say a doctor trained most of the time to a few basic techniques in some months, a few recipes far of course of the energy medicine.

Enter the energy

This is another concept quite central with regard to the practice of the digitoponcture and of course of the acupuncture (see chapitre 13).

Let us remember that when we act on a point, we are looking for before any to reach the Qi, the energy which circulates along the meridian. It **À retenir** should not be forgotten that this energy is the outcome of a mixture very subtle between the quintessence of the energy of the air and the quintessence of

269

the digestion of food bowl. And that this energy goes well beyond any materiality.

The energy that we are talking about in MTC is a Any other level, a level that we could qualify of metaphysics. It can only be felt. And this felt will be, not with our cognitive faculties, our Shen, as one feels a point hot or cold. This felt proceeded by what is called the "intuition", the intuition of the point. And that is what differentiates us totally of acupuncture and the modern digitoponcture.

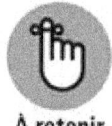

À retenir

This is not the patient who must feel a sensation, or if little. It is the practitioner who through a transmitter, in this case the pulp of the inch here, which must "feel" that the Qi is there, present. And when the Qi comes under his finger, it is at this time that we can say that he has "entered the energy".

How to Proceed

We have seen up to now the basic principles that underlie the practices of the digitoponcture. We have become aware of the importance to create little by little a "real hand of massager "Thanks to the opening of the Lao point gong and toning muscles palm prints. Let us now look at the different steps to put in place to restore the digitoponcture its true purpose, namely a pure technical traditional energy.

First step

It is the most important. We could call it "the step of the Visualization". I place in the framework of a practitioner of level 2 which has been mentioned previously. This practitioner will in some way draw on its own internal energy, on its battery of the kidney, to treat the other. If there was a well-kept secret in this practice, it is this step.

Before all our instrument of choice, like the needle for the acupuncturist, c is the inch and more specifically the pulp of the thumb.

Did you know that in the mapping of the cerebral cortex, the thumb is the area for which it is one of the most large projections? Certainly, we will be brought from time to time to use multiple fingers, or even the fist or the palm of the hand. But in the majority of cases, it is well the pulp of the thumb which will serve as the intermediary between the energy of the practitioner and the patient .

The Visualization, the great secret

There is a meridian that connects the area of the energy of the kidney with the area of the throat. It is the Meridian Zhong May who does not have a direct points on the surface of the body. It rises in front of the vertebral bodies up to the throat. Begin by imagining a ball of heat, energy, in the region of the Dan Tian, under the navel, to the inside of your lower abdomen. Whereas in a conscious breathing usual, the "belly fate" during the inspiration, here you are going to do the opposite: "I inspire, my belly retracts. I imagine then, like a straw in a glass of water, that the energy rises along the meridian Zhong May. I aspire this energy, I am fit throughout the inspiration. It comes up to the shoulders. I expires. My stomach relaxes. The energy descends along my arm, to arrive until the hands, and here in this case up to the pulp of my inches. "

When you apply the technique of visualization, little by little, to force of repetition, you will feel this energy as a stream Léger, a real flow of energy with a certain consistency. It is a little the sensation that you can have when you feel the "consistency of the air" by moving very quickly your hands open. You have understood that everything felt may be potentiated by the practice of the Qi Gong, of tai-chi, yoga or other traditional practices.

Therefore in summary: "I inspire, a flux of energy rises along the vertebral column from the Dan Tian to spread at the level of the shoulders. I expires and this energy descends to the pulp of the thumb. "

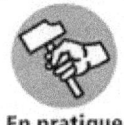

At the time of the expires, all the energy is concentrated in the area of the pulp of the thumb and not at the end of the thumb. It is therefore this wide area of the pulp which Between in contact with the point. At that time, the technique that we are going to use, like that that we can use with a stick of sagebrush in the moxibustion, is called the "Technique of pecking". As a bit of a green woodpecker which picote. It is to synchronize the breathing with the pressure:" to the inspires, I releases the pressure, to the expires, I support and so on. "To each respiratory cycle, it is the energy of healing that arrives at the level of the pulp of the thumb. I repeat, this technique is very powerful and it is therefore led by the Shen of practitioner, his mind. It is a pure vibratory flow, energy, all this worn by the visualization and the full conscience.

How many times must we repeat this operation? The Elders speak of 9-18 or 36 cycles of pressure-release. Everything depends on the number of points used, of the chronicity of the pathology of the direction that we want to give the treatment. In effect, especially on the points that we had called "points near", the more we will repeat the operation, the more we will get the energy to act on the point.

Second step

From this moment, what to do with his thumb? We have talked at length at the beginning of this course. It is essential to avoid falling into the trap of the "multiplicity", "10 000 Techniques". Do we need to go in one direction for toning, in the other to disperse? Should we start to the right or to the left depending on the sex ? Do we need to massage in the direction of energy flow circulating in the meridian or in the opposite direction? Etc.

You have understood that the first idea is to allow us to return to the Uniqueness, return to the techniques the oldest, in particular those advocated by the **Nei Jing.**

So here is the technique which has proven its worth for millennia, that we could qualify as a purely energy, which

272

provides substantially superior results with respect to a simple mechanical effect of a spot massage "Without Conscience".

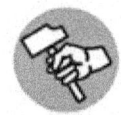

The technique of the "SMILE inside"

En pratique

In this state, you are going to issue by the intermediary of your heart" a clear thinking of healing," through what the tradition called the "SMILE inside". This emission of energy flow is therefore done in a state of pure detachment, without any effort. The practitioner has just only to imagine that the patient is in the process of curing, especially not to ask questions on the how. It is, I repeat, a continuous flow, thanks to the full consciousness which is done between the energy of the Heart and the pulp of the thumb. Yes, but this is. The duration of this emission energy of healing must be made at least for one minute. Recent research of the Quantum Physics talk about 69 seconds. During this period of time, there shall be no rupture of thought of healing. No interference thinking must not interfere with this flow of energy for the technique to be truly effective.

On the condition to have been practiced for a very long time the meditation as I said above, or the full awareness, few people are capable of such a concentration. It is for all these reasons that the technique of pecking"", which is therefore a first much easier, will be to focus, especially when one is young practitioner or self-taught.

Next to this technique of pecking, which sum any is very simple to implement, provided to give themselves the means, and there is another even more traditional than could be called a "streaming of energy flow of healing". It asks important knowledge and skills.

Some additional tips

A few tips to maximize this practice of the digitoponcture.

This is not a demonstration of force!

Before everything, and we have well understood, do we not somewhere in the area of "rude", but in the area of the pure

273

energy, the support must not be a demonstration of force. This should not be a mechanical action causing a sensation of pain in the patient.

As a technical pure energy, it is the practitioner who must intuitively feel what pressure it must apply on the point with the pulp of his thumb. And when it will become practitioner confirmed, there will be almost no more need of support for "enter the Energy" and act on it.

Not more that 3, 4, or even 5 points!

À retenir

Fundamental: the formula that you will be prompted to develop thanks to the methods of diagnosis of the MTC will never a countless number of points. According to the tradition, the formula will include any more than 3-4 or even 5 points, which will correspond to 6-10 points to massage.

There are two types of treatment: the salaries to referred preventive, that is to say of the treatments that we will have to practice on ourselves, or applied by a practitioner only in order to boost our body, our battery of the kidney to increase our immune defenses, our faculties of adaptation and our opportunities for self-healing. This type of treatment that we can call "treatment to referred Yang Sheng fa", or "preservation of health," will be on short periods of time.

The other type of formulas then corresponds to the therapeutic treatment to itself. In the tradition, hardly applicable in the cabinets, except if you practice on you-even some series that you will be prescribed your practitioner, it should make a cycle of nine days of treatment with a week of rest, followed by another cycle. Thus, two or even three other cycles can be provided in the light of the chronicity of the problem or the energy state of the patient.

Employ only a formula to the times

Another important point. It should be not to use a formula to the times. Some will want to change the point from one day to the other seeing that the results are expected. Do not forget that we are in a context of hyper-multiplication generating a notion of speed. The patient or the practitioner would like everything, suite. Let the time to time, especially when it is a chronic pathology. If your formula is "fair", the response to treatment will also be fair. It is only in the course of the 2e series that you can adjust your treatment according to the evolution of the symptomatology.

Do not forget: "It is the emission of the energy of your mind, with intermediate as your thumb, which is responsible for the timeliness of results. "

When you have developed a formula according to your own knowledge, assisted also by your intuitions, or that you use a formula "any made", before moving on to another point, you must feel that you have good" entered the energy", the Qi under your thumb.

Once more this sensation can not be quantified. It is part of the domain of intuition, of the sensation. Often we find in the texts the notion of "sensation of Energy Fluid and living". This feeling comes not from your cognitive faculties, of your Shen, but of your soul, your Hun, which is therefore located in the liver and which nourishes your heart.

When you become "competent unconscious" to force of repetition, you can rely on the sensitivity of your fingers. Touch the first zone in full conscience and stop you on the place that you collect "spontaneously", intuitively as the location of the point.

Very often you will feel a depression or a change of texture, consistency of tissues at this level.

Do not fall in the pitfall of the layman who merely to apply to the letter the measures that we find in the Treaties of acupuncture. These distances are data as general location. But he must know that this localization especially in acupuncture may vary from one patient to another.

In addition, our master told us that if we are wrong a little upstream or downstream of the point, this was not too serious. The everything and not to deceive of current of a meridian!

275

And of course, and I would not have of cease to repeat that it is you, as a practitioner, who must feel the point, this energy sinks and not by a detector regardless of what it is.

The contraindications

The few contraindications are call to the logic. For example, if the area where is located the point is reached by a skin disease as of psoriasis or eczema, we will not be able to "working" above. Similarly, in the case of pregnancy, it is better to avoid it, if it was not the knowledge, to deal in digitoponcture, especially if we use the points of ends. Too of action of "Sedation" can in effect do descend the fetus or risk of starting the work of way too early.

À retenir

A fundamental point to understand. If you-even as a practitioner are exhausted, or if you exit of a festive meal a little too watered, if you come, especially for men to have sexual intercourse with ejaculation, you may lose all the energy that you rest. And this is valid even if you treat yourself.

A corollary also valid especially for the practitioner of level 2. Since the processing consists, as we have seen, to tap into the energy contained in your battery of the kidney in order to treat the patient, it is fundamental to reload this that has been unloaded, and this, in a same day. I refer you to this to all the methods of preservation of life that we call "Methods Yang Sheng fa".

Such methods are all the more necessary for those who practice on a daily basis. Made the following experience. At the beginning of the afternoon, your language is dew, and theoretically without coating, if you are in good health. At the end of the day, it has a tendency to be pale with a slight white coating above. This signs a great loss of energy. If you're not careful, if you do not put in place this famous policy of selfishness salvateur, you will lose little by little your energies of protection and become permeable to external pathologies, to "external attacks". And this loss of energy will

276

also foster the emergence of "diseases internal say". And therefore you get older early.

Therefore, look well the chapters on the sleep, respiration, dietetics, the Qi Gong that you will find in this book.

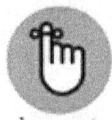
À retenir

Finally, a meeting should be a true act of Qi Gong, a act of full consciousness. It is not question of addressing to the va-quickly," between two doors". For that this state of direct transmission of energy between the patient and the practitioner can be done, it is very important to create a ritual of care, a space of care which can allow you very quickly to put you in the listening of your soul.

A few large combinations of points

Let us now look at a few combinations of points that you will be able to practice on you-even in case of need.

Formula 1: General toning

En pratique

If you had to remember a single great formula of general toning, that you can do according to the technique of digitoponcture, but also in moxibustion, this would be:

Table 14-1 Formula 1 toning General.

20DM, Bai Today	The one hundred meetings	At the top of the skull, in a vacuum at the apex of the two ears.	Great point of toning of the body and anti-fatigue.
36E, zu San Li	Three distances	Face antero-external of the LEG, to 3 distances of the knee joint.	Unavoidable point of longevity. Boosts the body as a whole.
6RM, Qi Hai	Sea of energy	To 2 through finger under the navel.	Invigorates the energy of the whole body and help to the uptake of the energy

			of the air.
17RM, Shan Zhong	The center of the chest	On the chest, on the median line joining the end of the two breasts.	This is the major point for toning the energy of the top of the body.

The purpose of this formula is to recharge your battery of the kidney. You should use it to each change of season, where your organism draws on its reserves to adapt. Especially at the entrance of the winter and to "The Rise of Spring". But also in all the periods of stress and major changes in your life.

It is important to follow the order of the points.

Formula 2: General toning

 Another formula very powerful general toning.

En pratique

36E, zu San Li	Three distances	Face antero-external of the LEG, to 3 distances of the knee joint.	Unavoidable point of longevity. Boosts the body as a whole.
6RT, San Yin Jiao	Crossing of the three Yin	The internal face of the LEG, to 3 distances above the medial malleolus, in a notch against the tibia.	Acts on the 3 meridians of the liver, kidney and spleen. Regulates all the lower furnace. Great point of gynecological disorders and sexual abuse.
11GI, that Chi	Pond of the curve	Decreased arm, to the outer end of the fold of bending of the elbow.	Point" anti-inflammatory" of the upper home, but also increases the effect

278

			of the other points.
4GI, He Gu	The meeting of two OS	In the angle top, between 1 and 2e metacarpal.	Among other things, large point which regulates the function of the three homes.
6RM, Qi Hai	Sea of energy	To 2 through finger under the navel.	Invigorates the energy of the whole body and help to the uptake of the energy of the air.

Formula 3: Anti-fatigue and for the neurasthéniques

En pratique When you are unable to start the morning when you are overworked, this can often generate problems of stagnation of blood and of energy. This formula can also be used in the event of neurasthénie more or less chronic.

Table 14-3 formula anti-fatigue and for the neurasthéniques.

1RN, Yong Quan	Gushing Source	In a depression on the soles of the feet when the latter is in bending.	It is the great point to boost the energy of the kidney, calm down the fire of the liver (insomnia 3 hours of the morning). The Taoist say it increases the life expectancy.
5C, Tong Li	Free movement	Anterior face of the wrist, with 2 fingers	Major point for all mental disorders. Point anti-depression

	above the ulnar muscle earlier.		and anti-excess of thoughts.
20DM, Bai Today	The one hundred meetings	At the top of the skull, in a vacuum at the apex of the two ears.	Great point of toning of the body and anti-fatigue.

You can also You massage point 1RN, in the morning at sunrise, during 36 respiratory cycles. But also in the evening before going to bed. This point then allows to restore the connection-kidney, heart, and to combat the insomnia.

Formula 4: Anti-anxiety

If you are in periods where the anguish and anxiety overwhelm you, a period that the MTC calls "the engluement the mind", when the energies especially Yin stagnate in the body, a very good formula to make itself:

Table 14-4 formula anti-anguish.

6CC, Nis Guan	Internal restriction	Face antero-median of the forearm, 2 finger above fold of the wrist.	Among other things, it regularizes the Qi, energy, by deleting the stagnations.
7C, Shen Men	Door of the Heart	Ulnar end of the fold of bending of the wrist, between the pisiforme and the ulnar muscle earlier.	It is the great point of insomnia, anxiety, nervousness and palpitations.
17RM, Shan	The center of the chest	On the chest, on the median line	This is the major point for toning

280

Zhong		joining the end of the two breasts.	the energy of the top of the body, but also calm the heart. It is the Xanax and the LEXOMIL Chinese !
3F, Tai Chong	Great abundance	In a depression in the angle top, between 1 and 2e metatarsal.	The major point of insomnia in 3 hours of the morning. It allows you to calm the liver and especially the spirit.

Formula 5: great formula for booster sexuality

Table 14-5 great formula for booster sexuality.

3RN, Tai xi	Great River	Internal side of the foot, in a hollow between the medial malleolus and the Achilles tendon.	The major point of sexuality (impotence, erectile disorder, premature ejaculation, libido to zero).
36E, zu San Li	Three distances	Face antero-external of the LEG, to 3 distances of the knee joint.	Unavoidable point of longevity. Boosts the body as a whole. Charge the battery of the kidney.
23V, shen shu	Shu point of the kidney	Put your hands on both hips: is located under the2, at a distance and a half of the spinal column.	Great point to strengthen the lombes, booster of the battery of the kidney and act on the sexuality.

4WD, Guan Yuan	Barrier of the Origin	To 4 through finger under the navel.	Great point of sexuality, but also to combat the sterility.
6RT, San Yin Jiao	Crossing of the three Yin	The internal face of the LEG, to 3 distances above the medial malleolus, in a notch against the tibia.	Acts on the three meridians of the liver, kidney and spleen. Regulates all the lower furnace. Great point of gynecological disorders and sexual abuse.

We could multiply the formulas to the Infinite. However, I refer you to everything that has been said in the chapter on acupuncture (chapitre 13), and in particular to the "method of choice of points according to the Pr Leung Kok Yuen" (Annex A). All these formulas can be practiced in digitoponcture. It is therefore a technique that will make you touch of the finger, it is the case to say, what is the energy IN MTC. It can be practiced by everyone and once more, it has that very little of contraindications. I think that before the practice of acupuncture, it is a very good method to address the "energy" and the methods of prevention and treatment by MTC.

Chapter 15
Moxibustion
For all
<u>In this chapter:</u>
"The discovery of a technique plurimillénaire
" That the practice at each change of season?
"

TEchnical plurimillénaire if it is, the Moxibustion is an integral part of the methods of prevention and treatment by MTC.
What is the moxibustion?

Le saviez-vous

It is an act of therapeutic or preventive measure which is to heat a zone, or a point located on a meridian of acupuncture, using among other a "cigar" to basis of flower of dried sagebrush called moxa.
This term would come from **mogusha** in Japanese which means "burn the grass".
In MTC, when we speak of acupuncture, very often the term Zhen Jiu. Zhen meaning metal, needle, and JIU meaning "a fire heats slowly".
In the **Nei Jing,** it is said: "If the acupuncture does not work, it is necessary to use the moxibustion. "
A proverb very known in China: "When the House has of the sagebrush aged three years or more, there is no need of Doctor! "
Manufacturing Mode
Another term to mean the moxibustion IN MTC is AI Jiu Fa, have "sagebrush", JIU "cauterize", "heat" and FA "method". In effect, it is sagebrush which will serve as a vector for heat certain points of the body.
The sagebrush is a medicinal plant to the full in the traditional pharmacopoeia. It has among others a very good calorific value and the smoke that it generates in consuming themselves is very fragrant. It is said that it invigorates the energy of the spleen.

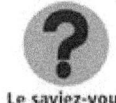
Le saviez-vous

Its smoke is much less desséchante that the cigarette, which allows the practitioner to be less exposed to secondary effects.

283

The Artemisia vulgaris, or wormwood, or "grass Saint-Jean ", is this grass that was burning at the Saint John to hunt the demons.

When it rises in flower, the stems are cut, met between them, dried the heads in the bottom to concentrate the beneficial substances. After a few weeks of drying, it removes the twigs and retains the leaves and flowers which will be crushed very finely. One thus obtains the "Velvet of sagebrush," which can be kept in the form of bundles for several years.

It then uses either in bulk or in the form of sticks: the famous "Cigars of sagebrush". For the manufacture, it takes of the WAD of sagebrush who will be wrapped very tight in of rice paper.

I advise you to take the traditional sticks, because often those found in the West are consumed too much too fast.

Action and indications of the moxibustion

Too often, there is a tendency to confuse heat a region of suffering with a hot water bottle, a lamp, a hair dryer and treat with a moxa. A moxibustion point is much more powerful. Of course due to the therapeutic virtues of the sagebrush, but also because the point of combustion will emit a certain energy vibration, heat a very particular which will be able to enter in depth in the body. But also thanks to the penetration of the therapeutic virtues related to the plant itself. To such a point that there are some "sticks of moxibustion" with a mixture of plants cleverly dosed to treat some types of rheumatism.

The main actions of such treatment are:

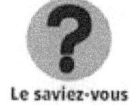
Le saviez-vous

" "Warm Up" the blood and energy in the event of internal cold.

" To circulate the energy.

" To invigorate the blood (among others by an increase in white blood cells) and unlock the stasis.

" Refresh the heat. This may seem strange to heat to refresh, but it should not be forgotten that if we are in the presence of a stasis of blood and energy, the latter generates heat and swelling. Since the action of the

284

moxibustion allows you to circulate, we can say that in some cases, it allows you to "refresh the heat".

"Some points can fortify the kidneys, sub-heard the "Charging the battery of the Kidney".

A few indications:

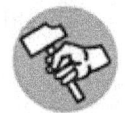

"

Moxibustion may be used by a practitioner for some rheumatism related mainly to wind and cold.

"Some joint pain.

"His action is also very powerful in the case of the collapse of the energy of the spleen with persistent diarrhea and a state of weakness and of internal cold which generate a weight loss very important.

"This technique can also treat some cases of sterility. We will take as an example a little further.

"And especially c is a great technique to boost the energy of the kidney, increase the immune defenses and the faculties of adaptation.

The different techniques

There are two major types of techniques, to know what the MTC calls the moxibustion direct and indirect moxibustion.

The direct moxibustion

The sagebrush in bulk is presented in the form of BOURRE of aspect very fluffy.

It can shape easily with the fingers to form of cones, of small pyramids or why not grains of rice. These cones can then be directly posed on the skin.

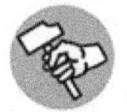

When the practitioner has chosen a point to "moxer", it moisturizes the skin and install this cone at the good location. Then he takes a stick incense and in turns on the summit. As soon as the patient feels a significant heat, it gently removes this cone for the replace by another.

In the tradition, we could repeat seven times the same operation. But this requires a lot of technical skill on the part of the practitioner to not burn his patient.

The indirect moxibustion

It is by far the most common.

It is relatively easy to obtain in the trade the famous "sticks of sagebrush". Some are covered with a thicker paper that it would be appropriate to remove. Other wear as pure name moxa rolls directly marked on the rice paper. This paper is to keep.

Then to the assistance of a lighter or a stick incense, you will turn on your cigar.

Attention Once lit, a moxa can no longer turn off. It is for this reason that any practitioner of MTC has in his cabinet what is called a damper. It is a small object in brass which allows you to turn off very quickly the stick. You can also to prepare a mold with an aluminum foil. Some even use a holster to cigars. Not a question to extinguish the sagebrush with water. And it would be too stupid to cut off the end.

When you use a stick "virgin, the Smoke starts immediately. During the second use, is formed, in the end, a cone of coal. At restart, as soon as a red dot appears, you know that it can no longer be off. But you will earn 2 to 3 minutes of smoke.

Attention To avoid burns, insurance being rather expensive at this time, you install on the skin of the patient the edge of the hand that holds the moxa. You then have a lot more precision with regard to the heating of the point. And in some cases, you can position your other hand, thumb and index excluded (what the Chinese call the mouth of the Tiger), around the point. Then you will find yourself if you heat too the area.

Always in the technique of indirect moxibustion, another possibility is offered to the practitioner, that of shaping a cone of sagebrush and the thread on an acupuncture needle. Once the card is inserted on one of the selected points, it will then be able to turn it on and let it burn until the end. The heat will then directly on the point of acupuncture. There are at the present time what is called mini-moxas which are much more practical.

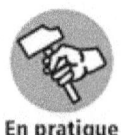

En pratique

286

The best technique

It is that of the pecking and not of the cherry picking as we often hear. For Dummies, of which I was a part: the woodpecker Picote, that is to say that with its beak, it tape always in the same place. The hen picks, that is to say that its head goes from right to left to search for its seeds.

Once the stick lit and well held in hand, you go Therefore heat the point. You can make slight rotation or not, but the smoldering is located at 2-3 cm from the skin. As soon as the person feels an excess of heat, you raise a little the stick, then you closer to New, where non of pecking"".

The entire operation lasts approximately 5 to 15 minutes. Everything depends on the indication posed by the practitioner.

Of course, from time to time, you tap the stick above an ashtray to remove the ash, like a cigarette.

At the end of the treatment of a point, the area must be well dew, almost red.

That practice with each change of season?

The changes of the season, especially if they are brutal, require a addition of adaptation for the battery of the Organization. Both seasons the more "dangerous" for health as the beginning of the winter, where energy is sinking into the earth and the beginning of the spring, if the SAP does not happen to fit by lack of strength, the tree dies. It is therefore preferable in these critical periods to help the body to booster its battery (rest, regular sleep, eat less: this is not for nothing that lent is located to the rise of spring...). Moxibustion is part of this arsenal of preventive.

Moxibustion of long life

We will see here a moxibustion which can be practiced by everyone, without any secondary effect, using a stick of sagebrush. It is the two points 36E, zu San Li, located on the outer sides of the leg," to three distances under the knee", such is the literal translation of the Chinese name of this point. Another translation much more symbolic: in the former time where the factors walked a lot, as soon as they felt tired, they stopped on the edge of the path for a massage or "moxer "this point. They could then make three leagues of more!

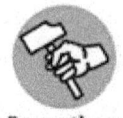

A little kitchen!
You will obtain the salt end of Guérande (avoid the big salt which can burst). Then in your **En pratique** supermarket or Asian store usual, buy a ginger root "young" (such as our new potatoes). In one of the Parties swollen, cut a washer of 2 to 3 mm of thickness, the size of the old parts of 5 francs. Drill it with the handle of a needle or a fork, of several small holes. Certainly, the holes will close, but this will increase the conduction. Then using a sharp knife, cut a slice of a length of 1 cm of a stick of sagebrush.

You, or the patient, are lying on the back. You fill in the navel of salt, until the area is convex. You install the slice of ginger above. And even above, the end of the stick of sagebrush. There is no more than to turn it on and let it burn until the end. Then you take the slice of ginger and spill the ashes in an ashtray. On the same

Slice, you can put a moxa. If you made a autopratique and an emergency is required, you take the whole tranche and you install it in the ashtray.

It is the purpose of this recipe? The navel is the point 8RM, Shen that, a point that it is not pique ever, but that we can heat up. It is rightly considered as the root of the Vitality. It invigorates very strongly the Yang, increases the blood and energy in the whole body. It is one of the major points of Tonic energy.

Why does it work? The salt is the flavor of the kidney, but it is also conductor of heat. The Ginger is hot and spicy. It wakes up the Yang and circulates. The sagebrush heats and trafficking. When making this kitchen? At each change of season to adapt to the surplus of energy that the body needs. But also in the states of large fatigues.

In MTC, this is a key point of longevity to prevent disease and maintain health. In tonic and regulating the energy of the spleen, it helps to fortify the organization as a whole. It is essential in the treatment of any kind of illnesses due to exhaustion. Moxibustion of this point is called therefore "moxibustion of long life". A book Classical Japanese mentions the existence of a family of centenarians whose members had the habit of heat very regularly with these points in the moxa. One of them has been able to live 242 years and more than twenty was centenary! This is not me who have said. I leave you to judge alone.

All Taoist who practiced the methods of longevity was at this place a small scar. It was not by four paths. After having manufactured with underfur of sagebrush a small grain of rice, it humectait the point with its saliva and posed the sagebrush above. With the help of an incense stick, it lit and Let burn until the end by avoiding to drill the phlyctène which was formed. Of our days, if a practitioner done this to his patient, it cost him dearly in damages and interests!

These points should therefore be heated at least 10 minutes each, with every change of season and when we simply feels tired.

A few precautions

When your practitioner has developed a formula after a proper diagnosis in MTC, and that several points may be heated, it must adhere to a certain order in the treatment. It is said as well that it is appropriate to begin to treat the side Yang before the side yin. It will begin therefore by the DOS before the chest, by the side sky (head and upper member) before the side earth (lower limbs).

Among the elderly and children, the time of moxibustion must be shortened.

It is said in the texts that after a session, you must not take shower or wash hands in cold water. On the contrary, it would be good to drink a cup of tea, or any other hot drink, to assist in the elimination of toxins.

Le saviez-vous

Do not play with the self-medication. Only a therapist trained to the MTC will be able to develop the appropriate formula, and will give you, why not, a stick of sagebrush to continue the treatment among you. This does not necessarily apply to the forms of toning data previously.

Use the real sticks of sagebrush and avoid taking the moxas called "without smoke" or "without odour". It is no longer of any in the Tradition and the little smoke that emerges is often toxic.

The smoke is dense and very fragrant. It must be done. For the firms, there are smoke extractors. I remind you that this smoke is much less asséchante as that of a cigarette, with respect to organic liquids.

If you practice in an apartment poorly isolated, your neighbors might think that you started to smoke a few Aphrodisiacs Herbs!

Contra-indications

You chauffiez you-even some points, or that this is a practitioner, it should avoid making such a treatment just after a large physical fatigue, a meal too important or a loss of seed for the men. Similarly, if you come to suffer a big annoyance or a great fear. The effects are then likely to be to the contrary.

Attention

Very important: the Moxibustion is not suitable to malignant tumors, especially when one is in a phase of accelerated development. In some cases, the practitioner will be able to help the patient to "rebuild" using certain points at a distance. But never to the side of the homes of the tumor. The action of dispersion of the stagnation linked to the Sagebrush and the heat then risk to disseminate the cancerous cells.

And of course, we will not cease to repeat, avoid any self-medication.

Chapter 16
Elements of
Pharmacopoeia

In this chapter:
" The theory of signatures
" The Four natures and the five flavors
" The seven types of order
" The galenic forms of requirements
" The art of combining the remedies between them

TheHas traditional pharmacopoeia Chinese goes back to the night of the time. It is one of the most developed and older than we knew.

Shen Nong, mythical figure if it is, was the discoverer of the virtues of tea and medicinal plants. For the little story, each time he is intoxiquait with a new unknown plant, he used the virtues of cleaning the tea to heal itself.

In short, he left one of the first compendiums of Chinese pharmacopoeia, the **Shen Nong Ben ca Jing, bringing together more than 360 species.**

With the acupuncture, the pharmacopoeia is part of the two healing methods and complementary in MTC, who do not seek the cooperation of the patient.

A drug, a formula is said Yao in Chinese. This can be a single product or a formula, a combination of several products.

Le saviez-vous

Most of these Yao are composed in majority of plants, then of minerals and a smaller proportion for animal products. The plant part constitutes 80 per cent of this Pharmacopoeia.

Indeed, it considers in a manner quite general that the action of the plants is more soft and therefore sufficient possibly when the disease is mild. In contrast, minerals and animal products are more toxic. They have of flavors and energies much more pronounced and become necessary when the disease is very serious.

We are going to see that a plant, a mineral or an animal product has to differentiate a nature and a flavor. But also a color, smell, a texture and a body or a meridian favorite target. This is also valid for all plant or animal products that we have in our base.

Some of these formulas are very known in MTC and will treat of the syndromes well individuals.

But there is another exciting aspect of this type of treatment. The one to adapt a formula at the discretion of the evolution of symptoms that the patient presents in the day to day. The practitioner will have to proceed to do this to an evaluation of the respective forces which are in presence. On the one hand, we have the right energy, the energy of Defense of the patient, what we called in the introduction to this book the Zheng Qi, energy right. On the other the attacker, "The strength of the Perverse agent", the 11th Qi. To evaluate this report of force, the practitioner will establish a diagnosis very specific in relying on the ba gong, the "eight rules". It is based on this type of fault finding that it is going to establish the bases of therapeutic way to combat the disease and paste as close to its evolution.

Two strategies will therefore s offer to him:

" Reconstruct the Zheng Qi, energizing the body so that it can again be autoguérir;

À retenir "Either disperse the agent perverse, disperse the Xie Qi, decrease the force for that the body can resume the above.

The theory of signatures

Before to go further in this study, we need to look at the fundamental of the Chinese Pharmacopoeia: "The theory of signatures".

In the West, as soon the [1st] century av. J.-C., Dioscorides is one of the first to convey this idea. **Simila similibus curantur, "similar care For similar".**

The idea of the signature was resumed at the Renaissance by PARACELSUS (1540). A simple direct observation of a plant allowed to discover the mode of employment. A gift to the man in some way, a present of God, to those who wanted to make the effort to see the hidden things behind the things. There would therefore be to observe the shape of plants, their color, the place where they grow, to deduct the applications that can be drawn. It is as well as the plants " sign "their use. "Everything the nature creates, he wrote, it the shape to the image of the virtue that it intends to attach. "

An example: the willow. This tree grows in the wetlands, to the edges of ponds and marshes. It must then treat the diseases caused by this medium. That is why Paracelsus advocated to treat rheumatism and the fevers.

But this theory goes back to the night of the time in China. It is even with the base of the entire Chinese medicine. It therefore stipulates that everything that has been created in the nature must in one way or another contribute to retain or regain a good health.

À retenir

Each plant has a form, an odour, a flavor, a color, a specific habitat. But also in a plant there has roots, bark, leaves, the seed, the flower, the rod. All this has a meaning, a "signature" that allowed the former to deduce the main indications as to their therapeutic properties and preventive measures.

For example since the night of the time, we knew that the walnut having the shape of the convolution of the brain and its color pearly could only have a specific action on this one!

There is a fungus very known in China, which has the form of a sea sponge and evokes the pulmonary alveoli. It is the tremelle in time zone (tremela fuciformis). This fungus has many similarities with the diaphragm, it was logical that it The testât in that sense. In effect, it "feeds" and moisten the diaphragm in dispelling the accumulations of mucus and opposes the sputum of bleeding. Even further, as these fungi are able to survive in very harsh climatic conditions, they strengthen the resistance to the cold.

One could cite as hundreds of examples of this type.

But, as it has been said earlier, this theory also applies to different parts of a plant. As an example, compare the effects of the seed of coffee and the sheet of tea. The coffee comes from the seed of the coffee. A seed is energetically very responsible, very concentrated. A simple SEED can give a baobab tree! Its concentration in energy will be "booster" by the roasting that goes "yanguiser" its effects. The coffee energizes the liver, fact fit the Yang To the top and prevents

293

sleep. Conversely, the tea comes from the emerging leaves of the Camelia sinensis. These properties are much lighter, air. It is for this reason that it is said in Chinese medicine that "the Coffee excites the mental While the tea opens this same mind".

Nature, flavor and place of action

That is the plant products, minerals, or animals, there will be for each of them essentially two important parameters which will determine their properties, their therapeutic actions we will as well talk about the "Four Qi", the "Four natures" and "Five flavors". It adds a third criterion, namely the place of action of the drug.

The four natures

The four Qi are:

ˮThe cold;

ˮThe cost;

ˮThe lukewarm;

ˮThe hot.

There join a fifth nature, a fifth Qi, which is the neutral nature. The pure neutrality does not exist. This just means that the flavor is very little marked. Here, the word Qi in two directions, the nature or the smell.

In the **Nei Jing, it is said: "In the presence of cold, use the hot; in the presence of heat, use the cold. "**

Drugs that improve or eliminate the symptoms of heat are considered to be of such a nature as cool or cold, as Huang Qin, the root of the Skullcap indicated in the case of fever with thirst and throat painful.

Of drugs capable of warm up the center, to disperse the cold will be of a nature hot or warm like GAN Jiang, ginger root.

 Drugs of nature, warm or hot allow to warm the internal, to disperse the cold, to assist the Yang, to reconstitute the fire and unclogging the vessels.

À retenir On the contrary, drugs of nature cool or cold can refresh the heat, disperse the fire, "cool" the blood, neutralize the toxins in the heat.

The costs and the cold are of a nature Yin, while the hot and the lukewarm are yang. But in the first group, the Yin can be of different strength: we talk of cold and fresh. As for drugs Yang where there is talk of warm or hot.

The fifth nature, the moderate nature applies to drugs that have not of action réchauffante cooling or obvious. In reality, there is still a tendency a bit hot or a little cold. This is the reason for which one speaks of "Four natures" and not five.

In our food, the Food neutral by excellence is rice.

The practitioner will always be careful to prescribe the appropriate drug to the effect that he wants to get. If for example it prescribed by error of drugs of high intensity (hot or cold) where a lower intensity (fresh or lukewarm) is required, there may be complications.

The Five Flavors

These five flavors will condition the effects of drugs and they allow the practitioner to change at will the formula of a product to adjust very precisely the effect that it should have. It differentiates the five flavors in two groups.

The piquant flavors and the mild flavor

The sweet flavor is included in the fresh flavor. This is for example the characteristic taste of ginseng. These two flavors are of category Yang.

" *The tangy flavor is a flavor which has a dispersant action on the Qi, energy.* It acts on the Qi because it is light. It is said that it favors the Qi. It is in addition a flavor which goes to the lung.

" *The sweet taste with respect to it is a flavor slowing. It slows down, calm. It is nevertheless classified as Yang because it has the property to nourish the body. It is the flavor that characterizes the foods that build the body as cereals and between other rice. It is transformed by the* spleen and gives the basis of blood and the energy. In reality, this flavor has as a property to do fit the nutrient species from the spleen. It promotes the work of the ascent of the spleen as well as its digestive function which allows him to extract the key nutrients in the food bowl.

Acidic flavors, bitter salt and

These three flavors are of a nature Yin.

" *The acid taste, sour to the property of focus, to be particularly useful to retain the liquid to the inside of the body.* It is a anti-action sudorifique. It also allows to reduce the loss of fluid by the excess of urine. It uses each time that there is too much fluid that comes out of the body. It has an action of constriction. That is exactly the reverse of the action Yang of the tangy flavor, dispersant.

" *The bitter flavor has for essential priority to combat the moisture.* It is a flavor that dries out the liquid. It is in more top down. It is a flavor that one must take when one wants to lower a fire that burns, even when one wants to foster the purgations, promote the stool.

" *The Salty flavor, it, is a flavor which softens.* It softens everything that is induratum in the body. Everything that represents a concentration of material in the body falls within this flavor. It also promotes the evacuation of stool by its action ramollissante.

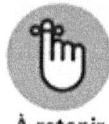

À retenir

So here are the essential actions of the five flavors. But do not forget the next thing is that in excess, a flavor turns against its target organ. We can then obtain the opposite effect to that desired. For example, the bitter fight against moisture. But an excess of bitterness (coffee, chocolate) turns against the body, leads to a state of internal cold, and therefore promotes the emergence of humidity!

Difference between flavor and nature

A food which presents a certain flavor also presents a certain nature. But this is not always "traditional".

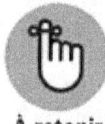

À retenir

The Qi, the nature of the plant, is assigned to the product itself whose origin is the sky, the part Yang down. The Wei, the flavor, it is the land that the gives. It is for this reason that the it is said that "the earth gives the five flavors".

And elsewhere this QI which is its nature, it is also the smell of the plant. There are plants that have a strong smell and very little flavor. Others have much flavor and very little odour.

That is why the traditional doctors screened their plants according to these criteria. They could even enjoy their effects simply by looking to see the shape and the Color (theory of signatures), in the feeling and then in the tasting.

The combination of these two elements gives a comprehensive nature to the plant that is therefore his IQ, its nature, its own character which can therefore be either Yin or Yang, be fresh, cold, warm or hot.

Let us take an example: the alcohol is typically of tangy flavor and its nature is hot. The mint is also a product of pungent, but cool nature.

The same for the sweetish flavor. There is a sweetish flavor of nature as hot as the ginseng. A sweetish flavor of fresh nature as the watermelon.

Some products can have at the same time one, two or even three flavors.

Basically, no product is neutral. Any product is necessarily rather Yang or rather Yin. We can talk about nevertheless to neutral products for certain foods such as rice, bread although it has a dominant slight Yang.

Place of action

Each drug is directed to a meridian and the body which corresponds to him.

In the **Nei Jing** It is said: "the acid between in the liver, the bitter in the heart, the spicy in the lung, the Salty in the kidney and the soft in the spleen. The acid part to join the tendons, bitter the blood, the spicy the Qi, the energy, the salted the OS and the soft flesh. "

À retenir

Little by little, the result of the experience, the knowledge of the places of action has led to better target the effect of the treatment.

Let us take the example of the asthma or dyspnea. Two bodies can be criminalized, the lung or the kidney. Once the component concerned found, we will choose the appropriate drug. If this is the lung and that there is a blockage of the Qi, we will take my Huang, ephedra, which has for a place of action the lung. If the cause of the condition is linked to the kidney, the practitioner will prescribe Ge Jie, the gecko, which reconstitutes the kidney and promotes the retention of the Qi.

Development of a formula

We are going to address this "the art of combining the remedies between them" in order to have a focused result more accurate than the use of a simple plant or another.

The eight therapeutic methods

These eight methods, still called Ba Fa in Chinese, are:

" The sudorification, Han;
" The vomification, you;
" The purgation, XIA;
" The Harmonization, IL;
" The warming, Wen;
" Cooling, Qing;
" The elimination, Xiao ;
" The toning, Bu.

These eight methods are a tool of first plan for the Chinese pharmacopoeia and they remain today used by the vast majority of practitioners.

The sudorification, Han

It is a method which is to cause sweating by opening of the interstitial spaces, the pores of the skin, what is known as the Ku Li. We can thus evacuate the perversity of the six climate excess residing in the surface of the body.

The sudorification, not only causes the sweating, but also:

" Expels The perversity toward the outside;
" Dissipates the perversity of the area;
" Relieve the energy and the blood;
" Harmonizes the energy of defense, Wei Qi, and the nutritional energy, Ying Qi.

 You can also use this method to push toward the outside of the perversity in the early stage of disease eruptive of the child such as measles,

En pratique

298

when the eruption develops difficult or slow to occur.

It can also be used, in the presence of edema more marked in the upper part of the body, in the early stages of disorders Pustular or ulcers or in the presence of a syndrome of Biao, area with alternating hot and cold.

Depending on the presence of heat or cold, of the state of the perversity or of energy right, of the physical constitution of the patient, it is possible to provoke the sudorification with products quills and warm or with products quills and cold.

We will see that it is also possible to combine methods of sudorification and toning.

The vomification, you

This method allows, as its name indicates, to expel by mouth, in causing the vomiting, mucus, foods or toxic substances that are stagnating at the level of the throat, chest, of the diaphragm or of the stomach.

In the **su wen, it is said: "What is in the top of the body must go through the top. "**

 If the vomification is time, a very effective method, it can cause, when it is repetitive, irritation of the esophagus and the throat. Its action very powerful **Attention** at the level of the diaphragm and the stomach can easily harm the true energy. It is a mechanism which is in danger of return against the patient. I am thinking here of the obsessive-compulsive disorders related to a blocking of the liver, the "bulimia".

Practitioners of later eras in **Nis Jing** have preferred to reserve its use in situations of acute clinical, to quickly evacuate the single wickedness of type fullness.

The Purgation, Xia

It is a method which is before any used when there is a stagnation of food or contents in the intestines or the stomach. But also, when there are fecal plugs, problems of heat (inflammation) type fullness, of clusters cold, blood stasis, clusters of tan or liquids.

In the **su wen, it is said: "What is at the bottom, it must be the pull and eliminate it. In the plénitudes of the center, it to drain toward the abdomen. "**

By and large, if we cannot evacuate the disease by the top, one uses Xia Fa in case of stagnation in the Foyer Medium or Lower to evacuate down.

It is of course the big method when there is of the constipation, the accumulation of dry stool, the blocking of the stool due to the accumulation of heat and the blocking of the TAN or liquids, the accumulation of blood stasis.

 Depending on the presence of heat or cold, of the state of the energy right or of the strength of the perversity, there are different types of purgation:

En pratique " The cold purgation, Han Xia;

" The purgation hot, Wen Xia;

" The lubrication, run Xia;

" The drastic bleed;

" As well as the simultaneous use of the methods of attack, gong and toning, Bu, and their combination with other therapeutic methods.

He should know that in this method, the diuretic action is secondary in the reduction of Shi and tan. The principle of the purgation is done in priority by the stool.

The harmonization, or regulating, IL

This method has the objective to reduce or to expel the pathogen by an effect said of "conciliation", he Jie, and harmonization. He Jie is a contraction of the expression meaning "harmonize the depth and to liberate the area".

It applies this treatment in cases where the perversity do is found more in size, but not yet in depth. The Chinese expression is **Ben Biao Ben Li, "half in the area, half in depth."**

This method allows therefore to harmonize the depth and liberate the area. It allows to harmonize all of the functional activities of the Organization in order to allow him to return to his physiological balance.

It treats the dysharmonies between the Zang, and the FU, the organs and the viscera, energy and blood, the Yin and the Yang. But also in the syndromes characterized by an imbalance between the cold and hot, in the complex syndromes where mingle disability and fullness.

We can apply this method in very many situations such as:

" The penetration of Han Xie, the cold perversity in the organization;

" The paludal syndromes, Naked Ji;

" The dysharmonies between the liver and the spleen, between the intestines and stomach, between the energy and blood, etc., in order to regain the balance and arrive to hunt the pathogen and restore health.

We can therefore consider that it is a neutral treatment linked for example to the psycho-emotional. It strengthens then the psychological balance.

In diseases where there is alternation between the cold and hot, the disease has a double aspect, the symptoms are contrary and it is then restored the balance as in malaria. But also in the Yin-Yang imbalances where there is no significant excess of Yin or Yang. It works on the two in a manner antagonist.

The warming of the LI of the internal, or calorification, Wen

This method is to hunt the cold and to restore the Yang using the principles as warm the depth, Wen Li, expel the cold, that Han, return the Yang, hui Yang.

In the **su wen, it is said: "What is cold, heat" or "treat the cold by the heat".**

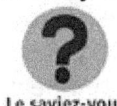

The syndromes internal cold may be due to the penetration of external cold directly in the depth, by the wrong employment of drugs of cold nature injuring the Yang energy.

Another case is the inadequacy of the original Yang leading directly to a internal cold.

In the localized stasis resulting in pain in the abdominal cavity mainly.

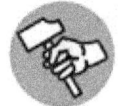 This technique may take different forms depending on that the cold is located at the level of organs or viscera, meridians or collaterals. It

can as well:

" Warm up the center and hunt the cold;

" Return the Yang and save the sick;

" Warm up the meridians and disperse the cold.

As the member of disability and cold are very often to be found together, it often combines the toning and warming.

The cooling, or clarification, Qing

This method is intended to deal with the syndromes depth, the Li, and heat, Re, tempering the heat and neutralizing the toxins.

In the **su wen, we can read : "What is hot, cool down" and "treat the heat** by the cold."

The heat can reside in the layer of the Qi, energy, in the nutrition or in that of the blood.

In serious cases, it becomes toxic. To re, it moves to the and can affect any organ or viscère.

 The cooling can take different forms such as:

" Temper the heat in the layer of the Qi;

" Refresh the nutrition and the blood;

" Refresh simultaneously the energy and the blood;

" Temper the heat and eliminate the toxins,

The field of application of this method of clarification is very broad. There is a rule that must not be lost sight of: "If in the stages of a affection of heat the Jing Ye, liquids Yin, are injured, or when the disability of Yin is accompanied to the conflagration of fire resulting in the appearance of the heat, it is imperative to maintain the Yin while tempering the heat. Then it cannot be use of drugs of bitter nature and cold. "

It is therefore a method for treating Re Bing, diseases of heat.

The elimination, reduction, dispersion, Xiao

This method aims to reduce gradually and slowly dissolve the formations concrete pathologies (TAN) which may appear at the expense of energy and blood or from the mucous Productions, food, liquids or parasites.
In the **su wen, it is said: "The hard, it must be split, conglomerates, it must be the dissolve. "**
Taken in the broad sense, these methods are designed to:
"To expel the mucus;
"To expel the humidity;
"To eliminate parasites;
" Regulate the energy;
" Regulate the blood.
It also means by Xiao, elimination, the methods which are used to promote the digestion of food and drive the stagnant, reduce the masses and disperse the accumulations.

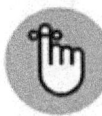

Let us recall that Qi Yu, the stagnation of Qi, is the point of departure for all stagnations and that it is directly linked to the liver, Gan. It is then produces a feeling of inner voltage, then the following signs may appear as pain in coasts, to the flanks, in the abdomen, difficulty swallowing, lumps in the throat, of menses disrupted in women.

À retenir

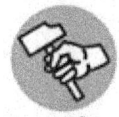

It is a method that we will apply by example For fibroids which correspond to a Qi Yu, a stagnation of Qi, with signs of Yu Xue. The color of blood is then dark. There is no blood clots. Qi Yu also includes the cysts of water.

En pratique

Xiao, the elimination combines with a slight effect Bu, toning, if one wants to circulate. By circulating, we help in the resolution of stagnations.

The toning, Bu

The toning aims to rebuild and to feed the energy, the blood, the Yin or Yang of the body, of an organ or a viscère, when those are in a state of disability or damage.

In the **su wen,** it is stated: "What is missing, it must be complete. "The toning allows therefore to find a balance.

In addition, when the right energy weakened is no longer able to resist the perversity in the eleventh IQ, or is no longer able to expel this perversity, it is possible to resort to the toning is as well to "support the physiological to hunt the pathological".

 From this observation, very many forms of toning may be exercised:

" The Yin, Bu Yin;

En pratique " The Yang, Bu Yang;

" The Energy Bu Qi;

" Blood, Bu Xue;

" The Heart, Bu Xin;

" Of the liver, Bu Gan;

" Of the spleen, Bu IP;

" The Lung, Bu EIF;

" Of the kidney, Bu Shen; etc.

If the Yin and the yang are all two deficient, or if the energy and blood are simultaneously insufficient, there is a need to harmonize at the same time the Yin and the yang and tone set the energy and the blood.

These different forms of toning are also found at the level of the five bodies.

The four roles of a plant

We will now see that even within a formula, each plant, each drug is going to hold a particular role.

In each formula, regardless of the number of products, the drug will enter in one of these four categories:

" The Emperor;

" The Minister;

" The public servant;

" The ambassador.

The product emperor is in relationship with the purpose of the prescription.

Depending on the purpose of the treatment, there will be one or several products that will be particularly concentrated in which the essential action will correspond precisely the effect that we must achieve.

These are therefore the products the most powerful in the action sought for the whole of the formula.

Very often, despite the number of existing products in Chinese pharmacopoeia, products which truly represent an action very precise and very powerful are not numerous enough. It should then be to add other products which may not have for essential effect the purpose of the treatment, but who among their therapeutic properties very many, have an indication in this direction.

If for example we want to tone the liver, the essential product may be a product unique. But we can add another product which is normally on the heart, but which has for secondary effect of toning the liver. It is a product whose action is less strong. It will be there to complement. It adds to the product Emperor. It is a phenomenon of assistance. That is what is called the Product Minister.

It may be considered that these two products are the two main points of the formula.

The third is the product Public Servant. It is a hierarchy in the Public Service Chinese. The role of this product is to prevent the negative effects of the main products.

The fourth type of ingredient fulfils two key roles. It typically assigns a diplomatic function, C is the product Ambassador. It is assimilated on the hierarchical Plan to a commercial, an intermediary. It allows different ingredients to be able to work together. It is a coordinator who made a link between the different actions of the other products.

It has a second role also, it is to lead the prescription in the body. It is in general the product Ambassador who brings the properties of precedents where they must act in the body.

These are the four types of products to which we will have to do. There will be talk of main products in the measure where they run the purpose of the prescription and there is talk of secondary products to the extent where they complement the precedents.

The seven types of order

We have therefore seen the four types of Yao, of drugs entering in a prescription. We know the nature, the flavor, the tropism of each plant. After a specific diagnosis (observation, palpation, questioning), we know what we want to achieve with a formula (the eight therapeutic methods). We know the hierarchy of the different components of this formula. We will now see the "seven types of order ".

We have successively:

" The large order,
" The small order,
" The order slow,
" The order fast,
" The prescription to single action,
" The Order to multiple action,
" The order complex.

These seven orders are justified on the basis of the diseases.

The *large* and the *small* order are mainly distinguished by the number of symptoms that one wants to take into account. Given a certain disease, if it is in a state relatively advanced, including many symptoms, it will be important to provide many products. An order small concerns the less serious illness and who have symptoms in a quantity less significant in number and variety. When there are 3, 4, 5 products, it is a small order. When there are 10, 15, 20 products, it is a great order.

As regards the order *slow* and *fast, here the decisive criterion is the toning and sedation.*

Le saviez-vous

When it was essentially a state of weakness, that one wants to toning, there needs to be a slow, by necessity, because it is not possible to tone up quickly. The order fast, it is the reverse. It is necessitated by the fact that the disease is yang, fullness, that it has a progression extremely fast. Even if it is not yet dangerous, it is progressing rapidly. It is the case in particular of seasonal diseases, diseases of the heat or of all diseases where c is a perversity which evolves very quickly. This is in principle not the case of a disease internally due to the emotions or injuries for example that progresses slowly and manifests itself gradually.

Single action and multiple action

The single action and *the action multiple* also relate to the different specificities of the disease.

" The formula *to single action* is generally composed of one or two products to action very fast. If for example, there is a certain disease which presents a serious developments and dangerous, it is appropriate to apply a single product against this disease, whatever the side effects of this product. It does not of reasoning. It is not expected of contrepoison. It employs one or two products that have all the same action. It is foremost a dispersant action. It considers that the order is an order strong and very violent. It is considered as being of type Yang. This order called "order Yang" is not due to the nature of its products, but to the action of the product on the Yang in the body.

" It opposed a *double order. It is an order that the is still called "Yin and Yang mixed." It is an order which also contains very few products, but where we give two products antagonists. And in this case the final effect is the obtaining of a result more slow.*

" *The Order* concerns complex diseases which are the result of the superposition of several diseases. For example, if the kidney is low, if the liver is bloated, we will combine two orders, one for the kidney, the other for the liver. If at the same time the Lung presents a certain pathological condition, we can add a third order. It puts the three orders together and are composed of a complex order.

Example of a formula: a simple cold

We are going to take to present an example of a formula that could be used during a banal "external attack", type cold simple, by the

En pratique aggression of the wind and the cold. In Chinese medicine, the cold perversity is easy to apprehend. The wind is the wind of the climate, but also everything that vehicle the wind, namely the microbes, viruses, etc. We will use a formula very well known in China, namely: GUI Zhi Tang, decoction to basis of ramulus cinnamomi, composed of five ingredients:

"**Ramulus cinnamomi, Rameau of the cinnamon tree: 10 g;**
"**Radix paeoniae albae, root of White Peony (root peeled and cut in tranche): 10 g;**
"**Radix Glycyrrhizae, licorice root skipped to honey: 6 g;**
"**Zingiberis Rhizoma 2001c, Ginger young: 10 g;**
"Fructus jujubae spinosae, the jujube: 5 parts.

Preparation

The first three plants are chopped and the five ingredients of the prescription are put in a liter and a half of Water, Reduced to soft fire up to obtain approximately 60 cl of decoction. It filter, we drink approximately 20 cc to warm temperature. After a few moments, it must consume a oatmeal of rice clear good hot, to strengthen the action of drugs. Then it must be cover warmly. A slight sweating must cover the whole body. It must not get out to large drops under penalty of injury to body fluids and aggravate the case. Very often, this single socket can cure the patient.

Explanations

In the light of everything that we have seen previously, are looking at a little more closely at this formula. It is therefore primarily intended to deal with the "syndromes of area" due to the attack of a wind-cold. When this "wind-cold" attacks the body, when it crosses the barrier of the skin because the pores, due to a internal weakness or a state of fatigue, have not been able to close in time, there will be the appearance of a conflict, a fight. The two protagonists are on one side the attacker, the "wicked" which may be more or less powerful. And on the other, the energy of Defense, the immune defenses of the patient. This fight is done at the level of the chairs superficial. The evidence that this struggle has well place are the symptoms that appear: headaches, fever, the congestion of the nose, etc.

In this formula:

" The twig of cinnamon-tree is the product Emperor. Its flavor is pungent and soft and its nature lukewarm. It has the effect of releasing the flesh and to expel the "wind" of the defensive layer.

" It is assisted by the root of White Peony which is the product a Minister whose acid taste and gentle and its cold nature have an astringent, having for effect to retain the Yin, do not cause a too heavy perspiration, but also to regulate the digestion.

" The young ginger, tangy flavor and warm nature helps the bark of cinnamon to mobilize the energy defensive and to hunt the wind. It also allows you to disperse the cold and to stop vomiting if they are present.

" The jujube, fresh flavor and warm nature strengthens the action harmonizing of the root of peony on nutrition and the blood. These last two including flavors combined are pungent and soft, products are officials of the formula. They have as a property of toning the energy of the spleen, conductor of the digestion of the food bowl and strengthen the defenses of the body.

" The liquorice root skipped to honey harmonizes the action of other plants so that together they can support the energy of defense and hunt the perversity. It is the product ambassador of this formula.

The combination of these plants allows therefore to obtain an effect reconstituting and an astringent effect. It allows to hunt the "perversity" and to restore a good level of immune defenses.

This is the example of a formula very old, well balanced and which, if it is applied to wisely, can give excellent results.

The galenic forms of requirements

The galenic forms are the different ways to prepare the requirements. In the course of the historical development of the pharmacopoeia, physicians were brought to create many of the galenic forms. Here are the presentations more traditional:

"The decoction, Tang;
"The pill, Wan;
"The powder, SAN;
"The medicinal pulp, Gao;
"The Wine medicinal, JIU.

The decoction

It is by far the more traditional. It is a preparation which consists of mixing drugs for the Make décocter, then to eliminate the solid residue to retain only the liquid which is then consumed.

It is the preparation the most commonly used, because it is adapted to the salaries of General Conditions as well as to that of acute conditions.

Le saviez-vous

The specific characteristics of a decoction are the speed of assimilation of drugs and the effectiveness with which the therapeutic effect can occur.

It has the immense advantage of lend themselves to changes and to allow therefore to adapt to the special features of the patient, to conditions encountered and to the evolution of the day the day of the symptoms.

Traditionally, products intended to be décoctés first had to be chopped. Of our days, used especially after sawing in slices so that their therapeutic properties can develop more quickly at the time of the decoction.

The pills

This form of preparation is to reduce the mixture of drugs in powder and then to the mix to different substances such as honey, rice flour, water, wine, vinegar to obtain a paste which is then formed in logs.

The particularity of these pills is to have a progressive action, slow and sustainable. It is one of the forms of preparation used the most at the present time.

In a general manner, the pills are adapted to the chronic conditions, but some can be used in case of emergency. It is also a form of privileged preparation with respect to the administration of drugs, very toxic, difficult to décocter, very costly or aromatic and that we may not cook too long.

En pratique

In current practice, the pills are most frequently employed are the pills to honey, water, basis of flour.

The powders

This preparation is to reduce the Mixture of medicinal substances in a dry powder and homogeneous. It can then be used by internal.

Once the products are finely powdered, they are administered in small quantities after infusion. They can also be crushed more grossly, cooked in boiling water and absorbed after filtering.

These powders can also be used externally on some pustules, or buttons, or certain areas sick.

The Medicinal pasta

The Pasta medicinal are obtained by the concentration of a decoction of the different Yao, drugs in the water or vegetable oil.

It can be found in many forms as the liquid extracts, the solid extracts, pulp décoctées, ointments, plasters or poultices.

The science of poultices is very used in TCM. There are compendiums of only pharmacopoeia intended for their use.

Le saviez-vous

In Chinese, are called Gao Yao. The basis used for the manufacture is a special soap in which substances are mixed or dissolved in such a way as to obtain a dough of color gray or black, which is then applied on a support in fabric or paper.

The whole is applied on the skin.

It remains strong at ambient temperature and softens to the temperature of the skin, which allows to the therapeutic action of drugs to express themselves fully.

This type of preparation is a job simple, easy to store and transport.

The poultices are very used to treat injuries and bruises, the rheumatic pain, abscesses. Some poultices can directly be used on acupuncture points.

The medicinal wines

The preparation of medicinal wines, or Yao Jiu, is to macerate of drugs in the alcohol of rice or sorghum. The clear fraction of the maceration is then administered by internal or used in external application.

This type of preparation is the most often used for treatments fortifying and nutritious, the treatment of rheumatic pain, as well as injuries or bruises.

In this category, we find the different medicinal dyes.

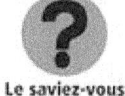

Le saviez-vous

The advantage of the alcohol in the fact of its nature Yang is to do very quickly disperse the different Yao, the different drugs that it contains, in the body.

Attention

Recent warnings

In China, the pharmacopoeia and medicinal plants constitute a "national treasure". The Pharmacopoeia is regarded as more powerful than the acupuncture. Even if a large part of knowledge that are his own stems from a traditional practice popular, with variations from one region to the other, doctors over the centuries have accumulated very large corpus of data in the form of a compendium, Ben Cao.

Some plants we are familiar as the Verbena, liquorice, the jujube. Several are however little or not known in our western cultures. It is therefore still unexplored territory for western scientists.

It is to be noted that the use of these formulas and of these plants is under-stretched a logical extreme and a great relevance. The study separately and try to discover the active principles and then to synthesize risk of us away from this theory of the signatures. Like a single substance often much too powerful, we would lose the effects inherent in this synergy of several ingredients that allows to avoid the effects too powerful and uncontrollable.

But it is obvious that it should not be to play the sorcerer's apprentices in the matter and that very lengthy studies are needed to become somewhat a conductor able to detect the smallest variations in the evolution of the history of a patient and to refine the day-to-day composition of a formula.

Chapter 17
Breathing in the center
Of all practices

OfYears the framework of the methods of preservation of life, methods say Yang Sheng Fa in Chinese and all practices which will follow, respiration, as we will see, is going to have a central place.

Why breathing?

The breathing is in essence, the fundamental element to implement to recharge the battery of the Kidney" (see chapitre 10).

The only problem is that, the Breathing being an element if obvious to us since our birth, we consider as ranging from itself and do not take the time to put it into practice.

And if we ask for people, since this morning, how many times have you breathed in full awareness, the most common responses are: "I forgot," "I will do this later", "I have not had the time", "I did not know that it was so important," "I cannot go to the Act", as many false alibis who do that delay our access to the full health and in a certain way to the fullness of a happiness constant.

À retenir

The breathing is so important that our master, the pr Leung Kok Yuen, told us the following things: "If, end-to-end, throughout the day, you do not breathe in full conscience 2 to 300 times, any other practice of health will then be virtually inoperative. "

Some points of reference

To understand the importance of this subject, it must have a minimum of benchmarks, knowledge of anatomy and physiology of respiration.

The breathing appears with life. At birth, you will take your first inspiration, which is an act Yin, centripetal in relation to the movement of energy and at the time of the passage, you will give your last breath, the complete exhaust of the Yang. Between the two, since your birth until the passage, you are not going to stop breathing.

But if one takes a bit of hindsight, we will very soon we realize that there are two types of breaths. On the one hand, what is called a unconscious Breathing, and on the other side conscious breathing. It is a truism to say: "If it exists, it is to be used! "

Conscious breathing and unconscious

That means *unconscious Breathing* ? This means that you do not know that you breathe. At this time, you are in train, I hope, to breathe, and you do not realize. I say "hope", because everything is done in our mode of life to give us situations where we stops breathing, where it starts in apnea. Tv and computer are part, with many other external or internal factors, these elements which consume so our mind that the body forgets itself to breathe.

As to *conscious breathing, it is interesting to understand that it is the only element internal physiological that we can make conscious instantly. For example, we can through the mental act on the heart beats for the increase where the slow down. For example some exercises from the yoga allow us thanks to mediation and the visualization to accelerate the heart rate to protect us by example of the cold outside thanks to the increase of the blood circulation. But all these physiological processes are slow to slow to install and will ask for tens of seconds to be put in place and a lot of training. On the other hand, when it comes to respiration, it is in the immediacy that I can make conscious. I inhale, I expires in full conscience. I come to overshadow the unconscious Breathing to make conscious.*

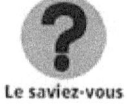

Le saviez-vous

The three major pillars of the life

To understand the importance of this breathing, we can say that in our life exist three major pillars of prevention.

"First pillar: our emotions and our mind which can actually be at the origin of internal pathologies. Little by little, by a bad management of emotions, we are going to be able to "manufacture" not to not a cancer, depression or any other pathology of self-destruction. The bad management of emotions can then shorten our life expectancy, but it will take several months, several years before it becomes a problem lethal.

"Second Pillar of the Vitality: eat and drink. Completely shut off to eat and drink, you will live another 5 to 10 days.

"The third pillar: respiration. Stop breathing, you do not live that 3 to 4 minutes.

The breathing is therefore the first outlet, the first source of energy which connects us to our environment and which allows you to operate the incredible complexity of our Organization. Without air, more of human life on this earth.

À retenir

In twenty-four hours, you breathe between 14 000 and 17 000 times, and this, since you are born. If considering a respiratory cycle is a inspiration followed by a expiration, you redeem on average 500 cc of air. In contrast, as soon as you are subject to stress, as soon as you are tired, in excess of thought, reminiscence, in excess of sadness, as soon as you have of the blockages at the level of the liver and therefore also your diaphragm, you do not redeem more than 200 to 300 cc of air.

When it becomes chronic, we can no longer speak of health, but just "survival" on a daily basis. You have lost any possibility of adaptation to your environment, your battery is flat, because it has no more fuel, and the first emotional shock which presents itself, or a sudden change in the weather, or even a stress which arises unexpectedly déséquilibrera you heavily on your cable of life. Your body will have lost the ability to send you of alarm signals. A disease may appear then brutally.

In this state of under oxygenation, under energy, your body emits when even a few reflexes of survival for recovering a little of this air vital. There is a lot at the depressed who have the DIAPHRAGM COMPLETELY BLOCKED: this are the sighs to repetition. Each time that you soupirez, you inhale STRONGLY, you bring a large amount of energy in your organization. It is a reflex of archaic survival. The yawning to repetition is also part of this type of reflex.

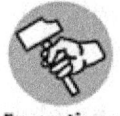

En pratique

To learn how to breathe, not even hard!

As in any initiation, we will try to create a mental image, in the occurrence here a "mental movie". It visualizes thus two large balloons in the chest that it brings together in a single. This balloon, you will inflate in inspiring, doing enter the air in your rib cage. But you decide a little arbitrarily not to move the thorax, a little as if you had a hand on top to prevent dilate. As this balloon inflates and that it is "trapped in this cage", it cannot then that descend, grow toward the bottom.

In reality, it is the diaphragm which is going to be pushed to the bottom. When it goes down, the mass of the abdominal viscera will be compressed. As this mass can not go in rear of the fact of the presence of the coasts and the vertebral column, it will have a tendency to "Exit" in front. It is for this reason that it is said that the "belly inflates". This is not the air that between in the belly!

Then in a second time, you "tuck" the belly. Suddenly, the abdominal viscera date back to top, support on the diaphragm. The fact of this compression, the two lungs are emptied and the expiration then occurs.

One of the great advantages of this mechanism respiratory, is to do work what is called the basis of the lungs. When one breathes only by at the top, it breathes only by the summits. However, it is necessary to know that all the toxins and pollution, waste, tend, the fact of the gravity, to go toward the base of the lungs. The simple fact of practicing this breathing allows all of these wastes to be mobilized and to be evacuated from the lungs.

The manner in which this movement comes to be described makes this abdominal breathing excessively simple to understand. I inspire, the Belly "fate" and I breath, the Belly "fit".

316

Often such as respiration reversed is become a reflex conditioning, some have difficulties to learn this natural breath. Then, an image additional mental: You receive a punch in the belly, which triggers a sudden expiration. Then the air between again in the lungs and the Belly "spring".

The Breathing abdomino-diaphragmatic

But next to that, you could implement what is called the "breathing conscious". Conscious breathing is primarily a "diaphragmatic breathing," often known under the term also "ventral breathing" or even "abdomino-diaphragmatic".

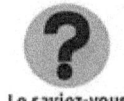

Le saviez-vous

If you have the opportunity to see a baby in the cradle, you can observe that it breathes only by the belly. Later, very many habits of life were finished by " reverse " our breathing. The layers of babies too tight, belts preventing any respiratory amplitude, some bodily Gymnastics We doing inspire by pulling the shoulders back.

All this has an impact not only on the amount of air that we inhale, but it does not work then mostly that the summit of its lungs.

Could we not say that the level of evolution not hardware, but of spiritual a people was directly linked to their clothing habits? Robes, gandouras," "dresses of the scholars, etc. The more or less large respiratory amplitude directly affects the oxygenation of our neurons!

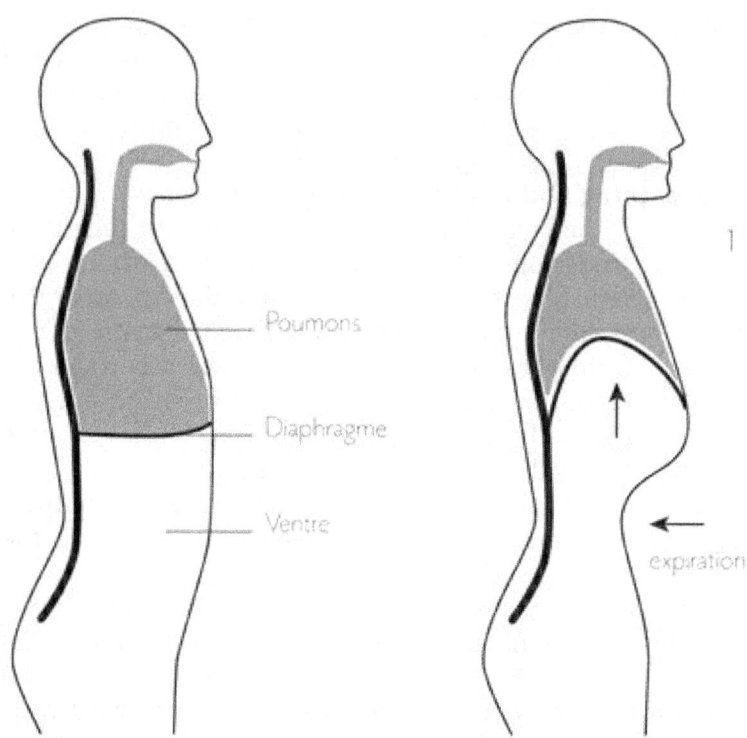

Figure 17-1 The breathing abdomino-diaphragmatic.

If we are talking of the diaphragm?

The diaphragm is in reality the main muscle of respiration.

However, these are the accessory muscles of respiration that have become the main muscles, among all those who have a respiration known as reversed. These muscles are among others the intercostal muscles or the muscles sternocleidomastoid muscles. This are the muscles that draw toward the top the coasts to open a little more the thoracic cage. They are visible at the time of the crises of asthma or among the respiratory insufficient. This is what is called in the medical jargon a "Draw respiratory". But it is the diaphragm which is the main muscle of respiration.

However, to be even more powerful in this type of exercise, it is necessary to know a minimum of his anatomy.

The diaphragm is a double cupola tendino-muscular that divides in two Our trunk, which separates the chest of the abdomen.

From there, it should view the next thing: the heart which is in the thoracic cage as well as the two lungs are "posed" on the diaphragm. Below the diaphragm, you have the liver-gallbladder, to the right of your abdomen, the stomach, the solar plexus to the center, as well as the part of the transverse colon and the Rate-Pancréas right, as well as the kidneys in rear. All these bodies are in direct contact with this pad tendino-muscle.

It is easy to realize that this area is fundamental. When, little by little, you'll unlock and do work your diaphragm, thanks to this breathing, hypotonic, it will find a certain force and especially its mobility. In effect, it will regain its amplitude. It can go up to 15-20 cm amplitude, between the movements of raising and lowering in the chest. We then speak of a release of the diaphragm.

The virtues of the ventral breathing

You will massage directly all these internal organs between other liver, true sponge in blood. And all of this by the raising and lowering of the diaphragm. That is the fundamental point of this breath.

You will avoid that stagnations persist and that they generate heat, the pain, inflammation, swelling, the transformation of waste as poisons to the origin of almost all the internal diseases.

À retenir

Another effect of this respiration, and not the least: a little more top, we saw that in the unconscious breaths we exchanged between 300 and 500 cc of air between the inspires and the expires. When we practice this type of breathing abdomino-diaphragmatic, we exchange between 3 000 and 7 000 cc of air, or 10 times more. At the time, we do not need as much energy. All the surplus will therefore we used to recharge our battery of the kidney.

The Sleep and respiration are the two main ways that Dame Nature has placed at our disposal for this recharge.

Once this respiration baseline well assimilated, we will be able to graft a multitude of exercises. Our master we had learned the three that I am going to present you expose.

Just a small caveat. At the end of a few days of practice, you may have of the frictions, Small contractures especially under the ribs. This is where attaches the diaphragm. It is quite normal.

Attention

This are simple contractures related to working a muscle which for too long has been left to the rest. Do not consult for as much!

Some will be afraid to practice by fear of "take the belly". But it is quite the opposite that happens. The more you "get out the belly", more the transverse muscles and other abdominal muscles will have to work for "return" This same belly. The result of the race, this type of exercise makes you lose belly.

The three years of the Pr Leung

These three exercises will act on virtually all of the Panel of pathologies that we not create to not by ignorance of the functioning of our body. This action will also be well, preventive and curative. Two exercises will lie on the ground or in his bed, and an exercise that you are going to implement throughout the day, and this, in any position.

A particularity as to the exercises that the will be practiced lying: for a better visualization, it will inspire by the nose and it will blow through the mouth to channel the breath. With respect to those charged throughout the day, the inspires and the expires will be only by the nose to prevent drying of the nasal false.

The breathing to wake up in full form in the morning

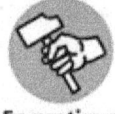

Better than the shower or coffee in the morning. This exercise must be practiced in the morning at sunrise before install the feet by earth. You go when even prevent your spouse before to avoid that it does not call for any of following the UAS.

En pratique

In effect, this breathing will be quite violent.

"I inspired at maximum of my possibilities quickly enough and I shall expire just as quickly by emptying completely the lungs. "

Avoid you raise in the minute or two minutes that follow: In effect, you will be temporarily shooté to oxygen, which may trigger some dizziness.

You will as well practice two sets of ten breaths aware.

First Effect: When you are going to breathe by the belly in a manner quite violent, making climb up and down your diaphragm, you will physically massage the liver and oblige the blood to leave toward the ends. If you practice this type of breathing every morning for a couple of days, you will see that your hands and your feet will start to warm up. It is the blood that sets out again toward the ends.

Second Effect: thanks to this inflow of blood very fast at the level of the brain, you will achieve much more quickly the state of full consciousness. It is the best way to wake up.

Third effect: the fact to mobilize the "belly" and the abdominal viscera, by these movements to and fro in the belly and in the diaphragm, will trigger what is called the "intestinal peristalsis" which has slowed during a whole night of sleep. There is then a large chance that you have at the time the desire to go to the saddle.

Therefore a simple exercise can you massage the liver, avoid its congestion, its problems of stagnation, but also all other internal organs and this, as soon as the morning. It leads you to the time ten times more oxygen than a breath unconscious, she wakes you up and also allows you to clean your intestines.

The Breathing For insomniacs

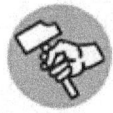

En pratique

Blow the candle to better fall asleep. This exercise will be the evening before going to bed. We will also be able to practice it during the periods of insomnia. Especially insomnia in second part of night again called "insomnia of three hours of the morning," which is directly linked to a stagnation of blood and energy at the level of the liver.

The evening before you fall asleep, when you are in your bed, you'll practice two series of ten breaths, but different from the previous ones. You leave quietly air to penetrate by your nostrils, without forcing the inspiration. Then you imagine that you have a candle in front of you and when you breathe out, the flame must almost do not move. The expiry will therefore be very slow and progressive. This expiratory time can be done in 30, 40 seconds, or even with the drive, a minute. You should never be out of breath. It is therefore appropriate to stop before arriving in the Apnea, blocking respiratory. On this exercise respiratory, you will be able to add a viewing. Can you imagine that the air you breathe is white, immaculate and nourish your body. The air that you will expire much longer is an air a little grayish, responsible of toxins from your body. It is all the waste of the body that are going. It is realized that thanks to this visualization, it could boost the elimination of waste by the expiry, especially at the base of our lungs. Remember, it is the mental energy, the power of our thoughts that direct all physical phenomena to the inside of our body.

When you make such a practice, another phenomenon will occur. If we had to speak here of fatigue in general, "I am tired", one of the major causes comes from the excess of thoughts. Our brain is in permanent boiling and our thoughts occur without interruption. It is a great cause insomnia, or at least this prevents us from having a deep sleep.

The whole purpose of this technique is to allow us to channel gradually all our thoughts on a single, namely the visualization of the respiration. It is a little as if you stop your computer Central, a little as if you disconnect.

À retenir

In a computer, you hear a noise: This is the fan which allows in permanence to cool the vital elements of the operation of such a machine. And the more you give work to do, calculations To perform, more the fan will rotate faster. If it fails, it is overheating and your computer grid. If we do not break through our breathing our "body-computer" and if our thoughts occur at a frantic pace, this "masturbation of the mind" will eventually produce a last symptom alarm signal: the burn-out. It is the body-spirit which at the end of a time disconnects. It sends you as the last alarm signal a profound lassitude, a pre-Depression until the burn-out requires you to refit complement. Respiration in full awareness of the kind that I have just you describe is the antidote to this state. In channelling your mental, you arrive gradually to only one thought : respiration. You are no longer that breathing.

Then you will see that you will fall asleep much more easily.

You can add a "ingredient" in this exercise: When you are in a period of insomnia, leave the air enter "without forcing", then the expiry is done very slowly. This represents a respiratory cycle. You are going to put you to count mentally these cycles, a little as we count sheep to fall asleep. A inspires and a expires equal to 1, and then a second cycle up to 10. At 10, you leave at 1 and you go up to 9. At 9, you leave at 1 and go up to 8 and so on... As a general rule, at the end of the third cycle, you are already returned in the Arms of Morpheus. The simple fact of channelling your thoughts on a single point, here the counting allows you sleeping very quickly. Made the experience the next time that you have this insomnia of three hours of the morning.

The breathing to manage his emotions

In the evening, 2 times 10 breaths, 2 times 10 in the morning, it makes us 40 breaths aware. Where are we going to put our 260 Other breaths in the day? This is where we come to a fundamental concept in MTC, "the full conscience".

In a day in reality, you have a plethora of moments that we could call "time death" and you think too much during these moments the dead.

In reality, in the day, you are quite capable of stop you, here, here and now, as do spontaneously the children after a period of hyperactivity. They stop, arise and one has the impression that they no longer believe in nothing, they are elsewhere.

For example you are at a red light, or in a plug, rather than leave you invade and phagocytose by your thoughts, you are going to say: "would like, I will take the opportunity to do so during 30-40 seconds 7, 8, 10, or even more breaths aware. "And this, that you are in any position, standing in train to walk, sitting in front of your computer, etc., you breathe quietly by the nose, without necessarily force its abdominal breathing, then you breathe out through the nose.

The breathing is ample, abdominal, but not forced and is done in full conscience. From the outside, the people do not realize your practice.

At that time, not only you exchange when even between 2 000 and 4 000 cc of air, 10 times more than a breath unconscious, but the day where you are able to stop you as this 10, 20, 30 times in the day by breathing in a dozen times in full consciousness to each time, so between 2 and 300 breaths, you will touch of the finger, you will progressively introduce you to: "Here and Now".

The simple fact to stop several times in the day can only be beneficial for your health. All the activities that you have in the day, in the morning at sunrise until the evening at bedtime, are activities which have an action that could be called as centrifugal to the issuance of your energy. You tap into your internal energy, in your battery, and you the issue toward the outside. One could say that it is the Yang which escapes from the body. So when you talk, think, move your joints, digest a food bowl, etc., all this request of the energy.

À retenir

If you do not take in the day, the time to recharge this energy that is escaped of the body, you would end up having to exhaust your reserves, by empty your battery. Conversely, if you stop from time to time 30, 40 seconds, each time that you breathe in full conscience 3 000 to 5 000 cc of air, you are in the process of recharge your battery you just to unload.

The master word in MTC, in the methods Yang Sheng FA of preservation of life is: "I discharge, I load, I discharge, I load continuously throughout a same day", while in our western way of life, "I discharge, I discharge, up to exhaustion of the morning until the evening. I try as well as to recharge the night by the sleep, during weekends or holidays. "But this is a Utopia, because your body at that time will be in dispersion of energy due to this excess of fatigue (MTC, c is the yin who is no longer able to retain the Yang) and you will not reach you reload. However, we learn here to We reload in a same day !!!!!

Why and how the full conscience?

You can reach the state of full consciousness, the here and now, thanks to the meditation. But it may be that the full awareness of those who meditate is not the same full consciousness which I am talking to you.

What then is the purpose of this full conscience? Learn how to manage our emotions! An emotion in Chinese medicine is to put in relationship with the energy of a software specific body and that is the energy of the heart that generates and regulates the whole of emotions. We then speak in MTC, the shen, of the Spirit.

Each family of emotion is therefore directly related to the operation of each component (see chapitre 2). If it is attached to study a type of emotion such as anger, sadness, fear, Reminiscence we could go as far as to say that you are the writer, the screenwriter, director and at the same time the actor.

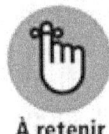

À retenir There is always the causal links in the crescendo of the emotion. But at the outset, there is a first image, which is juxtaposes a second, and then another and yet another. It is as well as takes place the film. The full awareness allows us to stop at the first image.

Spiritualité I breathe so I do not think more!

The full awareness of meditators is to arrive at a non-Total thinking. And who said then non-thought, said non-time. It is a little complicated to explain, but to make it short, we can say that the time exists because there is a before and after, the two poles Yin-Yang of duality. Because there is a past and because there is a future, there is between the two a "passage to empty", because two thoughts cannot be juxtaposed. Basically the full awareness, as defined at the level of our practices, does not really exist, because it is also the time. Neurobiologists have tried to give their own vision on the notion of time. They depart from the principle that we issue in permanence of thoughts.

Except that between two thoughts, there are a few milliseconds where there is nothing. The meditators try to gradually increase the duration of this vacuum between two thoughts to arrive to the non-thinking. We could call it the awakening. But as far as we are concerned, before to get there, we would have to generations and generations of "reincarnation" or hours of daily practice well incompatible with our current way of life. When we talk about health, preservation of the health, when we speak of full consciousness, it is: "I am here, I focus my thinking on a point for channelling and stop the flow of thoughts" and conscious breathing allows us to effectively achieve this state.

It is in this sense that one learns to manage his emotions, to do that in a family discussion, it does not pronounce a word assassinates capable of destroying a family. You are in full control and you do not play the movie until the end. You stop at the first image.

It is not a question to become beings" has-emotional", without emotion. Emotions are mandatory for a good functioning of the body and allow to feed, feed energetically different software components. On the other hand, it should not be that an emotion is too violent for a single blow or that an Emotion is always in permanently above the other.

We like this at our disposal methods of regulation of emotions and the full consciousness in fact part. This full conscience, you will learn through respiration, thanks to these multi-stops in the day.

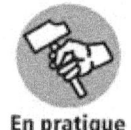

How do I enter the breathing in our genes

In any act of change whatever it is, you will pass by four successive steps. At the outset, there is

En pratique what we might call a unconscious incompetence which will then transform in incompetence conscience. Then you have the stage of Conscious Competence, until arriving to the jurisdiction unconsciousness.

"Initially, you had no notion as to the crucial importance that represents the respiration and of everything that you bring such practices. You did not have access to the knowledge and by the same token, you could not invent it.

"Then, pass on to this second phase which is the Incompetence Conscious. That is to say that now you know that it exists, you are still incompetent since you have not yet implemented. It is a step a little critical because to force back to next day the practice, you may forget it. And even persuade you that this does not work and why not, you return against the traditional teachings.

But if you request: Since this morning, how many times have you breathed in full conscience? I leave you to answer this question. You may then to make you feel guilty: "I know that I should implement this, but I do not get there. "If you then have the chance to meet someone who is able to explain to you what is the passage to the Act, self-confidence, and how practice, you'll spend in the phase of Conscious Competence.

"The Conscious Competence is the repetition, again and again, all of these exercises. But this is not done overnight. It takes about a year, to learn how to breathe in full conscience! You will practice, abandon, the reinstall, etc.

"At a certain time, you are going to reach the phase of the permanent self-regulation: is the Competence Unconscious. You do realize even more account that you practice this type of breathing, it will become almost automatic. And there, you will have made the real work of the initiation by being spent by these four steps. I hope from the bottom of my heart that you arrive all to this step.

Chapter 18
Dao Yin
Or exercises of Health
<u>In this chapter:</u>
<u>" The concept of exercises according to Traditional Chinese Medicine</u>
<u>" The two major types of practices of the Dao Yin</u>
<u>" The Art of Qi Gong</u>
<u>" Meditation, mode of employment</u>
The concept of exercise in MTC
What do we mean by physical exercises in MTC? Our Western culture was too much of a tendency to obscure the concept of internal exercise and when we speak of exercises, we immediately think of sports, gymnastics, or other external practices. We will see that there is a very important difference between the concept of Western sport and the Chinese exercises known under the name of Dao Yin IN MTC.
When we practice a sport, one of the first characteristics is that our mind, our spirit are totally mobilized toward a single goal to know defeat, Win, surpass themselves, when it does not become the object of a State narcissistic exacerbated.

Le saviez-vous

From the vision of energy in the body based on the Yin-Yang, sport is of a nature Yang: It has a centrifugal action on energy. When typing on a tennis ball, in a balloon, when short, it draws on its reserves, its battery of the kidney to produce this type of movement. But if we do not take care, the reserves may be squander very quickly, and the body break very quickly. A high level sportsman is to retire at 40 years!

Another requirement of the practice of Dao Yin, c is the very important concept of regularity, not to say of the everyday. In effect, the ideal would be to practice a half-hour of sport, walking or gymnastics movements, without reaching the stage of fatigue. We could say: "Too much sport of a single blow kills the sport. "However, in the West, we are too often of the practitioners of the Sunday, by jerking.

À retenir

Too often the sports practiced in the West promote excessive perspiration. At the beginning, a slight perspiration is beneficial. It is a transpiration of

328

surface that cleans the skin. In contrast, when it becomes excessive, it will "exhaust the heart". In effect, it will take its source in the organic liquids in the exhausting. An Antidote passenger will be the decision of drinks moisturizing as the green tea. All this will be developed in the chapter on the Dietetics.

The sport in too much of a tendency in the West to be separated from our daily activities. However, conscious breathing and certain movements can be practiced throughout a day.

When you are sitting for example, the fact to keep you well right without the support of a folder tones the muscles of your back and your belly. The walk in full conscience only concentrated on the respiration is another example of a "sport" daily. The same that climb the stairs rather than take the elevator. Thousand gestures of daily life can transform into external exercises provided of course to never forget the respiration.

Attention

The addicts of Sport

The muscles are to be put in relation with the software RATE IN MTC. Liver and spleen are in direct relationship. The excess muscle work causes secretion of endotoxin at the level of the liver which is responsible, in others, of the States of lack, of dependency. The sport practiced at high dose can become a drug. To force of practice Yang, the individual will deplete its yin. Yet the Yin, it is the ancestral oil, the oil lamp. At the end of the path, c is the early aging.

And a grand council! Never say: "I know my limits ! "It is already too late since you have already affected. It must learn the way of the JUST Middle, find a balance and avoid particularly changes in habit too brutal.

What is the Dao Yin?

Dao Yin is a term very ancient at heavy connotation of energy in its definition. Since we are going more and more toward the materiality, the term much more modern is YUN DONG: Yun to move and Dong, Move, Move. It is the modern sport as we know it.

We will therefore here the term Dao Yin who will be the precursor of another generic term, a little happening-everywhere, that we all know: The qi gong.

In the **Nei Jing, it is said that: "For all diseases of stagnation and accumulation, it is appropriate to the times to use the Dao Yin and Yao, drugs. " It was on a same pedestal these two practices.**

In Dao Yin:

Dao" means "Lead", "govern", but also "be directed". Attention, this is not the same DAO Taoists which means the track.

"**Yin** wants to say here "guide".

"So the Dao Yin implements some techniques for lead, guide the blood and energy. In fact, the purpose of these practices and to promote the free movement of blood and energy, to prevent blockages and stagnations can be put in place.

All the techniques met under this word also allow to recharge the battery of the kidney, therefore to increase the immune defenses and the faculties of adaptation and self-healing of the body.

The different types of Dao Yin

Dao Yin can be divided into two major types of practices. We will have as well the Dao Yin liabilities and the Dao Yin active.

Dao Yin liabilities

It is the therapist who runs, the patient, him, receives. What are all the techniques of massage, digitoponcture which we have discussed at length earlier. In effect, the therapist will be able to press the points of acupuncture, massage some special places, carrying out movements to and fro on the skin with the arms, pinch, Pull, rub, push, knead. But also make the friction, vibration, percussion. The different "manipulation" fall within this framework of the Dao Yin liabilities.

But there is another aspect of this Dao Yin liabilities. These are practices which consisted in letting go or to concentrate on a particular point. We will return there. What are all the techniques of meditation.

Dao Yin Active

It is the patient himself who must practice. To begin under the supervision of a master of Dao Yin or a seasoned practitioner, and then everything alone, once the initiation phase completed.

There are different types of Dao Yin assets which will be called by the following "qi gong assets".

A Dao Yin which concerns the movement of the body, the exercises known as "external".

These include the game of the five animals, Wu Qin Xi, put in place by a famous doctor of the Han Dynasty, Hua Tou. It is a qi gong external, but at the same time a martial art. It contains 10 movements based on the imitation of "five animals" (two movements per animal). As well, there is the Tiger which is about to pounce, the movement imitating the approach of the bear, the movement of the deer, monkey, the bird.

Later emerged the "eight embellishments," or "eight pieces of brocard ", Ba Duan Jin, commonly practiced in the Buddhist temples, in particular by the Shaolin Monks. This are eight exercises relatively simple to remember. Each fiscal year has a name very practical for that. Include: "support the sky with the hands to take care of the three households," "bander The CRA and aim the Eagle", "support the sky and rely on the earth to stimulate the Rate-Estomac a single gesture"...

Still later became the tai-chi-chuan, "boxing of the Supreme Ridge". It is a sequence that consists of 75 to 108 movements, depending on the different forms. It is at the same time a martial art and at the same time an external exercise of health. Several schools compete for paternity as the school Shen, the school Yang, the school Wu... Based on the rooting to land, the inverse of an exercise of physical force, it will be

331

characterized by a force flexible, dynamic. The body is in complete relaxation during the practice which ensures the fluidity of movement as well as their coordination. To make it short, we can say that it is the pinnacle of Qi Gong.

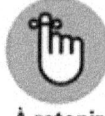

À retenir The tai-chi-chuan fact work not only the body but also the mind. It is an exercise of Meditation in Movement. When it is practiced in an appropriate manner, it can be very powerful to help treat and prevent many internal diseases such as cancer.

Then appeared the Wu Shu. When the movements, pathways are practiced quickly, it is a martial art. When the sequences are slowly, it is a qi gong external.

Attention There are still other Dao Yin external. For example those who are to direct and channel the breath on such and such a place of the body. We can still pair respiration with the emission of certain sounds.

But made attention. To practice this type of Dao Yin, it should be absolutely to be accompanied by a master at the time of the initiation.

Some sounds can heal

The **Nei Jing** has established the classification of five sounds, each corresponding to one of the five elements, of five movements. As well, it was the sounds:

"Gong, +/ - Our do which corresponds to the earth, the spleen;

"Shang, +/ - Re, which corresponds to the metal, to the lung;

"Jiao, +/ - MI, which corresponds to the wood, the liver;

"Zhi +/ - ground, connected to the fire, heart;

"Yu, +/ - The, connected to the water, kidney.

This type of Dao Yin is to issue a of the five sounds that, used appropriately, can act on the IQ of the organs, stimulate the circulation of blood and energy. The his Gong is the more serious, it is a very deaf. Going back in the range, one then has the its Shang, then in the middle, nor too acute, nor too deaf, the its Jiao. Regarding its Zhi, it is much more acute that Jiao and its the most acute is the sound Yu.

This is not for nothing that the acute tinnitus of type "Song of cicada" may appear when a weakness of the Yin of the kidney (the ears are the opening of the kidney in MTC).

In the past in China, very early in the morning, the masters of the methods Yang Sheng Fa, maintenance of the vitality, rose to go regularly to practice in the nature this type of Dao Yin. The important point in the emission of these five sounds is that these five notes must fit the Dan Tian, under the navel. It is the Qi of the Dan Tian which emits the sound, which rises in the throat.

The combination of all these Dao Yin is called Qi Gong At the present time. We will talk as well of Qi Gong calm and Qi Gong assets. These different types of practices bequeathed by the Taoists have as the first purpose, the maintenance of the Vitality. Practiced on a long period of time and with attendance, they bring a better-be both on the physical plane, that mental. These practices can also extend the life.

It should not be forgotten that one of the first goals of Taoism is to preserve its own health, the vitality of his body in order to be able to live for a long time, and thereby arrive at the full development of his Spirit.

The art of Qi Gong

Since time immemorial, in their methods as well preventive and curative, the different civilizations have put in place, series of movements which had as a vocation to go even further than a simple body gymnastics. In India, called this type of movements yoga. In China, originally called Dao Yin, the name the more common in the West is the qi gong. That is yoga or Qi Gong, their purposes will be the same: to combine the flexibility of joints, conscious breathing and meditation in movement.

 However, attention not to seek too quickly to achieve certain postures of yoga. If you start this type of practices to the fifties, your joints will of course be more steep, and you may trigger certain pathologies joints. We will see that the Qi Gong will be then can be more suitable for many people.

Attention

The term Gong sub-intends a direction, an effect, an effort and Qi is the energy. The Qi Gong is the mastery of the Qi, of the vital energy.

The qi gong. Everyone has heard of. But it is true that the there is a loses a little. In effect, there are thousands of Qi Gong, as well as Chinese masters and when you go to know the essential laws, you, why not, create your own series.

The goals of the practice of Qi Gong

We are going to see that such a practice is aimed at three goals essential to know how to keep the flexibility of its joints, breathe in full conscience to feed and circulate the energy in the body. And finally to stop our cognitive faculties, our excesses of thought which we tired to length of day.

Level 1: Conservation of the flexibility of joints

Look at this more closely and consider the following example: you decide to mount your two hands, arms stretched out in front of you, up to the vertical and the back on the sides, in such a way that the Hands espouse the shape of the body. It is a qi gong.

If you are viewing the movement of your wrist, it is sometimes in hyperflexion, then in hyperextension. Similarly, the Elbow will be at a time completely declined and another time extended. Finally, your shoulders are going to make a complete movement of external rotation. With a single motion, you just make work three joints!

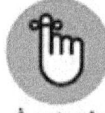 A good series of Qi Gong will be able to make work all the joints, in the aim to keep the flexibility.

But, as the body is traversed by a mesh of energy networks, this articular mobilization will also act

À retenir on the various meridians of the body and mobilize the energy. Where the name given to this type of movements, "IQ" wanting to say energy and "gong", movement.

Let us remember the chapter on the meridians. At the level of each articulation, we find six meridians, three Yin and three Yang. However, these meridians are directly in relationship with each of the internal organs. In retaining the flexibility of joints, we encourage the free movement of blood and energy at the level of software five bodies.

Level 2: The respiration in the center of the practice

In China, when we are going early in the morning in the public spaces, we see a very large number of practitioners and what resonates and a little disturbing the western, it is the extreme slowness of these movements! Modern life, while explosion of Yang, encourages us to implement practices that do not support the idle speed: it runs fast, always more quickly, it jumps. In short, we are trying to catch up with our shadow!

Resuming the same movement: When you mount the arm to the vertical, you inhale very slowly and trying to make a ventral breathing. When the arms collapsed on the side, you exhale while also slowly. It is for this reason that the movement is slow. It is fair punctuated by respiration.

A Qi Gong is before any led by respiration. To such a point that when the serial that you have chosen to practice has somehow become a "Competence Unconscious", a gesture automatic

À retenir

without involvement of the Shen, thought, you are no longer that "breathing".

And during a series that lasts 15-20 minutes, you have breathed more than a hundred times on the 300 cycles respiratory " in full conscience" that you should do in the day.

Not only the Qi Gong frees the circulation of blood and energy in relaxing the joints, but in a second step it can recharge the battery of the kidney, thanks to this hyperventilation.

Level 3: a meditation exercise in movement

This type of practice is still well beyond. Let us take the image of a sphere to represent the conscious, our cognitive faculties, the whole of the information received by our five senses, ego, our me and the inside another sphere, that of the subconscious with, to deep it, our spiritual soul, the Hun.

Our mode of life" "modern" has for consequence to create a true weave of conscious, a carapace preventing us to listen to the "Voice of the soul".

Once infected, the first two steps of the Qi Gong, it becomes a real exercise of "movement meditation". Little by little, to force of daily practices, we break this armor and we are creating a funnel between conscious and subconscious.

Our master taught us that each of us possesses a number of donations, and one of the consequences of these practices is to be traced back to the surface.

But especially, during the time of the practice, we stop to "think", we put in Standby our computer that is too often at the edge of the overheating, the "burn-out".

Little by little, to force of practices, you will learn how to live in full conscience and by that same again become the general-in-Chief of the functioning of your body. Thanks to "Here and Now", I am able to stop me at the first sign of a anger and to avoid trigger a mental tsunami.

Exercise of Qi Gong

En pratique

"1. Slightly bend the arms and lift the above the head, fingers and wrists casual. As soon as you start to lift the arms in front of you, inspire, and hold this inspiration until the arms are perfectly to the vertical.

2. Bend your knees, exhale and start to crouch. During the squat, keep the body right. At the same time, lower the arm and bend your elbows so that the hands go back.

3. Lower the hands along the legs. Raise-you, lift the arm and inhale deeply. Repeat the exercise ten to twenty times. "

Important: The movements must be carried out slowly and gradually. The Breathing must also be deep and regular as possible.

The first part involves the meridian of the bladder especially in the top of the back, where the points are controlling the lung, the heart and blood circulation. In the second part, it is the whole of the meridian of the stomach which is actuated. This Qi Gong prevents hypertension and chronic diseases. The physical movement activates the blood circulation and digestion. It improves the respiratory functions, strengthening the muscles of the chest and abdomen.

Should we be afraid of Qi Gong?

Often, false ideas are conveyed with respect to these practices. Some people are going to put in before the dangerousness of practices in Solitaire without permanently be directed. Certainly, there is a need at the outset a professor, a master who will teach us a series. But once the series well integrated, it is necessary to know to detach itself from the pole.

À retenir

The practice of the Qi Gong is a solitary act. There must be only one, face to itself, in close relationship with Mother Earth and the sky creator.

Can you imagine that, because the movement does not reach a certain perfection, we will "fall sick"!

In reality, if you are asked at the outset a certain accuracy, it is for you to be focused on the movement in order to disperse all ideas parasites. This allows you gradually to the vacuum in the mind. Then, the movements will have a certain "roundness" for that energy can circulate more freely, with fluidity.

But if at the outset, joint stiffness prevents you from accessing the proper movement, this has no species of importance. And even, the fact of the symmetry of the Movement, this can be an excellent way to recover the total amplitude of the articulation enraidie.

In reality, the Qi Gong can actually contain a certain "danger" if it is practiced in order to obtain something, a power, a gift. At this time, the Spirit is tense. Similarly, if we focus to bring the energy in such or such a zone of the body, and which is more, if we do not know to circulate the accumulated energy, this can generate stagnations localized.

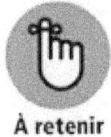

À retenir

337

From the time of the practice in order to maintain a good health, by releasing taken, by being in the felt, a Qi gong will only have positive effects on our health.

Similarly, we must not fall into the pitfall west of "Always Growing". No need to become a "collector of movements". To quote a phrase very known in the practice of martial arts: "I am not afraid of the person who knows a thousand techniques, but who has not practiced only once. But I am afraid I more than any one who knows of only one blow and who has practiced a thousand times. "

It should be fair to learn a series which "makes work all the joints, which act on all the meridians of energy and on all internal organs". Of the series very known in China as the "eight pieces of Brocard", the "Game of the five animals" obey these criteria. We talked about in the introduction.

When a Master has taught you a series, it is the one that you are going to have to practice on a daily basis, why not all your life. And one day, if you have the time or the inclination, you can introduce you to the "Tai chi chuan". It is as well a martial art that a "qi gong improved". To make it short, it is the "Pinnacle of Qi Gong". But to learn, it is appropriate to have a master, see once or twice a week and to give two or three years to master this art.

A series of Qi Gong can be learned in a few weeks.

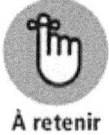

À retenir

The daily practice of Qi Gong can become the essential element in the battery of methods of prevention of Alzheimer's disease, in "the art of aging well," in the prevention of cancers and many other pathologies yet. By its joint actions for the Liberation of blood circulation and energy, charging the battery of the kidney, change of our profile mental and psychological, this practice will allow us to live the rest of our life, in all serenity. The single view of the centenarians, China, who practice on a daily basis and that we know they will not senile, should give us the envy to practice this "art of health" as regularly as possible. While being a meditation exercise in movement, the Qi Gong assets operate mainly on the flexibility of the joints and the circulation of blood and of energy. It is one of the reasons for which, it is better practice in the morning, with the jump of the bed. In effect the sleep, which has enabled us to recharge our batteries, has also had the result of us numb. This morning practice allows you to find our flexibility and especially to allow blood and energy to circulate to the ends, in particular at the level of the brain.

The Jumper of iron, between Qi Gong calm and active

There are parallel to this practice an excellent exercise that I invite you here also to put the most often possible implementation.

The four muscles of the most important of the Organization in direct relation with the energy of the kidney are: the quadriceps, the gluteal muscles, the lower part of the abdomen, and the puborectalis muscle. However, a single exercise can make them work all four, and well of other muscles again. It is the position called " The cavalier of iron".

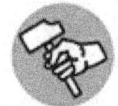

The position of the Jumper of iron, My Bu in Chinese, is done legs hand and on the other of the body in a wide position, the feet are parallel and directed to the front, the knees are bent and the bust is toward the front the more right possible.

En pratique

You must find a middle position between the hyperlordose and the hypercyphose. The top of the body remains free. 50% of the weight rests on each foot. You must have the air to be seated with the legs apart. It is a position that must become very stable. The more the feet are parallel, more the position is static. Attention not to descend too low at the beginning.

The rule is that we must not feel excessive tension in the knees. In some practices of endurance by kung-fu, we can go up to eat in this position. Very quickly, you will feel the aforementioned muscles become as hard as concrete. And in this position, you contract the muscles of the pelvic floor, as if you wanted to raise something of the earth with the testes to the man.

The energy level, it is said that "This exercise contains the internal energy of the Dan Tian the bottom away, by separating them from the surrounding energy". With this position opens the energy channel from the bottom, which is linked to the energy of the earth. The perineal membrane is relaxs more, which spontaneously produces its activation energy.

At the beginning, you do will keep this movement that a few minutes but with the training you can take a quarter of an hour or more. It is an exercise that you can do for example by brushing the teeth, or to many other moments in the day.

The meditation for all

We will now see another type of exercise capable to rebalance our character, our emotions, harmonizing the energies Yin and Yang in our body. It is meditation that is also called Qi Gong calm.

 Its essential role is to "feed the Yin" of the body, recharge the battery of the kidney. By practicing this Qi Gong calm very regularly, it progressively acquires the ability to control his spirit and energy, but it also gives to the Organization the capacity to autoguérir and to adapt to whatever situation.

À retenir

Meditation, mode of employment

The practice of meditation that we will discover could be called "the meditation of the middle". In fact, too often, we tend to go in practices complicated, not adapted to our western way of life, to our inheritance. And the fruit that we could remove such practices are far from being on the appointments and may even from time to time turn against us. This is the theory of the Shaver of Occam: The explanation or the simple practice of a fact has a greater chance to be true that an explanation or a practice complicated.

First point: Prepare

It is preferable to be dressed in clothes detailed, think of many relaxing its neck, would be this only by small massages or friction with the hands.

Just prior to sit, we should practice some movements, some stretching to relax his body.

It is also appropriate to take a few deep breaths to relieve the tensions of the body, to release the spirit of its concerns. Traditionally, we practice as well three deep breaths.

It is very important to forget his worries before to meditate.

À retenir **The second point: the good position**

When we begin this type of practice at an average age or advanced, there is no need to take positions such as the lotus or the half-lotus. In effect, the joints are often steep. These positions tend to block the circulation of blood and energy and to become very uncomfortable. It is the opposite of what we want to achieve in this type of practice.

"

It is better to just sit on a chair, the legs in a relaxd position, hips, knees and feet to 90 degrees. The En pratique dorsal column must be well right, the chin slightly reduced toward the chest to straighten the cervical spine.

" The chair should be neither too high nor too soft.
" The dos will not in contact with the folder.
" The eyes must not be lost in the far, but "watch without See "almost a meter in front of itself.
" It absolutely must be seated so comfortable and natural, relaxd, totally relaxd.

341

"Progressively the muscles of the shoulders, the hands, feet, arms, legs, face relax. One has the impression to issue then a slight smile inside.

Third point, respiration

It is the most important. It will be necessary to have previously learned to "breathe by the belly". The air absorbed in the chest will not dilate. We are going to push in the abdomen. When one expires, the abdomen is shrinking and the air is eliminated. In this mechanism, this are the lungs which expand toward the bottom, grow on the diaphragm.

When you breathe in this way, the relations between the organs are favored and especially, we fight against the Stagnations in blood and energy.

During the whole practice, our spirit does will therefore be concentrated on only one point, the respiratory motion. We will thus be able to free themselves from all thoughts.

Throughout the duration of the exercise, the inspiration is done by the nose and the expiry by the mouth barely ajar to better follow the exit out of the air.

It is very important in a meditation not to cause, but to follow his breathing.

Benchmarks for a good meditation

À retenir   The main purpose of this type of Qi Gong internal is to cultivate the inner calm which is yin to the opposite of the agitation which is yang. It is said that he "nourishes the Yin".

To force of regular practice, the character is changing. The Shen, the mind, the Spirit will calm down. It is a very particular, said of "full conscience", which is being put in place, state which allows the control of emotions by the Spirit, which is no longer agitated.

You can practice this posture two, three times per day.

If we had to choose, the best time to practice would be the evening. In effect, the end of the day

Le saviez-vous   is a critical time regarding the management of

342

emotions. The battery of the kidney is discharged during the whole day, and loses its role of control of "software organs". It is the hour of all TOC (obsessive-compulsive disorders) which range from bulimia, decision of alcohol or sweet flavors in excess. The parents have more patience with their children. It is the hour of the disputes, of conjugal violence. The revolutions, wars, conflicts of all sorts always begin the evening and that very rarely in the day !!!!!

Practice in the evening will allow to recharge powerfully this battery which then resumes the control.

The sleep of the end of the evening that will ensue will then be much more profound and repairer. This is a excellent exercise against the insomnia.

As to the duration of the practice, it may vary from one day to the other. A day that a few minutes and at other times why not a hour.

You focus therefore on the respiration, without forcing, you view, without the direct, the column of air into and out of your body. When appear of tensions or nervousness, it is important then to stop any of suite.

But the most important point is the everyday of the year for that this might have an impact on the character, the shen. Would it be only a few minutes of practice are sufficient to empty the spirit and to better respond to stress.

À retenir

And with a little training, you will be able to relax, letting go in any place.

It is at the price of such practices that we can achieve the longevity. In effect, this last is determined by the Preservation and the economy of the Ancestral oil. Not to touch it, it should be to have our battery recharged continuously. The Qi Gong internal is one of the exercises the more powerful to retain the Shen, the Spirit, in his body, and give our Hun, our spiritual soul, the desire to stay there.

Chapter 19
The Virtues Unknown
Of Sleep

ON cannot complete this part on the practices of the MTC without speaking of sleep. Sleep is a physiological act indispensable in our earthly life. In 100 years of life, we pass 33 years sleeping, more than a third of our life! It is characterized by a suspension of the vigilance, the conscience, what we have called the Shen in MTC, but also by a slowdown in certain metabolic functions (decrease in heart rate, respiratory, decrease of temperature...). All the muscles of the body will release. We can say that the man asleep is disconnected stimuli from the outside world.

Why is sleeping?

Sleep is the most natural way to recharge the battery of the kidney. It is the most effective method that we have inherited from Mother Nature.

In effect, always referring to the duality Yin-Yang, from the moment you wake up in the morning, all our acts of the day will have a centrifugal action on our energy. All acts of daily life such as talk, move, Digest, act, thinking and many others will be acts to Yang polarity. They will draw on our internal energy accumulated, in our battery.

But if we have not learned to well the recharge, if we sleep poorly, this battery is quickly going to unload throughout the day. And it is the fatigue which appears.

We have seen in the previous chapters that this battery was responsible for the self-regulation and the adaptation of the organism. If, at the end of the day, this battery is completely empty, our different software components will no longer be controlled.

In particular all TOC (obsessive-compulsive disorders) under the dependence of the Liver software will wake up. This is the moment when one starts to drink, where it rushes on its tablet chocolate, where one smokes more than reason.

But the anger belonging to the liver, as it is no longer controlled by the kidney, it is the time when the violence broke out. Have you noticed that the wars, revolutions do not begin that very rarely in the morning, but very often at the end of the evening?

A torture well known is to prevent a suspect to sleep. The batteries will be completely discharge. It is the ideal time to do confess or do a wash of brain. And if it takes too long, death can occur.

Tips for a good sleep

What position to take?

The best position is lying on the right side, the right leg elongated and the left leg folded slightly above.

If you lay on the left side, this is not too serious. You get tired just a little your heart which is compressed by the lung.

Some sleep on the back. But if their uvula, this small tab at the bottom of the gorge is a little swollen (power supply too loaded in Tan, in waste), c is the hum that appears, and your spouse was soon to make you back on the side.

"

Attention The "worst" positions is flat belly. Not only is this not a physiological position for your joints, especially of the neck, but you compress your rib cage and thus lose a large part of your respiratory capacity.

" The mattress must be relatively hard.

" The curvature physiology of the cervical column must be respected. Attention to the too big cushion.

" The well-ventilated room and not overheated. It is better to take a few blankets more than a superheated exhibit which dries the ambient air and exhaust (" hurts") fluids of the body.

Duration of Sleep

Le saviez-vous

It is said in the MTC that he should not sleep less than six hours per night and not more than eight hours.

"One hour more for a woman who, by its nature more yin that man, has need of more than recharging. We are talking here about the daily sleep and not that of the feast days.

"A child who is in full growth (the cell multiplication is directly put in relationship with the energy of the kidney) was in need of more sleep than an adult.

"A cerebral, of nature rather Yin, will need fewer hours of sleep that an athlete.

"An elderly person who does virtually more effort, among which the energy losses are less important, will need far fewer hours of sleep.

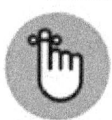

À retenir

But in a general way, an excess or a lack of chronic sleep is necessarily bad for the health.

The fact of sleep too long weakens the muscular system and by that same the software spleen. This can become the signature of a latent depression and have a harmful influence on the digestion of the food bowl and the transformation of food into energy.

A chronic deficit in hours of sleep prevents the Agency to rebuild its reserves. The immune defenses are dwindling, as well as the faculties of adaptation. Weakening of the protections of the body and diseases are at the end of the path.

It should also be to adapt to the rhythm of the seasons. In winter, the night being longer than the day, we will sleep more. In contrast, in the middle of the summer, we need fewer hours of sleep.

The Best Slots

If we refer to the day-night cycle, the day lit by the sun is the side Yang of the force. This is where the discharge its energy. On the other hand, the night is the side Yin of the force. It is at this time that we must recharge.

The best slots are located between 22 hours-23 hours up to 6-7 hours of the morning.

Starting from the principle that the optimal recharging your batteries is located around midnight (between 23 hours and 3 hours), if you lay all days to one hour of the morning and that you sleep your 8 hours, you lose when even a part of the recharging of the battery.

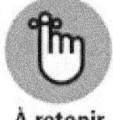

An essential element: the concept of regularity is a master word IN MTC. More than the slots, the danger comes of the rupture of rhythms especially when they are repetitive. It is difficult for example to recover in working three nights in a week and three days in the other. In the case of an obligation, it can remedy these "breaks" of PACE, in initiating the relaxation.

What is a sleep ideal?

When it is fully regulated, with a battery well recharged, a topic in good health must be able to fall asleep in the minutes which follow the sunset and wake up in full form without the aid of no alarm clock, the time that has been scheduled mentally the Eve.

There is another criterion in MTC. We must not remember his dreams.

It is considered that there are two types of Dreams: those to put in relation with the Emotions corresponding to the different software component. Another night activity: this is the information data by the Hun, the spiritual soul, housed in the liver. These are the famous "nocturnal intuitions".

Without s forward later in this type of consideration, it must know that remember his dreams may be the result of an excess of energy at the level of such or such a body. It is in fact part of diagnostic methods in MTC, with respect to the questioning (see chapitre 7).

When the person remembers some recurring dreams, he was asked to describe. If this are for example of violent dreams, warriors, surely it is the energy of the liver which is too tight. The erotic dreams with emission to repetition of spermatic fluid in humans will sign a collapse of the energy of the kidney.

It can therefore, thanks to the analysis of dreams, make a relational with the software components unbalanced.

How to prepare for a good sleep

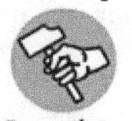

"

A basic rule: it should be put to bed when it is safe to have completed its digestion. To you to take the necessary precautions, knowing that a digestion lasts between 1:30 and 3 hours This aspect will be developed in the fifth part on the Dietetics.

" Then it is important to have the spirit to the calm. Therefore to avoid violent movies before going to bed.

" Do not fall asleep in front of the TV.

" Avoid Conflicts, discussions too bright.

What to do if you do not arrive at you fall asleep?

The three types of insomnia

" You do not arrive to you fall asleep. You turn in your bed. Often this state is accompanied by impatience at the level of the legs. This signs a weakness at the level of the Yin of kidney that no longer controls the Shen, the mind which is housed in the heart. It is the excess of mental activity which prevents you from sleeping.

" In another case, you fall asleep by depletion, you wake up, you sleep, and this several times in the night. This is called "insomnia of the average home". The food in your stomach "rot". You ate too much and you have not heard the digestion before you fall asleep.

" A third type of insomnia and what is called in MTC "insomnia in three hours of the morning," Second part of night. It is now before a table of blocking, stagnation of energy at the level of the liver. Very syndrome current in our western way of life.

These three types of insomnia can of course be combined between them.

A few small tricks

" Begin by practicing the exercise respiratory health that we had seen in the chapter on the breathing to combat the insomnia (see chapitre 17): breathe as slowly as possible, without any noise, in insisting on the expiry after a short inspiration.

" Fall asleep on a deep relaxation.

"Take your foot, it is the case to say: massage for 10-15 minutes your foot. You start by a general massage. You then you stop on some points. I refer you to the chapter on the digitoponcture. Emphasize these points 3F, 3RN and especially the 1RN. It is one of the major points of the sleep.

"In case of insomnia rebel, you can add the 7C, but the latter will be Massé rather in the morning. Or the 6cc you can do before you go to bed.

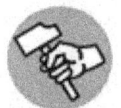

What to do in the morning?

Theoretically, your battery is recharged during the night. But the blood and energy tend to

En pratique stagnate because of the state of prolonged rest.

It is fundamental to stretch. As do the animals, you stretch on an inspiration very slow from the tip of the feet up to the end of the fingers.

You can also take great inspirations followed by expiries forced (see chapitre 17 on the respiration).

Please do not hesitate to you massage very quickly the whole body. Your hands will suffice for this, or a rolled towel to rub each zone.

And if you know of a series of Qi Gong, c is the time of the practice. This will completely freeing the circulation of blood and energy (see chapitre 18).

The relaxation to the rescue of sleep

The relaxation is indeed the great antidote to a poor sleep, a Sleep not recuperator.

But also, you can practice each time that you feel fatigue invade you. Normally you should never be tired. It is a symptom alarm signal of "too late". As much the prevent, or act as soon as it is issued.

Turn therefore to benefit the extraordinary virtues of the relaxation.

Ten minutes of relaxation well conducted

Le saviez-vous equivalent to three hours of sleep.

The relaxation is to release one by one all the muscles of the body, find themselves in a state close to the point of falling asleep.

At the outset, please do not hesitate to initiate you from a professional. Very many audio recordings leader of the relaxation sessions are at your disposal on the Internet.

Once you know you relax, you no longer need any support. In a few minutes, you get this state "second", this state of energy uptake optimal. You should also take the habit of making such sessions to the daily newspapers.

The two best moments in the Day are:

"

À retenir

After the noon meal. In effect the digestion of a Food Bowl demands a lot of energy. If your battery is not recharged, your body chooses to digest, but then you do more to "digest" the information in your work. Or it is the choice of the concentration, but your food rot in the stomach and in the late afternoon you still have not digested.

"*When you go home at the end of the afternoon.* You have emptied your battery throughout the day. It is high time to relax to avoid falling in all through self-destruction of your body. It is also an excellent method to have a falling asleep more profound during your next Sleep.

In short, in our modern societies, we cannot go without these techniques that have already been described there are hundreds of years in MTC.

Yin-Yang, sleep-wake: Learn to juggle with these two states. We will as well all the chances on our side to access the longevity in good health.

Part 5
The dietetics
Long life

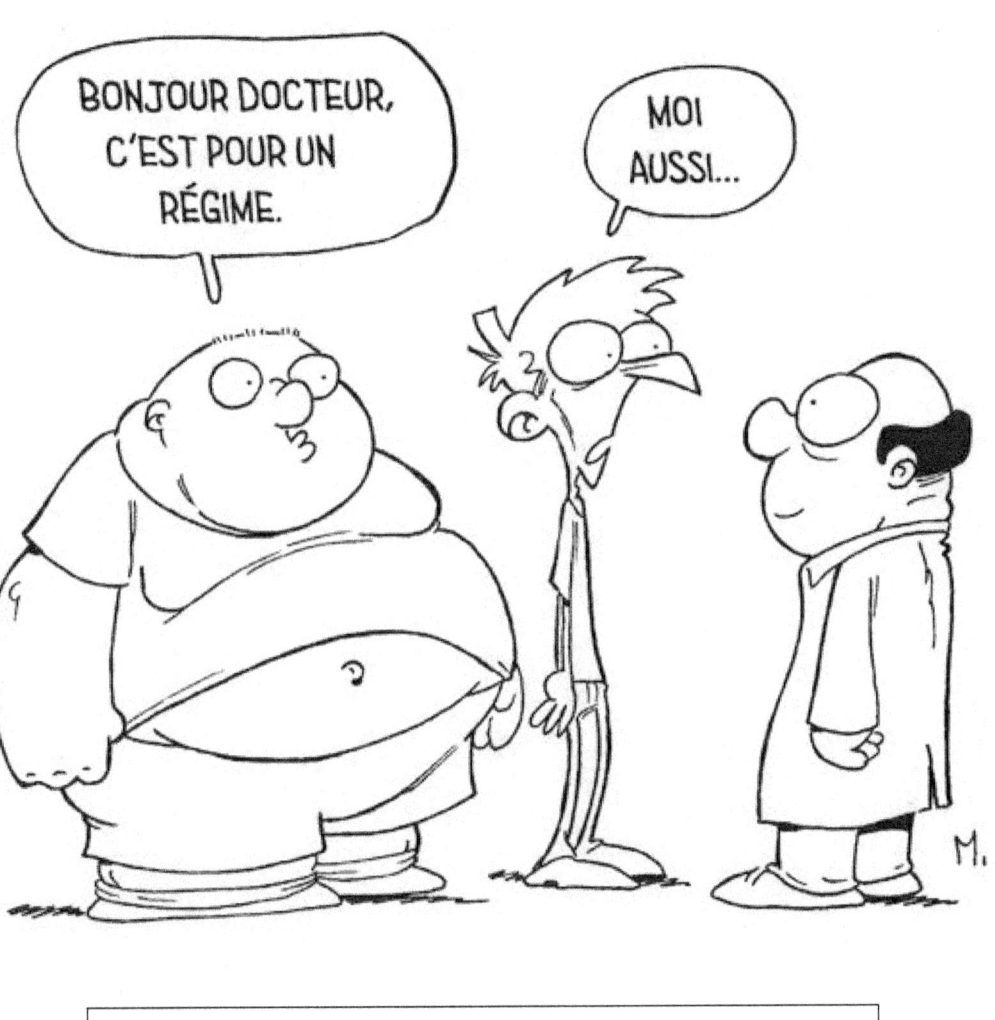

In this part...

This part dedicated to the dietetics of the middle you will learn to become the leader of the orchestra of your power supply, with food of the season and region. Not a question of "if enchinoiser" in addition to measure. And this, through nine rules unavoidable that well understood and applied as regularly as possible will not only of "make you lose large and swell the meager," but especially to stop tired unnecessarily your organization and to find a state of balance, good health on your cable of life. A chapter will be devoted to the problem if controversial issue of the hydration of the body. The data of the MTC in the material will help you to dispose of the errors conveyed in our modern world.

Chapter 20
The nine rules
TheA dietetics is of capital importance for the preservation of our health. The whole world is aware. But it is also an area where there are the more theories, the more often contradictory between them. The dietary systems to multiply at galore, but too often, they tend toward a certain radicalism which may put the health of the individual.

Unlike the modern teachings, the Chinese diet is not based solely on a physical representation and the biochemical human body. It takes account of concepts much more subtle, such as the concept of energy or the notion of symbiosis between man and the universe.

The Taoist philosophy which underlies the principles and the practices of the MTC advocates before any track of the middle and it is like that will be addressed here the Dietetics.

It is not a question here to go against your nature. From the Rules, to axioms of basis very easy to understand, we are going to deal with "the dietetics of fair middle" applicable to everyone. Well understood, it will not only find a good health, " to increase the meager and lose weight The Big". But especially to play a preventive role which is the very foundation of the MTC.

A caveat is in order. Whatever the accuracy and logic of the principles that will be set forth, you will need to keep you to change your habits too quickly. Let your body time to move from a state of imbalance to which he is accustomed over the

Attention

years, a new state of balance. It must be a period of a few weeks to sometimes several months to definitely change its bad habits. Want to change too quickly would be to make a reverse on a car which rolls to one hundred to the hour. Attention to the broken. Therefore, give time to time.

353

Attention

Most of the books speaking of dietetics in MTC are reserved to practitioners confirmed, able to make the correct diagnosis in their patient. These books speak only of dietetics therapeutic. This practitioner will then be able to make an order of dietetics at his patient, advising him momentarily to turn to such a flavor, such nature of food, why not such color.

This type of dietetics will be quite interesting to potentiate the effects of various treatments. The practitioner will be led to prescribe certain menus, to abandon such or such vegetables or fruit.

But, and this is very important, once the patient is rebalanced, he will teach him to expand its dietetics and return to the path of the just environment.

Let us take a simple example. You come to undergo an external attack, a "wind-cold" with all the flu-like symptoms that ensued.

Your organization has need of force to carry out the combat and reject the perversity. Your practitioner will tell you you put "green". That is to say not to consume during a week that rice and vegetables at every meal, without any other ingredient, and especially not of proteins that could bring an excess of heat in your organization. But once healed, you will need to resume a normal diet. Another example: you are of a nature Yin and decide to put you to eat only raw vegetables, which is more without the chew very long for the cook in your mouth. You will trigger of the pathologies of stagnation of blood and energy to more or less long term that may be very harmful to your health.

So pay attention to the self-medication food. You may, by lack of knowledge very specific information on the current state of the energy of your body to increase the imbalances, if this is to put you in a state of deficiency.

The dietetics that will follow will allow you to be the leader of the orchestra of your own western foods, season and region, even if from time to time we can afford to import certain products. But not matter to become Chinese for as much!

354

The special feature of the rules that will follow is that they are common to all the diet that we could qualify as traditional. With a few caveats according to the latitudes where we will find ourselves, we will be able to apply them in a few countries where we find ourselves.

A good dietetics at it alone is not enough to keep a good health. In effect, you can have the best dietetics of the world and even when "falling" ill. Why, then, have a good dietetics? Simply to stop tired unnecessarily our Organization, of losing too much energy to digest food that arrive in too large quantity in the stomach or which are unsuitable or unnecessary for the conservation of a good balance.

Remember the old adage: "Tell me what you eat, I'll tell you who you are. " Or what was said Michio Kuschi: "The man can eat everything, and yet he must maintain a certain order in what it consumes. This is a crucial point for the move to the development or decline. "

Finally, the word "regime" must be excluded from our language. This implies necessarily words such as "deficiency", "lack", "imbalance", "deprivation". And this is contrary to the conservation of a good energy balance.

Rule no. 1: Do the difference between festive meals and daily meals

Since the night of the time, in all the traditional dietary, the concept of holiday meals has been put in before. That is fêta Gods, Saints, anniversaries, the days highlights of a calendar, these days of celebration staked out and still beset the annual cycle of the five seasons.

These holiday meals are called Xiang Shou in MTC, the "enjoyment by the power supply". They have as a goal to "feed" the mental, the shen, the Spirit. We will see later that the daily meals, them, are used to nourish the body, to give him the necessary energy for its survival daily, but also be a help very significant in the daily recharge its battery.

À retenir

The festive meal allow reinstatement within them certain foods that we will be brought to exclude daily meals. These meals will thus have the immense advantage of allowing us to live in society.

355

Attention

Attention to certain modes, some currents of thought which advocate such or such a type of dietetics more or less radical. The dietetics is not reinvented. It is and always has been. To be too extremist, it can become for some a hell to eat some meals, if they are not safe, for example, of the origin of the foods that comprise them. They come to flee these holiday meals. I would not have to cease to recall that the energy of the fear is much more harmful than some deviations food.

In a month of meals, between lunch and the evening meal, we have 60 meals. We will see that it can be granted 8 to 10 festive meals per month, provided that the other 50 are dietary"". In the light of the next rules that will follow, we will see that the majority of people are between 40 and 50 festive meals per month!

In these festive meals that will last longer, this is the beauty of the provision of the Mets, the different smells, colors, flavors that will make this a festive meal.

But there is a corollary to this. If your state of mind is open, positive, you can at that time actually eat certain foods, certain associations which will be contraindicated in the daily meals. This will not harm to your organization, but to the contrary, it will energize and require to have of the peaks of digestion which he will be quite beneficial.

Conversely, if during these holiday meals you are not in your "plate", if you are depressed or confronted with problems that you mentally fatigued, then these same foods can become a poison for your body.

This division between the festive meals and daily meal thus allows to not sink in the monotony and especially not to make you feel guilty if you are prompted to make a gap. Still according to the inescapable law of fair environment.

Rule no. 2: know the great prohibited

We will now see a whole series of "prohibited". These are the foods to which it will have to carry a great deal of attention, because they are in the same unbalancing strongly the human being on its cable of life, when they are taken in excess. But, always in this vision advocated by the Act of fair environment, these "banned" can be reincorporated in the festive meal in the conditions seen previously. This vision has the advantage of you déculpabiliser when you transgress some dietary rules, and especially not you exclude from the community.

You said milk of cow?

Play the devil's advocate. Why a third of mankind, namely the Asian peoples, has never been enter in their feed, or then under certain conditions the milk of cow and all its derivatives? Why India has-t-she made the "sacred cow" and has put to the index the consumption of all its products, butter that they consume having nothing more to see with our butter?

Conversely, how can we explain the high concentration of fractures of the neck of the femur, in areas where the consumption of dairy products is at its maximum, as in the north of Europe?

A few points of mark: a baby of man at the age of 9 months weighs a dozen kilos, while a calf at the same age more than 200 kg. The proteins responsible for the growth contained in the milk of cows are much larger than those contained in the breast milk. With a little hindsight, we can see that our Organization is fact that filters. These proteins are going from month to month, year by year, Boucher all these filters, resulting in cardiovascular disease and many other yet. They are considered as the tan, of waste. It is as much energy mobilized in pure loss for that the body can eliminate them.

The other danger of these products is the following. When we are before any inflammatory phenomenon, a process of cellular hypermultiplication which is carried out in an erratic manner or excessive in certain areas: Chronic rheumatism, ball of fats, cysts, nodules, tumor process and others. All these pathologies may be akin to pathologies "auto-immune disorders". It is the body that in fact too to autoguérir. The simple fact of consume these products derived from milk of cow will increase very significantly the phenomenon of cell multiplication.

357

At the present time, very many cancer specialists who focus on this issue actually derive sounding the alarm and advocate the judgment of this type of products.

Why not do a test?

If I suffer from one of these pathologies, or multiple inflammatory pain chronic, why not do it myself the following experience. I stop the milk and all derivatives of the milk cow for three months. This is nothing in a life and I will see what happens in my body. I am first going to little by little sleep better and especially no longer have this sacred insomnia of three hours of the morning which is to put in a relationship with a filter clogging of the liver. Then, not not, my chronic pain will fade. First those located on the route of the meridians of the liver and gall bladder: neck, herniaires pain, pain in the knees... If I suffer from chronic sinusitis, **a fortiori** if they are due to seasonal allergies, this will have a direct impact. But I will make me realize also that, very quickly, this will have a beneficial effect on my mental, my concentration, my nervousness. Therefore, made the test. It will cost you nothing and will be able to "bring big"...

En pratique

How many times in my career, I have asked the total shutdown of these products to my patients who were suffering from rheumatoid arthritis, spondylarthrites ankylosantes, sinusitis, acute or chronic in repeat or other. And how many times have we obtained (patient and practitioner) spectacular results.

And of course, if you withheld the philosophy of this message, the derived from milk of cow must be completely stopped in the case of cancer or to prevent a recurrence.

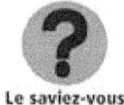

Good. We are epicureans (epicureanism elsewhere advocated by the Taoists), and love life. Well, between friends, nothing prevents us from consume the goat and ewe cheese, the less salty possible. Simply because the Cabri weighs the same weight as the baby of man...

Le saviez-vous

I just want to finish this connection by this terse response that we had done our master when we had asked for clarification on the dietetics of the child in the lower age. "I cannot answer this question because, for generations and generations, the child up to the age of two years minimum fed only to the milk of its mother" and a little further, we said "cow milk is for veal, breast milk is for the baby of Man"!

Will I transform into osteoporotic Gruyère if

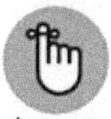

À retenir

I stop the milk of cow?
If I stop the milk cow, where will I find my dose of daily calcium?
Before all, we should not talk about decalcification, nor even of demineralization, but of osteoporosis.

When a word ends by the suffix -dares, this brings us back to the notion of proteins. This gives the strength to the bone of our skeleton, this are the bone spans that are fibers of proteins. It is on these bays that come to fix, not only the calcium, but also many other minerals. However, the substance of the problem is that, in certain conditions, can be install progressively a depletion of these fibers of protein. And, regardless of the quantity of minerals that can ingest, they are going to attach anywhere in the body, but not on the OS.

That said the Chinese medicine? "The energy of the kidney is the mother of the bones of the skeleton. "Since the millennia, Chinese doctors have put in relation the energy of the kidney and the bones of the skeleton. As far as we are concerned, this is relational done at two levels. The energy of the kidney was in effect under its dependence the fixing of minerals on the bone spans, but also the very production of these fibers of protein.

Let us go back to the basic question: Where do I find my calcium, sub-heard the minerals, if I stop the dairy products? He must know that all foods contain in a more or less large proportion. In particular, we find in the vegetables that come from the land, the main provider of minerals. The water that we drink is a mineralized water. Not all, but some of these minerals are completely assimilated by the body. Therefore, in reality, when we have a balanced diet, we have no problem with regard to the quantitative to the level of the contribution of minerals, and between other of calcium. And if you put in the head that your hypothetical future osteoporosis is due to this lack of minerals, you will fold on food supplements which taken in excess will be considered as a contribution of tan, waste, by the Organization.

Fault to be rejected by the body or fixed by the OS, they will come to harden your arteries and foster the emergence of calculations and other...

The real question is: How to recreate or maintain my bone capital, my capital of fibers of protein, bone spans?

"In the first place, we can quote a simple method, we still need to think about it and that this is possible: the exposure to sun at least 10 minutes per day. Remember the biology courses at the school on the rickets and the synthesis of the vitamin D. statistically, there are fewer cases of osteoporosis in the South, that in the North.

"Then, there is the setting in pressure of the OS. When you move, skip (Trampoline, "return of the Spring" in Qi Gong) you put the OS in pressure. This will compel then to rebuild its capital of fibers. Our modern dietary are made on the basis of food too smooth and too refined. Of the coup, one loses the habit of gum. But it also loses our teeth, because they are not retained by a bone tissue osteoporotic become.

"There is the third method, the more important, to shelter from this type of imbalance. It is the permanent recharge daily and the battery of the kidney by the implementation of the methods Yang Sheng, methods of preservation of life. If you learn how to breathe, to relax, to drink, to eat, to move, to make the love of adequately, you keep optimum recharging of the battery of the kidney. This will have a direct impact on the strength of your OS.

We can fully demonstrate in MTC that drink too much exhausts the kidney and promotes the osteoporosis. That Be permanently subject to fear, to the excess stress also depletes the kidney. He must be aware that a bad management of the stress has a much greater impact on your bone capital, that the amount of calcium that you could consume.

One of the visions of the life and death in Chinese medicine is a physiological decline normal to our ancestral oil housed in our energy from the kidney. When there is more oil, the Kidney" is off " and the Passage is done. It is therefore normal that in the fourth part of life, there has been much less capital bone.

Therefore, sun, movement and charging the battery of the kidney are the major methods for prevention of osteoporosis.

That is the saturated fat?

There are two types of fats in our food. Fats say saturated and those which are unsaturated.

The unsaturated fats

The unsaturated fats are able to divide at the time of the digestion and are indispensable. They provide energy, feed the brain, regulate the body temperature, regulate the synthesis of hormones...

These fats are found primarily in plants. The first vegetable oil, the more known in the world is the oil of olive. It is she who has the greatest range of therapeutic virtues.

But it is good, from time to time, to change and to turn to other oils as the walnut oil, rapeseed, sunflower, grape seed, sesame...

All oils are not created equal!

There is a vegetable oil which is saturated, which is considered as waste, tan in MTC, who "entartre"

En pratique the organization, c is the peanut oil. Pay attention to the aperitifs: a handful of peanuts gives the equivalent of a tablespoon of "bad" grease. But also the coconut oil, palm. To stay in good health, we should consume on a daily basis the equivalent of two to three tablespoons of unsaturated fat.

The saturated fat

The saturated fat lose their capacity to divide. In MTC, they are considered as the tan, waste, that the Agency must endeavor to eliminate. A minima, c is a unnecessary loss of energy to do this cleaning. On the other hand, if the contribution of these fats is excessive, this are all the filters of the body that will slowly but surely Boucher. Cardio-vascular diseases, scaling of the brain, arteries, rheumatism, different forms of cancers and other diseases are at the end of the path.

Where to Find Them? Mainly in the animal kingdom and their transformation: butter, cheese, cold meats, fresh cream, red meat, pork fat, etc.

Daily intake, or even bi-daily, of these fats and longevity are not good household. Reserve them for the feast days!

A single animal grease can still be divided, it is that of the duck or of the OIE. No, I have not said that the foie gras was to enter in the daily meals!

Le saviez-vous

Why flee fast sugars?

Here too, there are two major families of sugars: Slow sugars and fast sugars. We will leave momentarily from side the slow sugars which will become the basis of our daily diet.

On the contrary of slow sugars who will ask of the time for the organization to be assimilated, fast sugars are immediately supported by the blood, **via** the software Rate-Pancréas. Everyone knows the role of insulin to regulate the rate of sugar in the blood.

Take the Quick sugar will therefore temporarily put you in hyperglycemic state. The insulin secreted by the pancreas regulates very quickly this state.

But when the amount absorbed sugar, or of equivalent sugar, is too important and especially when this becomes a habit pluriquotidienne, the software Rate-Pancréas goes awry. Too much insulin is then secreted, putting you in hypoglycaemia. Hyper-hypo, an infernal cycle takes place with, at the end of the path, all stages of the pre-diabetes and diabetes. But also the scaling of the organization, because the excess of sugar turns in fat, Tan, in waste that can be stored in any part of the body.

If you revisit the cycle of the five elements seen in the first part, software, liver and Rate-Pancréas are in close relationship. When one of the two is misaligned, the other is also imbalance. However, the liver governs all the Tics, the Toc, the States of dependency. Very quickly, "without the knowledge of your voluntarily", you will become drugged sugar.

In the Chinese tradition, it is said, that we could consume five pieces of sugar or sugar equivalent to the daily, without that it is harmful to the body.

But that is. Everything is done in our western civilizations for you make totally dependent on this flavor through these famous "EQUIVALENTS sugars" which furnishes the endcaps of our supermarkets. Here are a few points to which show us the extent of the damage:

Table 20-1 equivalencies in sugar.

PRODUCT	Sugar equivalent
A chocolate bar	12 pieces of sugar
A liter of soda (black, orange or yellow)	28 pieces of sugar
A tin can the same drinks	11 pieces of sugar
Iced tea	14 pieces of sugar
A glossy Cornet	12 pieces of sugar
A tablet of chocolate	16 pieces of sugar
A slice of cake	7-10 pieces of sugar
A candy	1.5 piece of sugar
A tablespoon of jam, jelly, honey	4 pieces of sugar

In MTC, it is said that an excess of sweet flavor generates a "state of moisture" at the level of the software spleen, which can gradually be at the origin of the appearance of tan, waste more and more thick. This is the track open in the Onset of stagnations and obstructions.

But if we refer to the table of the five elements (see chapitre 4), we saw that the reflection, the " digestion of information", rehashing the past were to put in relationship with this software.

This excess of sugar will have an impact on the digestion of the food bowl, on the capacity of the spleen to pull the energy of the food. Very often ensue a state of overweight, and a "scaling quick" of the Organization. But the impact on the mind and emotions can take the first plan in this table, and these are the depressive states which are at the end of the path.

Do not be light...
You think you get out of it in taking the "light", sweeteners primarily to basis of Aspartame: it is **Attention** worse yet!!! When we speak of flavor in MTC, it is also of the qualitative, of the pure energy. Have you ever tasted a "sucrette" on basis of aspartame? Its mild flavor is 10 times more important than a normal sugar. This generates a energy peak at the level of the spleen much more harmful than that generated by a sugar Roux.

Last recommendation. As much you can stop the products derived from milk of cow of the day to the next if the heart tells you, as much the decrease **À retenir** of rapid sugars will take much more time. It will have to be done on several weeks, to find day by day a new balance, under penalty of you find in states of hypoglycaemia.

Flavors in excess, DANGER!

There are five large families of flavors in our food according to the MTC, each being to put in a relationship with a component software specific. Similarly, we have the five colors, the five odours, the five consistencies.

Table 20-2 The flavors related to bodies.

	Liver		RATE	Lung	Kidney
FLAVORS	AIGRE- ACIDE	AMER	SOFT	ACRE- PIQUANT	Salé
COLOR	GREEN- BLUE	RED	YELLOW	WHITE	BLACK
SMELL	Rance, fetid	Burned scorched-	Scented	Acre, raw meat	Decomposition
CONSISTENCY	SLACK	DRIVE	FIBROUS MATERIALS	FLESHY	CRISP

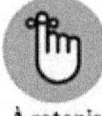

À retenir The rule is the following: there is no question of happen in such or such flavor. The Flavor "feeds" energetically the target organ with which it between in vibration. But taken in excess, it turns against the same body.

A flavor must not take the top permanently on another flavor. As well you should not say: "I am rather salt, acid rather..." of even a flavor must not be too pronounced, too powerful in the mouth. I refer you to what has been said on aspartame.

Excess of salty flavor

An excess of salty flavor is very detrimental to the organization. Belonging to the Kidney software, it will destabilize the latter, when it is taken in too large quantities.

It is said that "The kidney is the mother of the bones of the skeleton". It is also said that "eating too salty hurts the OS". This bad habit can lead to diseases such as rheumatism, osteoporosis, of low back disorders...

The "excess of salty flavor hardened": it is a great cause of malignancies or benign. The energy of the Kidney weakened, losing its ability to evacuate the liquids, is obviously a great cause of weight gain.

In the "cycle of the Five Elements", the kidney is the mother of the liver. The latter is no longer controlled," its Yin is no longer fed", the Yang risk of escape. It is a great cause of hypertension.

The standard is the following: bread without salt, it is bland and not very good. When one takes a good bread, we must not feel that he is salty. If this is the case, it is already too late.

 It should be absolutely to outlaw the saltshaker on a table, and never add salt on a dish.

Attention

Excess of acid taste

An excess of acid taste hurts the liver. However, the energy of the Liver governs all tendons of the body. It is among others a great cause rheumatism, stiffness, inflammation of the tendons.

The acid is found in excess in the fruit juice, the pizzas. Keep these dishes for the festive meal, but especially not on a daily basis.

Unfortunately, we find this flavor in almost all the flavor enhancers.

 Absorb a glass of warm water with a quarter of a lemon in the morning waking up, or well, the acidity contained in an orange is the standard. A

En pratique glass of orange juice brings you too acid taste!

Excess of tangy flavor

The spicy belongs to the Software lung. It is said that an excess of this flavor hurts the lung but also alters the internal mucous membranes such as those of the esophagus, the stomach or intestines.

The cells in our body need to swim in a pore fluid which will be "dried" by too much spicy. They will be fragile.

Excess of bitter flavor

We have already talked about the "mild" in the prohibited. Let us look now at what can generate an excess of bitter flavor.

This flavor which belongs to the heart has for property to the strengthening of the Qi. The Amer will for example, to strengthen the energy of the stomach. Does it not an aperitif (open the appetite) bitter to basis of artichoke for example to promote good digestion? But in the case of excess of intake of bitter flavor, it is said in the MTC that "the temperature of the body will decrease".

This internal cold will foster a slowdown of all the physiological functions of the body. This may be at the origin of constipation, weight gain by the retention of liquids, a transformation too slow food bowl...

Of stagnations will be able to install in particular at the level of the blood circulation and energy.

Gold in the West, we are very large consumers of this type of flavors, even if they are hidden by an excess of sugar. It is in effect the coffee and chocolate.

Le saviez-vous

Do we hear well: a coffee after the noon meal with a square of chocolate, by its nature Yang is quite beneficial to digest the food bowl.

But several cafes in the day, especially among the women who have a nature more yin than men, then become quite damaging.

It is therefore appropriate to have a power supply with all the flavors, provided that they are not too strong.

À retenir   Rule no. 3: adopt the single base

The classic menu of a Western is to take an entry, a main dish and a dessert. For all the traditional dietary, this is a festive meal.

The best way to take his meal daily is to opt for the single base where everything that you are going to eat is prepared.

À retenir

367

If we focus on the entries, it is the hour to eat, it was hungry and there is a tendency to rush on this the beginning of the meal. Gold in these entries, is either cooked meats, blocks, sausage or other. This being reserved for the festive meals.

But also of raw vegetables. We could think that it is a lesser evil. Certainly, the raw vegetables contain many vitamins. But the Chinese diet is not rational entirely on these bases.

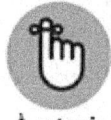

À retenir

Each food has an intrinsically nature: fresh, cold, warm or hot. Most vegetables are of a nature cool or cold, **a fortiori** if they are raw. However, if we compare the stomach to a furnace (the average home) for the cooking, the digestion can be done, it must be an average temperature of 38 degrees. This "cold" which between first in the stomach obliges the Organization to draw on its energy reserves to bring the temperature to 38 degrees and therefore begin the digestion.

In addition, as we hunger, we tend to serve copiously. However, vegetables contain a lot of fluids. These liquids dilute gastric juices and digestion is evil.

For all these reasons and many others, in the daily meals, it is preferable to go of entry.

Let us now to the bastion of desserts. It is most often of cheeses, to retain for those who take absolutely for the festive meals. Yet it would be better to prefer the goat cheese to those of cow, for all the reasons previously views and choose the least saline possible.

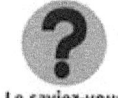

Le saviez-vous

The fruits as to them, when they come to the end of the meal, tend to block, to make stagnate the digestion. In the tradition, we do not eat the fruit after a meal, but between or before meals. Have fun to eat of the melon after a meal, there are great chances that you remangiez throughout the afternoon.

Do not try to you fold on a yoghurt. This are of dairy products to retain for the festive meals. The same for the pastries.

In conclusion, the desserts do not fall within the framework of a daily diet.

À retenir

Many nutritionists believe that we eat 30% more than the standard. With a profound vision, we could say that, from the mouth to the anus, we are only a series of process of digestion, assimilation, metabolism, of triage. The liver, stomach, the Rate-Pancréas, intestines are as many machines which, when they are too put to contribution, eventually wear out prematurely. A shortening of the life expectancy is at the end of the path. Remove entries and desserts in the daily meals allows you to eat 30 per cent less. It is as much energy to win to help the other functions of the body, among others the immune defenses, to be at the top. But it is also an excellent way to regulate its weight !

Rule no. 4: know the act of processing of the Cereals by chewing

Well understood, the rule that will follow will completely simplify the development of your daily menus.

When I was 10 years, I remember having had a professor of natural sciences which was come to class with a loaf of bread. It had shared between all the students by asking us to put a song in the mouth and chew. It was the famous experience of the transformation of cereals in slow sugars. At the end of a 20 chew, we had a taste of sugar in the mouth.

What is the best taste for children? Give them a quignon of bread to nibble, they you will be eternally grateful. This will allow their Discover the true taste of the sweet flavor. It is a very good way for that they do not like later fast sugars. In addition, this allows them to massage their gums.

Our body needs energy to operate. One of the essential goals of the power supply is precisely to provide him with this energy. The real source of energy is found to be in the transformation of the starch content in cereals and tubers, in slow sugars.

But remember the following rule: this transformation can only be done in the mouth, under the action of the saliva, on condition that

À retenir these grains are natures, that is to say simply boiled in water with the possibility to put very slightly from the salt or a net of olive oil on the pasta and nothing else. If they are mixed with the tomato sauce, butter, Gruyère, or any other ingredient, saliva is no longer to recognize the cereal and therefore loses a large part of its possibilities of the transform in sugar slow.

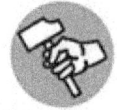 Remember that this action occurs only in the mouth, under the action of the mastication, and very little in the stomach. The transformation of

En pratique starch into sugar asks for a certain time. And it is necessary for this not evil of saliva. That is why, in all traditions, it is said that he must chew 20-30 times every bite of food.

If you chew like rice or nature of the bread, he turns into sugar slow and you effectively gives the energy your body needs. This energy Burns Foods and allows you between other keep the line. Conversely, if this same bread you used to saucer a flat, not only this transformation in slow sugar will not happen , but in addition, you will take the weight.

From this basic axiom, we will be able to develop the composition of the single base.

Rule no. 5: Dial the single base

In the base, you are going to put everything that you are going to eat during the meal.

In the first half of the base, obligatorily and at each meal, cereals. More conventional are rice, pasta, wholemeal bread, the bread to the HIS, the bread to cereals, potatoes. Less known, the sweet potato which contains a starch less aggressive than the potato and brings much more energy.

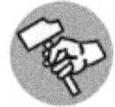 Complete rice

A small warning about the complete rice. Theoretically, it is a good thing, since in addition

En pratique to the slow sugars, it will give the fiber required for a good brushing of the intestines. But make sure you of its biological origin and that its last gangue does not contain insecticides or pesticides. Make sure you also that it is well cooked. And especially, chew-the well. For the transform into slow sugars, 30 to 40 chew are necessary.

For the bread, he must know that the wand Classic, the fact of the refinement of its flour, brings only very little of slow sugars. In addition, a crust too grilled, too "yanguisante", has harmful effects on the blood and liver. So choose other categories of bread as the bread full, at the ITS, to cereals. When you eat of the bread, you do not eat nor Rice nor pasta, and vice versa. And you don't just a slice, but the equivalent of half a plate.

What are we going to put in the other half of the base?

A meal on two will be vegetarian. To you to choir: at noon or in the evening. If you arrive to eat fairly early in the evening, it is better to take this vegetarian meal at noon, because the digestion will not erode the brain activity of the afternoon. It is up to you to choose your own pace.

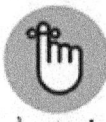

À retenir

These vegetables which therefore fall in the composition of each meal will play a leading role, thanks to their fiber, waste disposal, but also increase the work of blending of the stomach and intestinal peristalsis. In effect, the grain, where are going to be learned the slow sugars, are long to digest. Fundamentally, the allow vegetables to avoid the piles at the level of the stomach.

Then, your body has need of protein to feed the muscles and the flesh. For vegetarians, it will need to learn to use soybean and its derivatives, ensuring of course to their provenance biological. As regards the GMOS, avoid falling down in which radicalism being used by the fear that they generate eventually be more harmful to health than the product itself.

TOFU

Le saviez-vous

Traditionally the tofu is, among other things, an excellent way to replace the meat. But there is a rule that the Western know little: it must be cut into small dice, thus increasing the contact surface and cooked for a very long time to that it can actually be digested and that it does not come to generate a state of cold to the inside of the stomach.

Similarly, soybean sprouts traditionally don't eat raw but bleached, i.e. to undercooked to mitigate the coldness of their nature.

For those and those which have the habit of eating animal products, it is obvious that it is necessary to restrict the contribution, this would be only a meal on two.

This is equivalent to a week of meals, to once of red meat, once or two of fish, once of white meat, once lean ham and finally once again an omelet. The latter is much more digestible than the eggs to the flat, the hard-boiled eggs or to the hull, that we will retain for the festive meals. And of course not at the cheese, but for example with fine herbs, fungi.

This you can amply in protein and thus you do not risquerez clog your organization.

In some dishes, the vegetables may be mixed with animal products or soy. But do not forget: cereals and tubers must be consumed natures.

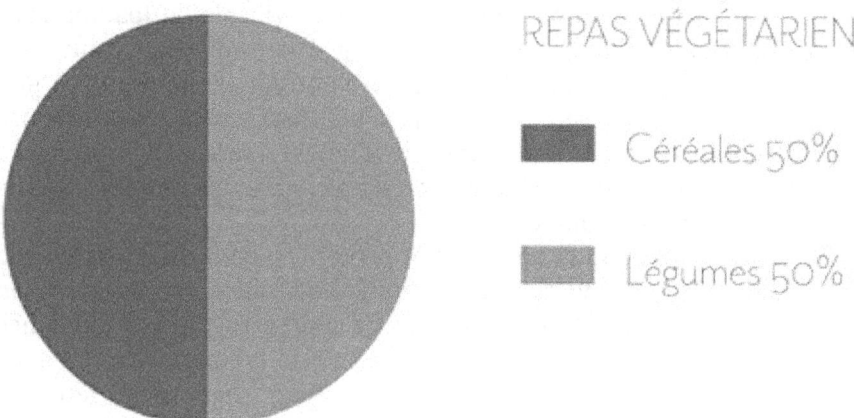

Figure 20-1 composition of a vegetarian meal.

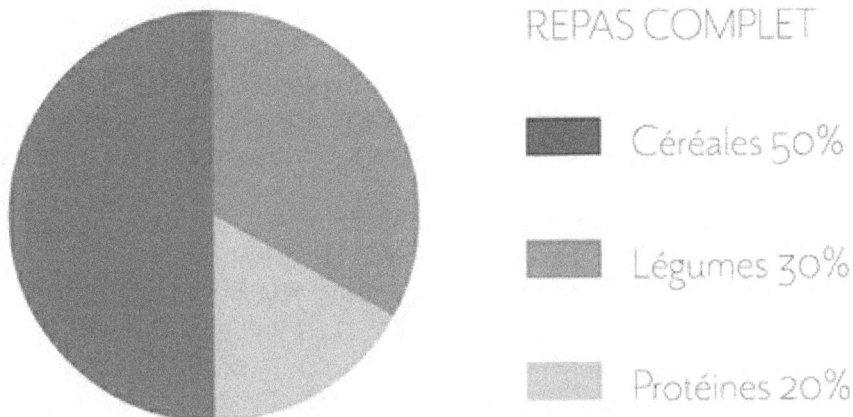

REPAS COMPLET

Céréales 50%

Légumes 30%

Protéines 20%

Figure 20-2 composition of a complete meal.

The legumes, the "3 in 1"

That this is the red beans, black, white, broken peas, chick peas, peas, lentils, soybeans, all these legumes can become our friends, if we consume wisely. It is a source of protein Very appreciable able to replace the meat. But also a very important contribution in slow sugars, low glycemic index. Finally, their high fiber content is fundamental to digest and improve the intestinal transit. A true "3 in 1".

Yes, but that is! All these legumes fermenting very quickly, and their main role in MTC is to clean the intestinal villi by the "Internal Wind" that they generate. We are for the "Rehabilitation of Pet" IN MTC. It is only in our civilizations puritan that issuing some noise disturbs. It goes all otherwise in India, in Africa or in China... However, there is the reverse of the medal. If you are under the influence of emotions internalized, if the energy of your liver is blocked, at best, these legumes will make you Roter. At worst, this will you bulging very quickly with all the pain that ensued. The legumes Yes, provided to be in good mental health.

Le saviez-vous

Rule no. 6: Learn to eat well

This is the keystone of this dietetics of fair environment.

You start by taking one or two spoonfuls of rice, pasta or a bite of bread. You take care of the

En pratique

373

chewing conscientiously, up to feel a sweet taste in the mouth.

Then, eat one or two spoonfuls of vegetables, meat, fish.

These dishes can be cooked with herbs, all the spices of the creation, olive oil. This flat has the taste, while avoiding the flavors too pronounced.

Then, you resume of cereals and so on.

The STEW is it part of the dietetics of the Middle?

Yes, according to all the preceding criteria. We still need to know the EAT. You ask the right questions: y a-t-it of butter, cheese, meats, milk, sugar, rapid, in this dish? Not. It is the meat, the less fat as possible, which has cooked very long. The vegetables are carrots and onion. Let us not forget that the real stew, c is a kilo of carrots to little of beef. Of course, the vitamins have in part been eliminated by the long cooking, but many other components equally important are present in the flat. You rattraperez elsewhere for vitamins. Finally, the sauce, it is a wine that has lost its alcohol and the binder, it is of the flour or cornstarch.

It is therefore **a priori** a dietary meals. But it is the way in which we are going to eat that it might not be at all. Recognize that you eat this dish with pasta. If you mix everything in the base, you not only lose this aspect dietetics, but in addition you are going to take the weight. The height would be of saucer then his plate with bread. The best way to proceed is the following. You use half of the plate with cooked pasta to the water, very little salted and a net of olive oil to avoid that they do not stick together. In the other half, you put your stew. You eat and Chew one or two spoonfuls of pasta, then you go to the stew and so on. This is not serious if at the end of the meal of pasta are mixed with the stew. Three quarters of the cereals will be transformed into slow sugars, vital energy.

When we look more closely at it, all the traditional civilizations operate on this principle. Let us look at a few examples.

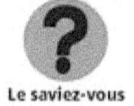

"

The real Couscous in the desert is eaten in the following way: The wheat seed form a pyramid in

Le saviez-vous

the center, and the various dishes are prepared all around. It draws with the fingers in the seed, it in fact a dumpling which will be extensively chewed. Then we pique in the various dishes and it returns to the seed.

"Hindus make their galette of wheat that they avoid broil. They chewed a few bites to then be used in other dishes. But they do not use this galette for saucer.

"The Asian, almost a third of the world population, have always opted for the sacrosanct bowl of rice that accompanies their flat. With their baguettes, they take of the rice that they chew vigorously then they bite then in the different dishes. It must never mix the rice with the other ingredients.

It is not that complicated that to prepare such meals. You turn for example in one half of the base of the rice and in the other, green beans still a little crunchy cooked with a little garlic and parsley. A chicken thigh is also possible or the white fish. There you have a meal dietetics.

Another plate may be composed of pasta and Macedonia of vegetables. A good piece of wholemeal bread, of the omelet with herbs and mushrooms can enter in the framework of the Dietary meals.

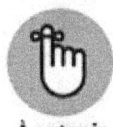

Breakfast at the center of controversy!

À retenir

King's meal or not? Everything depends on the orientation that you want to give your life! You have just to sleep 6-8 hours to recharge your battery of the kidney for the day. Perhaps you have done a few exercises to the alarm clock to increase this recharge? And there two solutions are offered to you:

"**You either decide to do a breakfast pantagruélique. Let us remember that a depleting digestion of half the battery of the kidney to be conducted to his term. As the latter is theoretically well recharged, you will digest this hearty meals. But that energy lost for nothing!!! You prefer at this time the earth to the sky.**

"**Either you made a breakfast frugal. A few fresh fruit of the season and region. Or even the muesli wet with hot tea or soy milk hot. Or well two or three slices of bread complete, without butter, with two or three tablespoons of honey or jam. This breakfast then brings enough energy to hold until the noon meal without cutting, empty your battery for the Digest. It is said that it is self-sufficient. You prefer then the energy in your organization.**

A common rule for a good number of centenarians: A small breakfast, a noon meal, a taste of 16 hours and a meal in the evening just as frugal. "Eat Too much brings us back to the earth. Do not put the quantity of food at the center of its concerns connects us to heaven, to the spiritual". The future belongs to those who eat little! Enjoy to invest on the quality rather than the quantity. With regard to the Danish pastries and other, this will be for the breakfasts of celebration!

Rule no. 7: Retain the rule of three hours
This rule could also be called the "Act Anti-nibbling".

 It is said: "For three consecutive hours, after the last bite of a meal, you should not put this would be only a single mouthful of bread in your mouth. "

À retenir A digestion can be compared to a washing machine. The prewash is done in the mouth with chewing and saliva. The stomach is the drum of the machine. The last bite of your meal swallowed, a whole process of digestion is going to walk. All this under the control of the software Rate-Pancréas.

The washing powders and fabric softeners will be incorporated into the food bowl: this are the gastric juices, pancreatic, saliva, the bile a little more low. Then produces a rise in temperature: A digestion will done at 38 degrees. It is the illumination of the "Average Household". Where the need not to lose too much energy that is drawn from the battery of the kidney to Do not eat too much food of cold nature, veggies and to avoid drinking cold.

All this is followed by a period of breaststroke, mixing, before the lower port of the stomach no opens and that the assimilation begins.

All these operations last between 1:30 and 3 hours. Everything depends on the quantity of food ingested, if yes or no you have well-mâché, your state of mind at the time of the digestion, the amount of energy you have...

What happens if you start to nibble? It is a little as if you had invited a number of guests and that two or three people come to add to the unexpectedly. Then you decide to add rice on a rice already during cooking. Result: The first rice will be inedible because too cooked, and the second will be just as much, because not enough.

That is exactly what happens when you Munch. Your stomach is never empty. In small clusters of food, stagnations occur in the stomach. The energy of the spleen loses all discernment in the yard of the food bowl. At the end of the path, c is the Scaling, weight gain and large fatigues.

This act is therefore at the center of the practices of longevity, at the center of the methods of preservation of life, methods Yang Sheng Fa IN MTC.

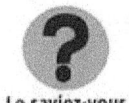

Two types of saliva?

There are two types of saliva in MTC. That which is secreted during the chewing of food. This are the glands parotidiennes who participate in its development. This saliva is directly put in relationship with the software Rate-Pancréas. It contains some elements promoting the digestion of food bowl. The other saliva is secreted in the language by a special gland. During the exercises of Dao Yin, when you touch the language in the upper Palace, you will force this saliva to be secreted. It is then called "liquid gold." It is in relation with the energy of the kidney, and invigorates it. The kiss lovers, who promotes the secretion of this saliva, increases the libido! The platonic Kiss has no place in the sexuality in MTC...

Le saviez-vous

Rule no. 8: Follow the Law of the nine days

This rule will allow us to vary the most possible our food and we dispose of the Pizza, kebab, the sandwich, steak frites daily.

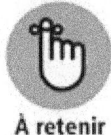

À retenir

It is said that: "nine days of suite, you should not remanger the same vegetable, the same fruit or the same protein. "

Since in nine days, between the noon meal and that of the evening, we have 18 meals, we will be able to eat twice a same food.

Several reasons for this. We have fallen into the through where the nutritional composition of a food is a view to the magnifying glass. While the MTC speaks of flavor, color, nature of a fruit or vegetable, therefore of pure energy, nutritionists speak of calories, minerals, vitamins, fats, proteins, carbohydrates, etc.

This vision makes us lose sight of the whole of the interactions of these different elements within a same food. And the temptation is then great to supplement by the famous "food supplements" such or such lack assumed.

We have thus lost sight of the "intelligence" of our organization, capable of capturing the different elements which it has need, for its proper functioning, the food bowl and even, in some cases, make reservations. And all of this is under the control of the energy of the Rate-Pancréas software, conductor of the digestion of food bowl.

If your battery is recharged, it is your body itself which makes the self-regulation.

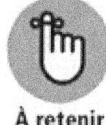

À retenir

We insist, in this rule, on the need to consume fruits and vegetables of the season and region. In effect, each of them is considered as a real "alicament" with his organ-target Meridian, its nature, its flavor and color.

If the season of the tomato is spread from July to September, this is not the fruit of the Chance. Of Nature slightly cool and acid taste and soft, it allows to produce the organic liquids, to rehydrate the fluid compartments, dissipate heat and to calm the liver. It is therefore quite specified for the Nature Yang of the summer. On the other hand, if we take all the days, these virtues will return against the organization, and weaken the Yin of the kidney.

Thus consume of tomato two to three times, for a period of nine days, is quite beneficial.

If you do not have an idea, you can rely in table below. You redécouvriez the extreme variety of fruits and vegetables of the season and region.

Table 20-3 fruits and vegetables according to the seasons.

Spring		Fall	Winter
Garlic, Artichoke, Asparagus White, asparagus Green, eggplant, Chard, beet, Carrot, celeriac, White cabbage, cauliflower, Kale, Kohlrabi, cabbage Red, cucumber, Zucchini, Cresson, Endive, spinach, Bean, Fennel, lettuce Roman, lens, Turnip, onion, sorrel, Sweet potato, small White onion, small Peas, leek, Peas Gourmand, pepper, Potato, Radishes, radish	Garlic, Artichoke, Asparagus White, green asparagus, Eggplant, Batavia, Bette, Red beet, Blette, broccoli, carrot, Celeriac, celery-branch, White cabbage, Cabbage, Brussels, Chinese cabbage, cauliflower, Kale, cabbage Roman esco, Kohlrabi, red cabbage, Cucumber, gherkin, Squash, zucchini, Cresson, spinach, Fennel, Bean, Green beans, lettuce Roman, lens,	Globe Artichoke, eggplant, Chard, Beet Red, blette, bolet, Broccoli, carrot, Catalonia, celeriac, Celery-branch, boletus, Chinese cabbage, Brussels sprouts, Cauliflower, kale, red cabbage, pumpkin, coprin Hairy, squash, Cresson, endive, spinach, Fennel, Lettuce, chews, corn, turnips, onion,	Beet, Broccoli, Cardon, Carrot, Catalonia, celery, Cabbage, white cabbage, cabbage Of Brussels, Cauliflower, Cabbage Curly, red cabbage, Chinese cabbage, Pumpkin, Squash, Cresson, crosne, Endive, spinach, Chews, turnip, Onion, sorrel, Parsnips, sweet

long, Curly endive,	corn, Mesclun, turnip, onion, Sorrel, sweet potato, Pâtisson, small onion White, small peas, peas Eat-all, Leek, pepper, potatoes, pumpkin, radish, radish Long, salsify, tomato	parsnips, sweet potato Soft, Foot of Sheep, oyster mushroom, Leek, potimarron, Pumpkin, radish, rosé Meadows, salsify, Jerusalem artichoke, Trumpet of the DEATH	potato Soft, dandelio n, Leek, apple Of earth, pumpkin, Radish, salsify, JERUSALE M ARTICHOK E
Apricot, almond Fresh, pineapple, Lawyer, banana, Blackcurrant, cherry, lemon, Date, strawberry, Strawberry Of wood, raspberry, The fruit of the Passion, Kiwi, tangerine, Melon, mature, Apple, Blood orange, Grapefruit, Papaya, Plum (Quetsche, queen-Claude),	Apricot, bilberry, almond, Lawyer, banana, Brugnon, Cassis, Cherry, Lemon, fig, Strawberry, strawberry of wood, Raspberry, fruit of The passion, red currant, Kiwi, lychee, mango, Melon, Mirabelle, mature, Bilberry, nectarine,	Lawyer, chestnut, Lemon, clementine, Quince, dates, Fig, fruit of the Passion, khaki, kiwi, Lychee, tangerine, Mango, brown, Bilberry, hazelnut, Nuts, olive, orange, Papaya, fishing Of Vine, pear, Apple, Plum	Pineappl e, lawyer, Lemon, clementi ne, Dates, fruit Of the passion, Guava, Grenada, Kaki, kiwi, lychee, Tangerin e, Mango, Orange, Blood orange Grapefrui

| RHUBARB | Papaya, watermelon, fishing, Pear, apple, plum (Quetsche, queen-Claude), Grapes, rhubarb | (Quetsche, Queen Claude), grape | t, Papaya, pear, Pomelo, apple |

With regard to the protein, since a meal on two must be more or less a vegetarian, it is very easy to change. Once the omelet, chicken, of the gilthead bream, tofu, of lean ham, etc.

À retenir

The consumption of cereals and tubers is not in this rule. Certainly, we can vary our grain, but before the existence of the means of transport present, where there was water, c is the rice which prevailed. At the center of the continents, it was the wheat. Remember however that the rice as a "cereal of the middle" is the most to even to bring good energy whose body has need.

Table 20-4 A few examples of vegetables with their virtues IN MTC.

		Indications
ALGAE	- Cold nature and salty flavor - Refreshes the internal heat, help the thyroid function, drains the system	- Fatigue, constipation, hypothyroidism, goitre - Cough with thick mucus, asthma - Edema, obesity, rheumatism, high blood pressure (HTA)
ARTICHOKE	- Cool nature, bitter flavor and soft - Nourishes the Heart and calm the spirit - Stimulates the	- Lack of appetite, state of overwork, anxiety - Digestive laziness, chronic diarrhea, liver

	liver/VB, antitoxic	disorders, gout, kidney stones, diabetes.
ASPARAGUS	- Cool nature, bitter flavor and soft - Moisten the lungs, dispels the glaires - Refreshing and blood thinner, lowers blood pressure	- Bronchitis, dry cough, HTA, arteriosclerosis - Digestive parasitosis, constipation - Recommended in case of fire inside
EGGPLANT	- Cool nature, fresh flavor and astringent - Purifies the heat, circulates the blood, calm the pain - Tonic of the stomach, GI, antiseptic - Calm the Spirit	- Hepatitis, abdominal pain, diarrhea, irritating, hemorrhoids, state of nervousness
LAWYER	- Cool nature, fresh flavor and bitter - Stimulates the digestive functions, invigorates the general energy, calm the Emotional Heart	- Flatulence, bloating intestinal, bad breath, pregnancy, growth, convalescence, overwork, nervousness, anxiety, stress
BLETTE	- Nature fresh, sweet taste and tasteless - Hunting the heat, frees the toxins in the skin, dispels the hematomas, stops the hemorrhages, invigorates the heart, calm the spirit	- Anemia, heart weakness, fatigue, overuse, chronic constipation, drunkenness, cystitis, dermatosis, irritability, measles, herpes
BEET SUGAR	- Neutral nature and	- Anemia, neuritis,

	fresh, sweet flavor - Nutritious, quickly charges in energy of maintenance, refreshing, promotes menstruation	cancer, influenza, agrees to subjects exposed to stress Yang
BROCCOLI	- Cool nature, fresh flavor - Soothes the heat of the bronchi in summer, purifies the liver, improves the view	- Urinary difficulties, irritability, presbyopia, conjunctivitis, influenza, bronchitis
CARROT	- Cool nature and Yin, mild flavor, slightly bitter and pungent - Stimulates the appetite, tones the digestive capabilities, invigorates the battery of the kidney, eliminates the stagnations	- Fatigue, physical and moral, growth disorders, bone demineralization, dental caries, peptic ulcer, laziness of the Vb, hepatitis, parasitosis, intestinal worms, dermatitis, chronic cough, asthma, angina, decline, night vision, urinary retention, urinary difficulty, water retention, overweight
Celery	- Nature cool or cold, fresh flavor and slightly bitter - Consolidates the kidney, stops the bleeding, invigorates the stomach, the RT	- Overwork, convalescence, sexual fatigue, HTA with headache and dizziness, obesity, insomnia, anger of children, irritability of

	and the Vb, tempers heat, improves the urination, decrease the TA	menopause, aphthae, laryngitis,
The Paris mushroom	- Cool nature, fresh flavor, astringent - Stimulates the appetite, invigorates the energy, detoxifies the blood, stops the diarrhea, reduces the Tan, calm the spirit	- Lack of appetite, diarrhea, cough Grasse, hepatitis, measles
CAULIFLOWER	- Cool nature, fresh flavor - Lubricates the intestines, tones the Pancreas	- Slow digestion, lack of appetite, constipation
Pumpkin, squash, courgette, pumpkin	- Cool nature and Yin, mild flavor - Removes the heat, dissipates the moisture - Stimulates the pancreas and lungs - Calm the pain, neutralizes toxins - The seeds and seeds kill the parasites and the toward	- Intestinal pains, diabetes, intestinal worms, cystitis, asthma, bronchitis, insomnia, anger retracted, frustrations, hyperactive Fetus
Green Cabbage or red	- Nature cool or cold, fresh flavor and bitter - Nourishes the skin and lungs, heals and lubricates the mucous	- Cough Grasse, asthma, skin disease, frostbite, injury, insect bite, burning, fever, flu, constipation, hot

	membranes of the stomach and intestines, quiet heat, infections and the nervousness	flushes, rheumatism, stomach ulcer, intestinal infections
CUCUMBER	- Cold nature and Yin, flavor sweet and bitter - Refreshing, soothes the thirst, promotes the circulation of the water	- Swollen Tips, conjunctivitis, redness and pain throat, febrile condition, blood temperament, too Yang, anxiety of children
Chinese cabbage	- Nature cold, fresh flavor, slippery - Refreshing, diuretic, promotes perspiration, lubricates and heals the digestive mucosa	- Peptic ulcer, constipation, abdominal bloating, vesicular laziness, conjunctivitis, inflammation of the throat, influenza, fever, cystitis, urinary difficulties, overuse, stress, ++ Yang temperament or hyper Yang
CRESSON	- Cool nature, fresh flavor-bitter, vegetable of been, very Yin - Removes the heat, Waters, moisten the lungs, promotes urination	- Dry cough, dry mouth, aphte, herpes, perlèche, fatigue, poor appetite, hair loss, skin diseases, water retention, irritability, anger of children, temperament Yang
ENDIVE	- - Cool nature and Yin, mild flavor-bitter, vegetable of Winter	- Fever, disorders of the appetite, convalescence,

	- Removes the heat, improves digestion	hepatitis, overweight, calm the effects of Yang
Spinach	- Cool nature, flavor bittersweet - Invigorates all organs, lubricates the intestines, nourishes the blood, sealed the thirst	- Thirst, short breath, convalescence, drunkenness, diabetes, constipation, hemorrhoids, urinary difficulties, conjunctivitis, bad night vision, anemia, Demineralization, stress, physical strain and moral, excessive food, obesity
FENNEL	- Warm nature Yang, tangy flavor - Warms and invigorates the kidney, disperse the cold, balance the function of the stomach, the regulates the respiration, favors the arrival of rules and increases the milky secretion	- Chronic back pain, swelling of ankles, urinary incontinence, battery exhaustion of the kidney, bloating, stomach pain with the sensation of cold, flatulence, diarrhea, lack of appetite, painful rules
LETTUCE	- Cool nature and neutral, bitter taste sweetish and - Invigorates the energy, mobilizes the stagnations of blood and Tan	- Nervousness, irritability with palpitation of the Heart, insomnia, puff of heat, constipation, hepatitis, diabetes, abdominal pain of the rules, abscesses of the breast, acne, furuncle,

		stitching, burn, conjunctivitis, subjects bilious and Yang
Chews	- Cool nature and yin, bitter flavor and soft - Nourishes the Heart and Lung, lubricates the intestines, sedative action and tranquillisante	- Nervousness, sleep disorders, temperament Yang, cough, chest tightness, atherosclerosis, constipation, intestinal spasm
TURNIP	- Cool nature and Yin, bitter flavor and soft - Refreshing, mobilizes the stagnations of food, removes the moisture, purifying, breastplate, calm in the Emotional Heart	- Fatigue by stress, nervousness, anxiety, noises in the ears, bronchitis, angina, cough, cold, obesity, gout, renal calculation, eczema, acne, burns of the skin, frostbite, abscesses, alopecia areata of the Child
SORREL	- Cold nature and Yin, flavor acid, astringent - Refreshes the blood, hunting the heat, diuretic, pest	- Diarrhea glaireuse and painful, difficulty urinary, vaginal discharge, red eyes, hot piss
Sweet potato	- Neutral nature and Yin, mild flavor - Improves the functions of the stomach and the pancreas, strengthens the physical constitution, dissipates the heat, purifies, promotes the	- Functional colopathie with alternating diarrhea and constipation, diabetes, hepatitis, cholecystitis, skin lesions, bad night vision, lack of Breast Milk

	rise of milk	
DANDELION	- Cool nature, bitter flavor and slightly sweet - Improves the functions of the liver and the VB	- A disorder of the liver/VB, conjunctivitis, dermatitis, insect bite, Verrue, obesity, cellulite, excess food, the beginning of the flu, colds
LEEK	- Nature lukewarm, tangy flavor - Invigorates the kidney, strengthens the Yang, circulates the energy, dispels the stagnations of blood, diuretic, neutralizes toxins from the intestines, causes perspiration	- Cold, blow cold, nausea, belching, excess alcohol, low back pain, gout, urinary tract infection, pain cardiac region, atherosclerosis, obesity, impotence, ++ for topic Yin
Potato	- Cool nature, fresh flavor - Improves the functions of the stomach and pancreas, lubricates the intestines, promotes the diuresis, calm the inflammations	- Pain and stomach ulcer/ duodenum, constipation, regurgitation, nausea, lesion of the skin
Black radish and red	- Cool nature and Yin, flavor sweet, pungent acrid and - Deletes the digestive stagnations, improves	- Slow digestion, lack of appetite flatulence, calculation or laziness of the Vb, migraine, cough, asthma,

	respiratory capacity, dissolves the bronchial mucus, calm cough, diuretic and allergy	pertussis, bleeding from the nose, gout, articular rheumatism
RHUBARB	- Nature is very cold and Yin, bitter flavor and soft - Removes the heat and toxic, promotes the circulation of water and food in the digestive tract, promotes the menstrual flow	- Dry constipation, abdominal bloating, stagnation of blood with pain and pelvic congestion during the rules, state of heat with fever, headache, redness of eyes, mouth ulcers, crisis of hysteria or great anger
TOMATO	- Nature slightly cooler, acid taste and soft - Product The organic liquids, waterproof thirst, invigorates the stomach, facilitates the digestion, accelerates the transit, calm the energy of the liver, dissipates the heat, combat microbes and the Intestinal mycoses	- HTA, redness of eyes, headache by excess heat, pain throat, loss of appetite, thirst, dry constipation, bad breath, excess of meat, food poisoning, pain lombes, knees, gout, convalescence, state of fatigue

Rule no. 9: Moisturize his body without tired his kidneys
What is the role of the drink?
Our organization is comprised of 70% of water distributed according to the Fluid Compartments specific.

The development of these fluids is the result of a very complex process. At each level of the body, the liquids ingested are processed in pure and impure. The pure elements mount and the impure elements descend.

It is the software Rate-Pancréas which performs this sort. It is said in the MTC that: "The energy of the spleen affects the quality of the production of organic liquids. "

These liquids to lubricate and nourish all tissues, organs, the tendons. The tears, saliva, the Intraocular fluids, in-ear, the synovial fluids, blood, lymph, cells, whole is bathed in these liquids.

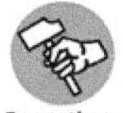

A balance between inputs and outputs

And if we were talking about water balance? The water, except when it is transformed into grease, or lymph fluids or other, is not stored in the body.

En pratique In daily life, there must be a balance between the inputs and the outputs. In addition, all fluid compartments of the Organization is constantly renew. It is therefore necessary to The Daily of hydrate intelligently his body.

At the level of outputs, we find the urine (1.5 liter), the sweat, the evaporation of the skin (0.8 to 1 liter), faeces (0.2 liter), the air that we breathe out which is very humid. We are therefore losing between 2.5 and 3 liters of liquids that we absolutely must reconstruct. Let us now look at the entries: the food that is wet, especially if we consume fruits and vegetables as we should do each day (0.8-1 liter), the degradation of foods (0.4 liter), the air that we inspire which is responsible of moisture. Some people in the insufficiency of energy of the Kidney can take the weight when it is raining or that the air is very responsible in moisture. The skin can promote penetration of fluid, especially when we take too of baths without adding the Prior of the salt to rebalance the osmotic pressure. There is no more to balance the inputs and the outputs that a liter to 1.3 liter provided by the drink.

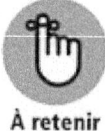

The most important thing to understand is that there must be a balance between the inputs and the outputs. And this balance must be found in **À retenir** such a way that the bodies are not depleted, Do not

390

overspeed precisely by a surplus of these fluid intake.

The great Rule

We must know that the way to drink is one of the fundamentals of the dietetics, common to all traditions. Because of the lack of knowledge and deep visions, we do not know drink and this can have serious consequences on our health.

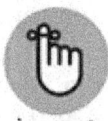
À retenir

The rule is the following: "a person normally constituted, in average climate conditions, should not drink more of a liter to 1.2 liter of liquids on a daily basis, to condition of drink in small quantities fractionated, never a big bowl of a single blow and avoiding drinking during a meal, except a few sips of hot tea, or for the Epicureans a good glass of red wine by small lampées throughout the meal. "

If we consider the kidney organ as a machine to filter the waste and not the liquids, like any machine, it has been designed with a certain ability to work. The Chinese tradition speaks of a daily intake of six bowls of liquids, either approximately 2 liters. This quantity takes into account not only the various drinks that we eat, but also of the liquids contained in the food. This is equivalent to drinking an average of one liter of liquid.

Attention

If we increase this fluid intake, we are going to necessarily put this machine in the overspeed. During the years, nothing will happen. But will come a time where the machine will run out. It will lose its ability to eliminate. A part of these liquids will remain in the body and promote weight gain by the retention of water.

In some cases, this phenomenon can occur very suddenly, in a few months. During a great stress for example (divorce, change of life, death of a loved one). There are seasons of life as the menopause or the premenopausal in a woman who promotes a natural weakening of a certain quality of the energy of the kidney that can come to add to a pre-existing imbalance. If it does not change its habits water, then it can very quickly take the weight.

Yes, but this is. It is all the energy of the kidney that will be reached by this excess of fluid intake. And the consequences are going to be much more important and insidious as one might think. We have seen that the energy of the Kidney governed as MTC not only the filtration of liquids in the goal to eliminate waste, but also the immune defenses, faculties of adaptation, the immense potential of self-healing of the body, the fixation of the calcium at the level of the OS, the different marrow, brain including.

In addition, the energy of the kidney plays a very important role at the level of the memory, the control of the fear, the anguish and the confidence in itself.

À retenir

Forcing people to drink to length of day 2 liters of liquid per day is likely to have serious consequences on the physical, but also on the mental health of the person.

According to the theory of the Yin-Yang, when the machine kidney is fatigue, C is the yin which decreases, favoring the increase of the Yang, therefore an excess of heat. This appearance of heat will not only foster the multiplication local microbial that can be at the origin of Cystitis, vaginitis, but also a evaporation of liquids and therefore a thickening of the latter. This are the kidney stones that will be at the end of the path.

Therefore leaves to hit your deep beliefs, the MTC explains that an excess of fluid intake contains many more disadvantages than positive points when we speak of the preservation of health.

Of course, it should be to modulate this rule according to the circumstances. It is obvious that if you are in full urinary tract infection or that you are in the process of eliminating the calculations, it will agree on time to drink much more than a liter. But this may be a double-edged sword. In effect, if after the crisis, you continue to drink 2-3 liters of liquids in daily life, the same causes produce the same effects, you will create a new ground conducive to the emergence of such imbalances.

En pratique

Five glasses with mustard in ras are a liter! Let us take a simple example. The Ministry of Health advocates to drink according to the following diagram, throughout a day: breakfast, a large bowl of coffee, chicory or tea, and a glass of orange juice. In the morning, a glass of water. At lunch, 2-3 glasses of water, at the taste a cup of tea nature or milk, chocolate or chicory. At dinner, a plate of soup and two glasses of water and in the evening a herbal tea. Placed end to end, it is two and a half liters in everyday life! Look around you. At breakfast, the half-liter is very quickly reached. In the restaurant, a tin of black Drink carbonated and two or three glasses of water to side, this fact already almost a liter!

All traditional peoples are familiar with this rule of hydration. When you go in India, Africa, and obviously in all Asian countries, you drink only in small glasses, in small cups. You have the impression to drink throughout the day, but this are each time to small quantities. It is far from our "MUG " Western.

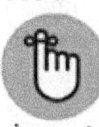

Drink too much is as harmful as play to the camel, namely remain several hours without drinking. Do not forget one of the Rules princeps of prevention, À retenir it is the regularity.

The different types of beverage

In passing by the soups, alcoholic beverages, fruit juices, teas, herbal teas, water, are doing a small tour of the various proposed drinks.

Alcoholic beverages

In the alcoholic beverages, we have the alcohols the "hard", wines and beer.

The alcohols drives are reserved for holiday meals to brighten up his mental, with all the precautions that are required. A beer between friends, or when it is very hot poses no problem. In contrast, as always, taken in excess c is a drink which is returns against the organization. The mixture of cold and gas will very quickly make bulging the stomach. And as this is not a cut-thirst, the more you drink, the more we thirst.

As for the wine, there is a side the rosé wines, white and the other the red. Leaves to disappoint many of you, the white and especially the rosé contain too much sulfuric derivatives and assault excessively the liver. A cooked in the Dew wine gives you headaches very acute.

Le saviez-vous

In contrast, the red wine, taken in small lampées throughout a meal, may be considered as a drug allowing you to digest your food bowl and even to descale your arteries. But you are not required!

Of course, the alcoholic beverages may not become our daily drink.

Fruit and vegetable juices.

Fruit juices and vegetable juices have the drawback of cut the long fibers which the body absolutely need to digest well. No Dietary tradition has never put in before. If we take the example of orange juice, or several oranges are necessary to fill the glass, it exceeds the quantity of acid. However, too acid taste turns against the energy of the liver.

The water

Of course, it is the first drink that comes to the idea when we talk to hydrate the body. Except that the fresh water goes down immediately in the small intestine and obliges us to urinate for nothing. For that it might nourish the fluid compartments, it should be taken at a temperature of 38 degrees. What admittedly is not very good !

Then, we will turn to the herbal teas. But he must know that each plant, that this is the thyme, verbena, the Mint, etc., has a medicinal virtue specific well. As soon as it is taken on a too large duration, not only does it no longer has the expected effects, but it turns against the body. This cannot therefore become our drink in the daily.

Attention

394

It is a disease at low noise, linked to a overconsumption of soda, that they are yellow, orange or especially black! Considered the "foie gras human", this pathology would reach more than 6 million French! The name learned is the fatty liver. Outside of the sedentary lifestyle, junk food, several factors directly related to consumption of soda are to put in question. A soda under a few forms that this either contains, for a tin, the equivalent of 10 to 12 pieces of sugars fast!

In MTC, it is said that this imbalance totally the software Rate-Pancréas, conductor of the digestion of food bowl. It is a major cause of the occurrence of pre-diabetes, diabetes and cardio-vascular diseases, but also mental illness and emotional as the Depression. However, there is a very close link between this software, and that of the liver. Not only this surplus of sugar will "fatten your liver" as a goose that we gave. But as this software to under its dependence all tics and TOC of the organization, it is a real state of dependence which is going to install, identical to what occurs for any drug. The most destabilizing accumulations of all of these beverages is a certain Drink carbonated black. The black color belongs to the energy of the kidney in MTC. When it becomes excessive, it imbalance at the root of the functioning of the body. All the more that the quantitative between in game and that very quickly it is more of a liter of this drink which is daily ingested.

In addition, this drink has an acidity close to that which is secreted by the wall of the stomach to digest the food bowl, 2.5 pH! It is not surprising that this either at the outset a very good medicine for the tourista! But taken daily, this completely destroys your acid-base balance. Excess of acid, sinew and liver are not good household. This are the rheumatic pain that appear. Finally, it contains some plants which are already of the drug. In short, with all this cocktail clashing, it is not surprising to see put in place such an epidemic! And you well understand, obesity that follows is only the tip of the iceberg.

The soups

The soups can enter in the quota of liquids daily newspapers. Moreover, in the tradition, we prefer the clear soups to soups mixed together. The quantitative is very important. Not more of a rice bowl. All ingredients beneficial are present, without a too-full of liquid does Vienna injure the energy of the kidney.

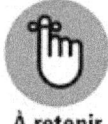

À retenir

While it could be the ideal drink to moisturize his body without tired the energy of his kidneys? We will see that there is a universal beverage, known since the night of the time, consumed by more than half of the population of the world: it is the tea and more particularly the Chinese teas that are adapted to our temperate climates. This beverage may actually be taken a whole life in daily, and hydrate very strongly the body without generating exertions of the battery of the kidney.

Chapter 21
The Chinese teas,
The drink of long life
<u>In this chapter:</u>
" <u>The Virtues of tea</u>
" <u>How to properly prepare the tea?</u>

POur the MTC, this drink represents a kind of panacea both by its therapeutic virtues that preventive measures. It is the daily drink of billion people on this planet. Extensive studies on the tea are made by the Russians and the Americans. Some go so far as to say that the tea could become the drink of the third millennium with regard to the prevention of cancer and many other pathologies yet.

The Categories

Before any it is important to know that the Chinese teas have very little in common with the other types of teas indians, ceylanais, Himalayan and others.

The tea comes from the Camelia, of the same family of those who grow in your garden, but the camellias that are used to make tea in China are very different from those that grow in India and in other lands. They are called elsewhere Camelia sinensis.

Le saviez-vous

Unlike the other types of tea, they have no aggressive action on the liver which result cause of iron deficiency. They do not energize the Spirit. You can take in the evening without that this prevents you from sleeping.

Green, black tea, oolong

There are three kinds of Chinese Tea: green teas, oolong teas or half-fermented and black teas that the Chinese call red teas, the fact of their color of infusion.

In reality, it is the same sheet which has suffered the different preparations.

If there picking the more young leaves of tea and let them dry in the hours which follow in the sun or in front of a source of heat, it is of green tea. The Dom Pérignon teas is the white tea, harvested only once in the year in climatic conditions specific. In view of its high cost, it is preferable to consume during a festive meal!

When we left to ferment these same leaves a few days and that they then dry, c is the tea half-fermented still called oolong.

Finally, if they are left to ferment much longer for some, a full year in a cellar, they take the appellation of black tea.

After the fermentation, they can be dried and soak up the smell of some of the bark. It is then a matter of black tea smoked.

He must know that all the categories of tea have a very high power hydrating. This power as we will see is one for three or one to four by report to the water!

A tea for each time

En pratique

This are the green teas which should be consumed the more often. But do not succumb to the current mode. At the beginning, take pluri-daily in this category of green tea could be detrimental to your health. In effect, they are cool nature, and consumed even hot, if it is cold outside or you are in the weakness of Yang, a quantity unreasonable of green tea could generate stagnations of liquids at the level of the stomach, be indigestible. To introduce you to the Chinese teas, it is better to begin by the oolong teas.

We should have at home the three kinds of tea. In the morning, you choose the tea of the day according to the following criteria:

"If it is hot outside, if you feel you are in full form, then you choose for the green tea.

"If you need to lose a bit of weight, that your liver is somewhat "throttled", that you do not digest not very well, it is then the black tea that suits you.

"When you hesitate, you then take the tea of fair environment, namely the oolong tea. It is as a general rule that you are served in the Asian restaurants.

It will teas as our wines. There are dozens of brands, as well as producing families. To you to progressively refine your tastes and learn to fully the taste.

Their virtues

Since time immemorial, the Chinese knew the therapeutic and preventive virtues of teas. It is Shen Nong, the "Divine reaps", one of the Three Emperors mythical of China, which was one of the Fathers of the medicine. It is one of the first who strongly advised to boil the water before use in order to clean it up.

According to the legend, one day, resting under a tree, leaves came to fall into the simmering water. It testa this infusion, and was surprised of powers conditioners thereof. The drink "tea" was born in the year 2737 av. J.-C.

Shen Nong said then: "Tea awakens the moods and the thoughts of the wise. It refreshes the body and soothes the mind. If you are shot, the TEA will make you the force. "

We are going to see some virtues of this "Drink of long life", data by the tradition, but also by the modern research.

The tea made "fit the spirit"

Le saviez-vous

It is said in all the Ben Cao, the compendiums of Chinese pharmacopoeia, the tea made "fit the spirit", the shen, wakes the mental, lightens the ideas. In some way, it makes you more intelligent.

If one refers to the theory of signatures, by comparing the coffee and tea, coffee comes from a seed. A seed has a very strong concentrated energy. It can give a baobab tree. At the outset Yin, this seed has become Yang by the roasting. It will give a peak of energy very powerful on the energy of the liver, and the Heart, generating insomnia and nervousness.

On the contrary, the sheet of tea in full development has a Air Nature, light. Its action is much slower. Of where this concept to raise the spirit without generating a peak of Yang in the body.

A smart mouse!

The Japanese have put in place a scientific experiment to prove the statements of the tradition. The elements: a labyrinth, a piece of Gruyère at the exit and at the outset a batch of mouse only hydrated at the water. The goal is for these charming beasts to find the exit to eat this cheese! On average, after many passages, they were five minutes to find the output. New experience, even Protocol, new labyrinth, new batch of mouse, but this time only hydrated with Chinese green tea. At the end of the experience, they do that two and a half minutes to find the piece of gruyère. They are more intelligent! The TEA allows to put continuously the spirit in a state of wakefulness. And as we should consume in small quantities broken down throughout the day: more need of coffee in excess!

The TEA eliminates waste

On the contrary of the COFFEE, TEA allows you to circulate , to make disappear the clusters of food, dissolve and eliminate fat. It also allows to eliminate waste and toxins present in the body. This is especially the black teas who will have this action of "cleaning".

It is one of the only plants which has as joint action to promote the elimination of stool and in the same time to be very slightly diuretic. By making "flow", it promotes intestinal peristalsis, but also the elimination of waste in the urine. By his action of lubrication, it allows the advance of the contents.

It contains certain proteins able to encompass the "poisons " at the level of the liver and reject by faeces and urine. It thus allows to eliminate the toxins and poisons in some medicines, in certain drugs. But also to act on the effects of pollution, on certain substances found in suspension in the water or radioactive substances contained in the air. By this action, the TEA allows the body to resist the cancers due to iatrogenic substances.

 The TEA allows among others to assist in the elimination of nicotine and is therefore quite indicated for smokers.

Le saviez-vous

400

The tea has the property to dispel the emanations of the alcohol. Its nature "fresh" will oppose the hot nature, Yang, of alcoholic beverages. Green tea concentrate is capable of very quickly dispel the state of drunkenness, but also allows you to hunt the hangover of festive tomorrows.

The hydrate tea

À retenir

The tea has a very strong power hydrating. To persuade, there is only to observe the skin of Asian, African women who has an advanced age continue to have a skin is very smooth. When you have dry mouth, you thirsty, especially when it is hot, or after a prolonged effort that triggered a strong sweating, when appears the symptom alarm signal that is the thirst, if at that time you rush on the cold water, which more is gaseous, you will very quickly sweat and especially, the more you drink more you have thirst. You are going to trigger what is called La Ppie.

The effect of the tea is the opposite. It favors the production of organic liquids, reconstitutes the saliva and removes the sensation of thirst. The Tuaregs in the desert only Drink hot tea and not more of a liter to 1.5 liter in a day, despite the 40 degrees in the shade.

The tea also allows to moisten the lung. However, it is said in the MTC that the skin belongs to the lung. It is, among other an excellent anti-wrinkle!

Le saviez-vous

The tea, on the condition to be bu in small quantities broken down throughout the day, enables to reduce the nausea of the pregnant woman.

The modern research have shown that the Chinese tea contained a tannin, called Dan Ming, substance in large quantity in young leaves of théiers. When this product Between in contact with alkaline products, toxins or heavy metals, it is assembled to the latter to form an insoluble compound which can then be easily evacuated by faeces and urine. It is said at that time that it allows to neutralize the toxic substances, to protect the intestinal mucosa and the stomach, to prevent problems of ulceration, prevent the dental chalk.

The Caffeine contained in the tea is, on the contrary of the coffee, very slow to act. It is for this reason that the tea is not energizing, does not bother. Once its effects dimmed, one does not feel fatigue.

Method of preparation of tea

What water choose?

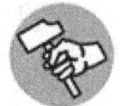

En pratique An experience to do! Take two transparent glasses, with the same amount of tea. Pour the boiling water above. In one of the glasses you will put the mineral water, or outcome of a charcoal filter, or better still a filter put in by-pass on the tap of your kitchen, reverse osmosis. In the other of the tap water. At the end of a few hours of infusion, the tea of the first glass remains translucent. This is not the case for the second glass. The tea is disorder and a oily deposits is located at the surface. If the tea becomes your daily drink, prefer a water "clean".

What container?

The teapots in land, bronze, are to be reserved for the black teas. A teapot Do not wash never soap. The successive tannins eventually in culotter the walls. There are as well in china teapots centenarians.

The teapots in porcelain are to book the green tea or white.

But to the use, prefer teapots made of transparent glass. You will be able to appreciate the color of different teas, since all teas can be infused.

How do we prepare for it?

Two modes of preparation: the tea ceremony, a ritual very precise, different depending on the categories of tea. Each tea has in effect a temperature and a infusion time which he is clean. This is not what we are talking about here.

We will attach to see how to make the tea can, little by little, without any precipitation, become our daily drink. We will see that in reality, this will not be that of the hot water with a few leaves inside.

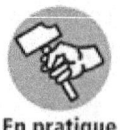

En pratique

The simplest way is to proceed in the following manner: in a teapot in Pyrex transparent, you put two pinches of tea between the thumb, index and the major strained, without that this does not exceed between the three fingers (and not more!). And this, for three-quarters of a liter of boiling water. It is necessary to know that the daily tea must not be strong in taste. It is normal that it remains clear, translucent. This is what differentiates it from the Indian Teas. Then, you boil the water. As soon as the first bubbles appear, you pay in the teapot. However, if it is of green tea, you will have the prior "wet" with water at ambient temperature, to avoid that it is "burned" by the hot water. Once the water is paid, the leaves will rise to the surface, and then at the end of a few minutes go back down to the bottom. A dozen minutes after, the tea is drinkable.

How the taste?

If you are at home, on the same tea, you can repeat the infusion two or three times in the day. It is said: "The tea of the first infusion begins to give the taste of tea. The second gives a feeling very smooth and pleasant at the level of the palace and the throat. The tea of the third infusion is more pungent. He announced that the Dan Ming, the tannin, appears. The real medicinal effects of the Tea Act at that time. "

The other solution is to prepare your Thermos of tea, the ideal is to get a thermos double-wall of treated aluminum, for that there is no exchange of ions with the drink. There is among all specialized resellers in tea. You can as well the keep warm a whole day.

Certainly, at the end of a few hours, it darkens very slightly, because of the dust of tea will be continued to infuse. But this to the advantage of being more convenient to use and enable you to see the amount of liquid that you can eat in the day. There is not a country in the world where you can boil the water and prepare a thermos. More tourista at the end of the road, since the bébêtes are killed!

Some additional tips

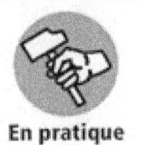
"

403

En pratique

It should be to avoid drinking tea boiling. This could irritate and burn the mucous membranes of the throat and the esophagus.

"To the reverse, a tea do not drink never cold, under penalty of the Make indigestible and make him lose its therapeutic and preventive virtues. And turn to the index "iced teas "any loans which contain the equivalent of 12 pieces of sugar and which have obviously more nothing to see with the tea, if this is the name!

"Do not forget the rule: "Drink in small split quantity without flooding his body. "

"You do not need to add any ingredient in tea. Obviously not of "tear of milk" to the English mode, or lemon!

"The sweeten is totally unnecessary and even discouraged. You lose a lot of its virtues.

"And do not add any plant in the Infusion! It is this last which would take the top in the light of the effects very subtle tea. Let us take the example of the Jasmin Tea. It is a plant pungent and which acts on the surface of the body. Taken in excess, it can easily give of the hives.

"Do not drink the tea of the standby. The proteins will become denatured and it becomes indigestible.

"Do not discard the tea leaves. This is an excellent fertilizer for your plants.

"A last Council. Do not change your habits too sharply. Start by a few taken, then, little by little, take this drink a dozen times, in small glasses Arabs or Chinese, throughout the day. This will become an act of full consciousness, an act Qi Gong. Like the respiration, stop as well several times to think, to stop his central computer will allow us to live more and more in the full conscience. This full conscience is one of the major conditions to learn to manage our emotions and thus become Zen.

Attention

When a western goes in the desert to follow a caravan of Bedouins, he has any interest to bend to the local rituals. The Bedouins have the habit of consuming the famous green tea with mint by small glasses throughout the day, warm or hot, and little more than a liter to 1.5 liter while it is 40 degrees in the shade. Of course their efforts are counted. But when the same! They import the green tea from China since hundreds of years. It is, indeed, a beverage very sweet, but this quick sugar is immediately supported by the Organization, without creating peaks of insulin, to give the necessary energy to avoid any overheating in internal. The mint of spicy nature and fresh causes a very slight sweating while cooling of the body. In the manner of a bottle of water that they would surround a moist cloth to keep the freshness of the beverage. In the same perspective, by 40 degrees in the shade, the Bedouin fully cover their body of cotton fabrics in order to avoid the evaporation of the organic liquids.

But be careful not to get accustomed to the mint tea in a temperate climate. Not only the sugar would resume quickly its perverse effects, but the excess of Mint would eventually "wounding the energy of the lung" and turn against the body. Without counting the adverse effects of a surplus of sugar fast. On the spot, the Western who do not bend to these rituals, **a fortiori** if it made a rally, or that it is spending rashly its forces, is obliged to drink 3 to 4 liters of water in the day, when this is not more. The result of the race, when he returned to him, the energy of the Kidney collapses and it loses its immune defenses, and ages at an early stage.

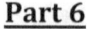

Part 6
The part of the TEN

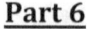

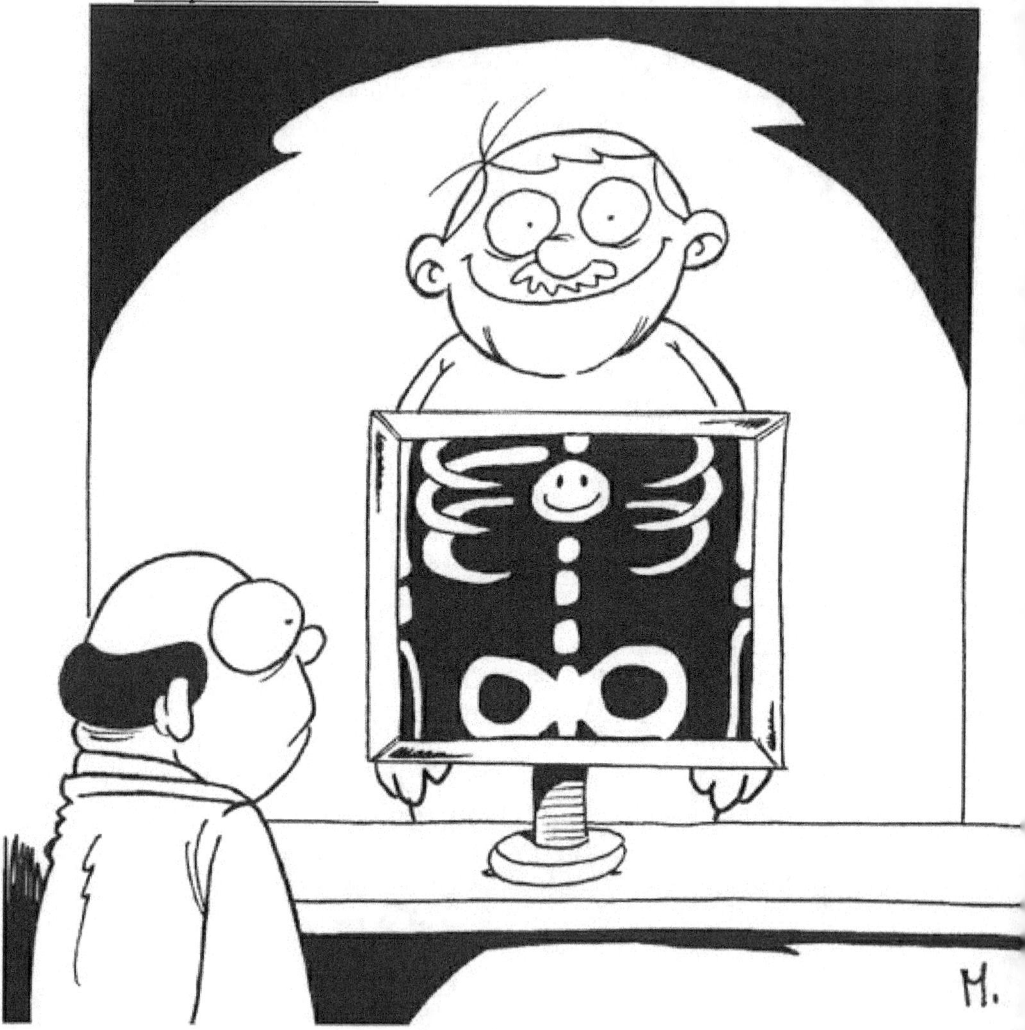

In this part...

The life may not be that if we breathe, if we eat and if we believe. These are the three main pillars of the Vitality. We are therefore going to divide this part in three times ten commandments, advice or rules which will help you to find a new balance and a new impetus on your cable of life. We will begin by a charter in ten points to learn to manage our emotions. Then what must be put in place in the morning and evening to reload permanently its battery of the kidney. As to the Dietetics, we will see an essential aspect, namely the ten reasons why it should be to learn to chew. You can have the best of the dietary, if you do not chew your food bowl, she ends up losing all its value.

Chapter 22
The Charter in ten points
To learn how to manage
Our emotions

EN MTC, it considers that the emotions are poorly managed are at the origin of the emergence of virtually all internal pathologies. Does not speak-t-we not of the "destructive wind of emotions"! We had seen in the theory of the five elements that the five families of emotion fell in resonance with the software five bodies. Let us remember the couples anger-liver, sadness-lung, fear-kidney, Reminiscence-Spleen and joy-heart.

An emotion is pure energy, without physical consistence, without smell or color. It "feeds" the component to which it belongs. It is not a question here to become beings "empty" of any emotion because without them, we would not be human beings. But if a particular emotion comes to take the front of the scene continuously, or if it becomes too brutal, then it is destructive to the body, and turns against its target organ. Let us look at the ten fundamental points which will allow you to keep your balance on your cable of life and you will always feel well "Here and Now".

Relativize

Facing a test of life, a source of fear, a "thing" that disturbs your habits of life, it is the field of your mind that ends up to be captured by this negative energy. The problem is there, in front of you! It You seemed insurmountable! It darkens day and night your field of vision! It becomes fixed idea which rotates round, as a fly which tape to windows without being able to get out. But if you reculiez of your field of vision this "thing", this "fixed idea," without consistency, without material, without smell that torments your heart.

If you put in perspective what seems to be a test of insurmountable life, history to see everything there is to side: Your blinders will progressively by fade. And if you repeat like a mantra: "There is no problem considered insurmountable which could not be divided into several small problems which, each taken at hand, will be surmountable. ". Or again, what they say to length of day the

408

Burkinabe and still others: " There is no problem! "How many tests" without issues" have you had in your life and who, a few days, a few weeks or months after were returned to oblivion. Therefore relativize, diminish the importance, allows you to dissolve at the root of these emotional waves to avoid that they become déferlantes destructive.

Get out of the theater stage

The Taoists often compare the life of a theater stage. Each of us, in this scene, plays a particular role and each role is essential for the game of life is balanced. The primary role in the scrubber of scene, everyone must give the best. When a grain of sand comes to put in this part, it is the whole spectacle which suffers. However, there is a corollary to this vision. How many theatrical scenes play in the family, or between "friends", where the players will insurgent, if invectivent, se hate, swallow their bile! How many umbilical cords not cut! How many dominated that finish in depression, in the blocking of the energy of the liver, in cancers! A solution: exit the scene of theater, become spectator. The assailants, in the absence of the respondent, will eventually choose another target, since yours becomes transparent. And in a single moment, all your nodes will dissolve.

Watch without emotion, watch without judgment, listen without answer. But all this can be done only by the issuance of an energy very powerful, the basis of relations of our humanity: altruistic love, love free without obligation to return.

Wait for the storm to pass

We have seen in the first part that life was the duality Yin-Yang, and that nothing could have of existence on this earth without that its opposite complementary-do not existed. We must do there! Happiness cannot exist without the misfortune, the Laugh without the cry, the joy without the sadness, the States of grace without the states of disgrace. On our cable of life, of the tests arise of the INVISIBLE.

These are the tests that we are destabilizing and which are likely to make us fall to the bottom of the chasm. Nobody can escape it! When they arrive, accept to cry, spend nights of insomnia and take nothing for us stultify. In MTC, sadness combat the anger, according to the cycle of the five elements. It is an emotion of self-regulation necessary. Flee those who tell you: "Thou art a man my son, you must never cry. "You eventually make "amputees" of love. Espouse This old adage: "The one who touches the bottom of the river has more chances to propel themselves to the surface than that which remains between two waters. ". To force readings, understanding of the "things of life", to put us in the listening of our soul, we understand a day that there is not fundamentally of tests negative. Only the tests that we are evolving. And then after the storm comes the beautiful time!

Work the forgiveness

It is one of the central points in the Confucian philosophy. Forgiveness is the antidote to the anger, these two words could not coexist. We know that anger, this emotion to trend Yang belongs to the liver in MTC. The side Yin of this emotion, the other side of the same coin, that advocate all religions, all traditional philosophies including the Taoism, this total gift that you made to the other or to yourself (per-donnare) is a real medicine. It allows to eliminate little by little this "emotional virus "so devastating than is the energy of the anger, when it becomes excessive.

It is the history of the type that is being railroaded in the street. Several cases of figure are possible.

Its "aggressor" is much lower than him, insolent limit. He did not even apologize. It is the anger extériorisée which then takes the top. This can go up to the pugilism. The more the Yang of the Liver Monte, the more the Yin is depleted. When these situations arise, this can become one of the major causes of high blood pressure. This energy of the Anger is there, Tapie in the heart of the person. And at a greater emotional storm, a internal wind very powerful can stand up. It is stroke or heart attack which are at the end of the path.

Its "aggressor" is much stronger than him. A sense of inferiority, resentment, anger interiorized appears. Indeed, he knows that if he responds, it is going to fight to flat seams. If this situation is repeated, this emotion, as a fire that smolders, one to which Ronge the apple, will be at the origin of a multitude of pathologies of blocking and stagnations especially at the level of the energy of the liver. In MTC, c is one of the major causes of the appearance of breast cancer in women, especially when it is located on the lateral side of External this body, where passes the meridian of the gallbladder. A solution to get out of this situation which may seem often without outcome, to eradicate this virus: the forgiveness.

Four reasons to forgive:

" It did not express, and therefore it was unnecessary to get angry.

" It is knowingly that you has rushed. You have a few notions of "philosophy of life", in particular the Law of Causation which said: "The One who voluntarily done evil to other sends a negative energy, that will sooner or later in full figure. "You do not want, but that is what is going to happen. Everything is a question of time.

" You forgive also, because you now know the damage of this virus emotional. It is in some sort of "the selfishness salvateur". The Buddhists call it "endure". This is not of the cowardice. Quite the contrary. It is a genuine force, not given to all the world.

" You forgive, but give him also of extenuating circumstances. It is the fault of its condition of life, its bad education, his karma, etc. It is the empathy. You can even try to help to change. But all the world is not a saint. If you join this vision of things is, at the beginning of the work, a hundred times a day that you will be prompted to forgive. Little by little, it will become "Competence Unconscious". You do not leave that grew up.

Dissolve the fear of death

And if the meaning of our life was to understand our death, to give him a sense? We have the opportunity as a human being to have the faculty to meditate on this inescapable deadline. Then, do not rely to the next day! The meditation which allows us to put us in the listening of our soul can give us of screaming understandings. The reading of ancient texts, some initiations and the help of masters can we be a very great help.

In MTC, the fear of death is the emotional Cause first of the emergence of virtually all internal diseases. That we give him the name of fear of the disease, fear of suffering, fear of aging, it returns to the same.

Let us not forget that the energy of the Fear literally drain our battery of the kidney, which is the source of our vitality. We have seen in the first part, this metaphysical concept on the basis of the understanding of the MTC, namely, the concept of a spiritual soul and body soul. These hosts somehow do not seek to live in a house tidy and clean to want to stay there. And if one of the great sense of life was to put us in the listening of our soul, the one who knows everything, which is able to give us the intuitions of life through our meditative practices, relaxation, Qi Gong, culture of the present moment. And if the meaning of life was to feed our soul by this envy intuitive to learn, understand, read, write, and this until our last day. By giving this meaning to our life, little by little the concept of death dissolves to give birth to that of a passage. This passage, where the physical body, emotions, our ego, attachments-repulsions will disappear more or less quickly, but where the soul will follow its path.

This are the teachings princeps of Taoism, but also all the philosophies and religions. Then, attach us to love the life, for, when our time will be completed on this earth, love the death.

To achieve the full conscience

And if it was the great secret to learn to manage our emotions? The full conscience is different from the state of emptiness that are looking for the Buddhists. It is a state of mind that is acquired to the force of pluriquotidiennes practices. You can call it: "Here and Now".

How to reach this state? In the first place by the meditation. Yes, but that is! That is capable in our modern world to devote several hours per day to this type of practice. The simplest method for beginners is to learn throughout the day

412

to ask twenty, thirty seconds, without thinking of nothing, or at least be concentrated on a single point.

In the course on the respiration (see chapitre 17), it has been advocated to stop 10-15 times in the day, during a 30 seconds, to breathe in full conscience. In the course on the tea, to chapitre 21, we have seen that we must drink in quantities split and in full conscience our small glasses to tea. When you relax one to two times, 10 minutes in the day, meditate 5 minutes per day in a seated position on a chair, practice 15 minutes of Qi Gong: all these daily actions allow you to be there, here and now, you create a superego, a "Jiminy Cricket" who sees you act. It is an entity immaterial, without consistency, without smell or localization which sees you reading this text. Use it to stop you to the first image of a film emotional which is in you. If we take the example of the anger which belongs to the liver, before a word which kills do so of your mouth, before hitting or insulting someone, you will be able to direct the film which is built, to play a role without that it does hurt Vienna neither you nor others. You can stop at the first image and even the transform.

Not to lose in the meanders of the negative judgment

This is not a thin case that to unlearn to judge! I am not talking here of the altruistic judgment, positive, the side Yang, light of the force, but this judgment permanent negative on all and all things. Imagine a world without slander, without criticism, without charge, nor déblatération, without Gossip: There would be no more large-thing to say in family meals. We would then be in the need to relearn how to speak of the essential, "things of life".

Do not forget that teaches us the MTC: "What thy heart emits, thy heart receives. "To force of emissions of negative energies, it is not surprising to find themselves in situations of negativity, evil-BE or suffering. It is this quantum physicist Russian who was taking as an example the visit of an exhibition of painting. At a time, a table you dislike. Yet if it is, is that it has at least liked to someone, would be this only to its author! Instead of spitting its venom, judge negatively, you only have to spend your path and feed your eye of a table which is on the same vibration that your cable of life.

413

As a kaleidoscope, any ultimate truth has in it a thousand and one facets, a thousand and one ways to apprehend. Exit out of the dark side of the "force" to go to the light of the positive thoughts. Accept the contradiction as an essential element of the dialog. But this request here also a lot of selfless love and the progressive abandonment of the carapace of his ego.

Recharge the battery of the kidney

There are a thousand and one methods to learn to manage his emotions, but almost all come from outer brackets. Since our early childhood, we have been led to believe that we were the effects in the appearance of all our ills and not the causes: "If I am under the influence of recurring anger, sadness destructive, of chronic fears, it is because of the other and I am not there for nothing. "And if we look at the other side of the lens?

You do more without knowing the importance in MTC of this famous battery of the kidney, center of the self-healing, self-regulation and the adaptation of the organism. When we implement all practices to bring it to the daily in its rate of recharge maximum, it is the agency itself, which autogère at the emotional level. Either by elf-regulatory the software component to which corresponds the unbalanced emotion, or by putting forward an emotion capable to control another one.

If one morning at sunrise, you have a sense of sadness, it is just a self-regulation that emits the body to calm a state of anger excessive. I refer you to the cycle of the five elements (see chapitre 4) where we can see that the combat sadness the anger. If you come to undergo an important emotional trauma, your body, thanks to the battery of the kidney, will be in a position to put forward what is called "a state of Resilience", a state of amnesia targeted. But even more, some time after, your body will rid itself of its " emotional waste", able to rise to the surface in the periods of weakness. That is the purpose of the methods Yang Sheng Fa, prevention in the MTC. We could go as far as to say that a true practitioner in MTC does not cure his patient. It restores to the body of the latter the ability to autoguérir, by circulating which is stagnant and helping to recharge its battery.

Adopt the internal smile

We have seen that the heart, while being the master of the five emotions, had the same energy vibration that the joy. Not the false joy which ignites the stages, but this joy characterized by the permanent smile. In a first time, it is fundamental to relearn how to smile. Why not take a Ice as witness and work on a daily basis the "Smile of the buddha" or of the saints? Little by little, this smile will be part of your personality. External, this smile is intériorisera. It will call "The smile inside".

In MTC, called this state "the heart open". It is our ability to smile continuously, to admire the good side of the world that surrounds us, to adopt a positive attitude toward all things, to satisfy everything, to never complain. A common point to very many centenarians, it is to see the draw on their faces the "wrinkles of the smile." Having such an attitude allows you to calm down the fire of the emotions, "Feeding the Heart", unlock the circulation of blood and energy.

Adopt a new philosophy of life

The Pr Leung, in his Testament philosophical, we had bequeathed the following text: " Change progressively your power by following the advice. Slowly start to do the exercises Chinese in adapting them to your needs. And especially, adopt a philosophy of life, a way to see the things that put the emphasis on the following points:

" Rendez-vous responsible for your actions and your choice.

" Extériorisez-you and get involved in activities and thoughts altruistic. These thoughts must lead on actions that are larger than you, are enriching and make you more fort morally.

" Do you use to resolve as quickly as possible conflicts in order to avoid the loss of energy emotional. Fair or unfair, good or bad, whatever your decision, that it make you lose or win, try to find the best solution to your point of view as quickly as possible and proceed to something else.

" Live fully the rest of your life. If you have committed an error, fix the error and continue to the suite.

"Do you accept, do you like, follow-you. Know how to say "yes" or "no". Be attentive to your internal prints and enjoy them. Be comfortable with yourself when you are alone.

"Love his entourage is an absolute necessity if we want to be able to live in society, which contributes to promote health. "

Chapter 23
The ten practices
Day-to-day
Longevity in MTC

OfYears This chapter, you will have access to ten daily practices intended to recharge your battery of the kidney to prevent all types of pathologies physical, mental or emotional. These practices will also be a tremendous help for the healing of these same pathologies. It is not question of spend hours and hours to cultivate our ego, our narcissism, our navel gazing, to become drug addicts of the gym. But just to incorporate in our day, a series of fundamental actions to implement to retain the balance of life.

Yes, but I do not have the time! To Meditate: a day of 24 hours can be divided into three times eight hours. As well we have eight hours for sleep, eight hours for work and eight hours to care for self and others. We will see that even in the Metro or in the car, we can take care of itself.

Expanding our field of vision. And if we consider that a day is to the image of a whole life! In the morning, to the rise of Yang, a new life begins. Its peak is at noon. Then at the end of the afternoon, the Yang begins to decline doing his place in the Yin. In the evening, it is falling asleep. The Chinese call this a small death. It is like this that will happen the beginning of our passage. Then, the other facet unknown to the life occurs during our sleep. And again in the morning, another life restarts, with its batch of tests positive and negative, of emotions, meetings, readings... In this day-life, we must find a balance between the Yin-Yang, between the selfishness salutary and altruism, internalizing and externalizing. The practices that will follow will have to integrate harmoniously within the framework of this day-life.

Conscious breathing in the center of practices

In the morning at sunrise, in the evening before going to bed, throughout your day, respiration should become a real **leitmotif. Ask yourself on a daily basis the question: "How many times have I breathed in full conscience since this morning? "You can practice a thousand and**

417

one things for your health. But if the respiration does not follow, all the rest is of almost to nothing, except perhaps to allow you to survive (see chapitre 17**).**

The Sleep, the other facet of the VITALITY

Take care of his sleep is an essential aspect in the methods of prevention in the MTC. It is the most natural way that has given us Dame Nature to recharge our battery. If you sleep 33 years in 100 years of life, this is not for nothing (see chapitre 19).

The relaxation to the rescue of the blows of the bar

As soon as you feel the dawn of the signal of alarm that emits your body, namely the fatigue, all business cessantes relax a few minutes. Do not forget: 10 minutes of relaxation well conducted equivalent to 3 hours of sleep. The two best moments to relax are after the noon meal and toward 17-18 hours. Observe the rules of the Sleep and you do not wear that better (see chapitre 19).

The Movement is life

Practice daily, during 10-15 minutes, a series of exercises which are mobilizing all your joints, act on all meridians which are in relation recall it with the internal organs. And why not initiate you to the practice of a series of Qi Gong. It is a very great legacy of the MTC to enable us to achieve longevity in good health (see chapitre 18).

Massage-you again and again

Take a moment in the day to massage the bottom of your back, your neck and any other place of stiffness and pain. Why not in the morning in his bathroom. As it is said: "There is never better served that by itself! "In the evening before bedtime, massage your feet a dozen minutes. And if you know a few fundamental points at this level, such as the 1RN, 3F, 60V, the 3RN, do not hesitate to practice a automassage in digitoponcture to their locations (see chapitre 14). It is an excellent way to achieve a state of relaxation general and against the insomnia. The end of the end is to have a massage. The Massage releases, fact energy flow along the meridians, acts indirectly on the stagnations of internal organs.

The meditation for to listen to the voice of his soul

There is no need to set the bar too high at the beginning of the practice. In position sitting on a chair, 5 to 10 minutes of meditation can transform your life. This type of Meditation allows us to divest ourselves of the carapace of our ego, supplied in continuous flow by our five senses, by too much information. Little by little creates a funnel" between this armor that is our Hyper-conscience and our subconscious the more profound. Do not forget, one of the great sense of life and put us in the listening of our soul (see chapitre 18).

The regularity, keyword of the longevity

Like the regularity of the cycle of the seasons, the day-night cycle, our organization is fact that cycles (blood circulation and energy, digestion-assimilation-evacuation, etc.). We need points of regular mark that punctuate our day-life. Do not hesitate to plan our day in the morning at sunrise, planning bounded by fixed schedules and regular as to hours of sunrise and sunset, hours of meals, hours of certain practices such as Qi gong, relaxation or meditation. However, do not become the slave of these "schedules"! Too regularity kills the regularity. I refer you to the concept of "enjoyment" developed in the part on the power supply.

A good muscle tone in daily life

Not need lock you into rooms for this or to do sport up to exhaustion. A regular sport is necessary for the conservation of health, but it is on a daily basis that you should work your muscles. Mount the stairs slowly and in full conscience to muscle your legs. Practice the position called the "cavalier of iron" (see chapitre 14) when you brush your teeth or dry your hair. This is an excellent way to tonify the four muscles are the most important to the energy of the Kidney: the quadriceps, the glutes, the abdominal muscles down and the perineum. A few "ABS" by here and there, a few slow movements in muscular tension extreme, a dozen of the pumps at the height of a bathtub, will be very effective to maintain a good muscle tone, the guarantor of a good blood circulation and of energy in the body. But all this means of course that you have the will, the determination, the confidence in you and the changeover to the Act. But that is another story...

The walk of long life

The walk is considered in MTC as one of the first antidepressants. It frees the thoughts, circulates, avoids the stagnations, invigorates the energy of the spleen, conductor of the digestion of food bowl. Each time you need to move from one point to another, opt for the meditative walk, walking of "full conscience" (see chapitre 17).

The return of spring

There is an exercise known to all practitioners of Qi Gong: "The return of spring". Without taking off the heels, it is to give impetus to a movement of vertical shaking, self-maintained by the swaying motion of the shoulders. The swing hand exclusively of the hocks, without that the shoulders are not tight or raised. Once the movement driven, the body enough relaxd, like a spring, this movement will not seek no more muscular effort. You will feel your eyes move in your orbits, your lungs in the thoracic cage. Your breathing must not be directed. It must be done simply. It adapts to your pace. The effects become visible at the end of two or three weeks of practice. The more visible occur at the level of the metabolism of the cells of the skin. The face takes a fair complexion rosé, because the blood circulation is regularized, where the name of "return of spring".

These shocks are mobilizing all your fascia, your plans of landslide, favoring the elimination of waste and the liberation of the stagnations. The immune system is discharged of toxins and by that same fortified.

This exercise improves the overall state of health, stimulates the sexual functions and promotes the loss of weight. In short, a true exercise of long life and what is more, free. More need to invest large sums in devices that will produce the same result. The few contraindications are obvious : pregnant women, during the period of the rules when they are important or as a result of layers, in case of pain in the knees or the Lombes. I do not have the time? This exercise should only be practiced twice a day and during a period of only two minutes! And if you can't, made of jump rope or the trampoline!

Chapter 24
The ten reasons for
To chew

NOu can have the best possible dietetics, bio and all the rest, but if we do not réapprenons chewing, instead of gain in energy thanks to daily meals, c is the battery of the kidney which will gradually be depleted. The energy of your spleen, conductor of the digestion of food bowl, in the absence of prédigestion of food bowl in the mouth thanks to this chewing, will produce an additional effort and "usera" prematurely. Look around you. It chews 4 to 5 times, it devours without even knowing what we have just swallow and it gobbles up again. While according to all traditions, it is 20 to 30 times that we should apply mastic our bite. In MTC, we are going so far as to say that it must apply mastic to the soups! One of the signs that we find in many of the centenarians, this are the masseters, masticatory muscles located at the level of the cheekbones that are very developed.

A direct action on the energy of the body
To realize, digestion can mobilize more than half of the energy contained in the battery of the kidney (see chapitre 2). By chewing, not as a turtle or as this child who does not stop chewing a food that he is unable to swallow, but quickly 20 to 30 times each bite, you avoid unnecessarily lose energy. You make it easier for both the work of the stomach. This is the time of the digestion which is shortcut. You avoid the postprandial fatigue, the States of somnolence of after meals.

The analysis of the food bowl
The saliva is "intelligent". It is able to recognize each component of the bite of food. But also a subtle energy present in the color, smell, the nature, the flavor of the food. From there, she gives orders accordingly at the digestive system to a better digestibility of the latter. Thanks to this same chewing, you no longer need a booster cushion of taste. You will recognize for example the taste of different categories of rice as would a goûteur of wine. It is one of the reasons for which the MTC advocates the regime dissociated

in a same meal. This will allow the saliva to distinguish even better the components of the bite.

The saliva transforms the cereals in slow sugars

We know that the purpose of a daily meal to the inverse of the festive meal is to nourish the body in energy and by there even to help the recharging of the battery of the kidney. The saliva, thanks among other things to some enzymes that it contains, hydrolysis, transforms the starch content in the Cereals, tubers and pulses into maltose, in slow sugars. When we mâchons long bread or rice, we feel gradually this sweet taste in the mouth. It is this taste that we call "mild flavor" IN MTC. I refer you to the basic rule which is to eat cereals and tubers "nature" in the mouth, without the addition of any other ingredient, for that this transformation is optimal.

The saliva, grand cleaner food bowl

Of slightly acid pH, saliva contains certain substances capable of neutralizing poisons and small bébêtes reactions. For example, eating raw vegetables bio or his garden, is good! But this can only be done if we "cooked" this vegetable in his mouth thanks to a long chewing to warm the nature too cold of these foods. The saliva will also allow to destroy parasites and small eggs clinging to the leaves. It is thanks to the saliva that the wounds of the mouth heal very quickly. It is this same saliva, which plays the role of a natural antiseptic for small wounds or skin bites.

Chewing promotes the renewal of organic liquids

When we mâchons sufficiently our food bowl, it is a half-liter of saliva, which is found in the stomach. It is one of the reasons for which it is unnecessary to drink in excess during a meal. Because the digestive juices and the efficiency of digestion are reduced and the time of digestion lengthened. This saliva is made up of 95% water, drawn from the organic liquids. Good mastication obliges to regenerate these same liquids. It is a great way to oppose the stagnations of blood and energy in the body.

The saliva, a powerful lubricant

The saliva has a great power humectant, but also of lubrication of the digestive tract, esophagus and intestines. It therefore facilitates the swallowing, especially when one is in the presence of this that the MTC calls the "syndrome of the nucleus of plum," whose origin is in the blocking of the energy of the liver under the effect of internalized emotions. Often found among women, the fact to chew extensively promotes the lowering of food, thus avoiding this sensation of ball in the throat.

Combat depression!

Two reasons for this. The own of a depression is to be folded on itself. If it comes to persuade him to chew at length his food bowl, we defeated in part the nodes of its emotional straitjacket. In addition, we saw that there were two types of saliva, a belonging to the energy of the kidney and the other in the spleen. When we mastiquons our food bowl, it is this last which is secreted by the parotidiennes glands. By requiring the Agency to secrete this saliva, it regulates indirectly the software spleen. However, it is said in the MTC that the spleen governs the reflection, the fact to rehash the past, emotions that when they are in excess contribute to the onset of the Depression. It is for this reason that in some ancient texts of MTC, we find the aphorism in shortcut:" chew helps fight against the Depression. "

Lose weight

The fact chew at length takes more time. It gobbles up less of bites, while being more quickly sated. In addition, we have seen that the software Rate was the conductor of our digestion. If you ask him to provide a excessive work by a too big effort of digestion of food BADLY chewed, it will weaken. It follows an internal imbalance which causes a abnormal weight gain. In contrast, swallowing food" prédigérés" in the mouth, in smaller quantities, it will harmonize the action of this software. In the space of a few months and without "regime", we can find its ideal weight.

Chew away from the Dentist

The fact chew allows you to put the OS in pressure. However, it is one of the only means to foster the creation of fibers of protein, on which come to attach the minerals to give the strength to the bone. However, in MTC, the teeth are considered as the end of the bone. If these are not maintained by a solid bone, they become rickety and fall easily. There is a Taoist exercise which consists of slamming of the teeth a hundred times in the morning, to combat this problem of heaving. But chew at length allows you to lead to the same result.

An act of full consciousness

Before that chewing does not become unconscious competence, water will be passed under the bridges. We should consider the chewing as an act of full consciousness. We should not speak during the daily meals, to allow us to concentrate on our food bowl and the chewing. But let us be realistic. As conscious breathing, to learn to chew is very easy. But the regular practice is any other. We practice, and then is forgotten. Then one restarts... It is a good education on "the fickleness of things". But the fact of repair continuously the book on the profession will help us to acquire this status if important IN MTC of "full conscience", "Here and Now".

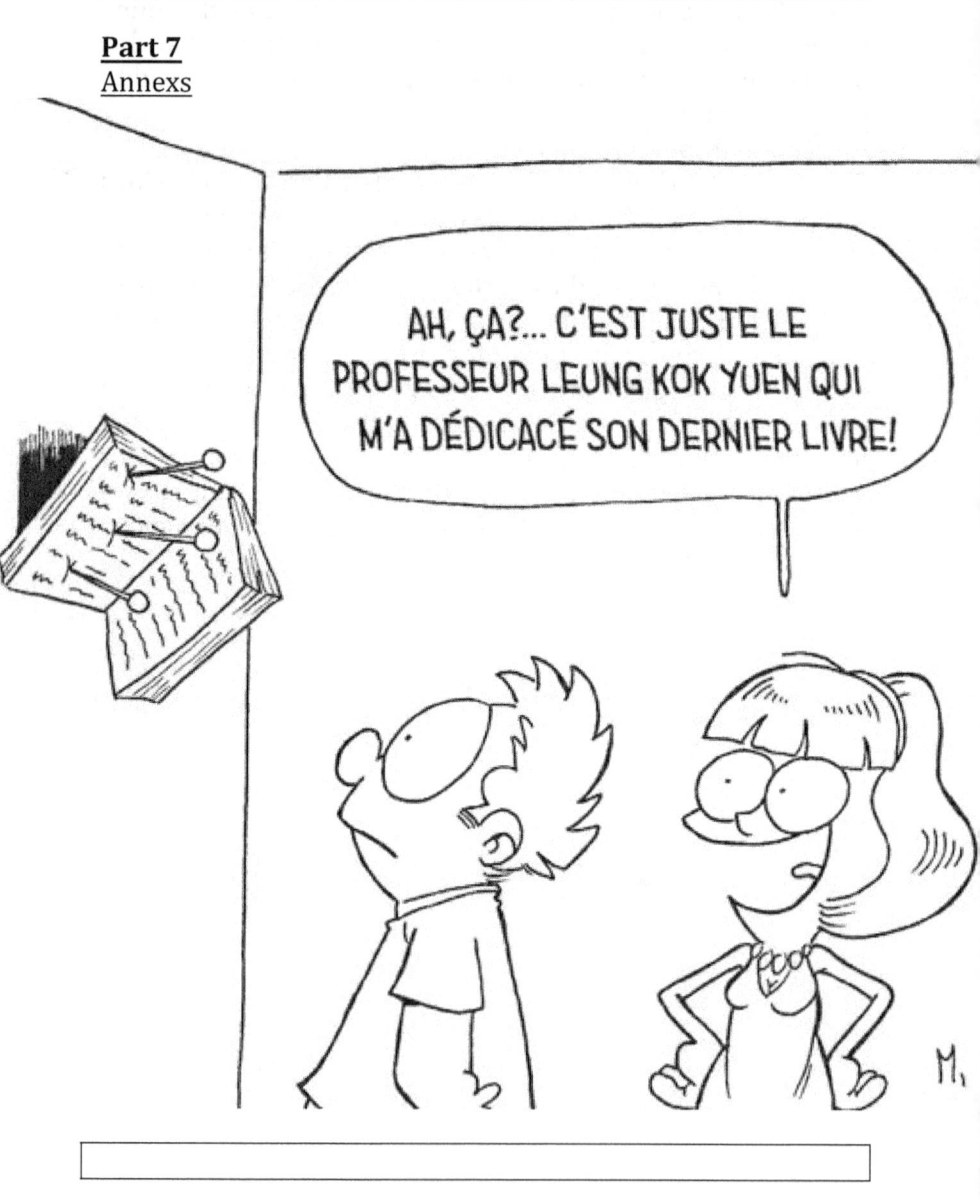

In this part...

Annexs A and B are more technical, and reserved for practitioners, or future practitioners of the MTC. The Pr Leung Kok Yuen has bequeathed to his students his technique of poncture closest to the tradition. Let us not forget that it was Grand Master in acupuncture and regarded as such in China, and then in the United States. There you will also find the grid of choice of points which will allow you to deal with a few pathological situations. If you have the profound vision, you will see that this education is a real treasure.

For all null, the Annexs C and D provide useful addresses and a glossary of the most commonly used terms in the MTC.

Appendix A
The Technique
Of poncture of
Pr Leung Kok Yuen

NOu have seen in chapitre 13 **an introduction to ancient techniques concerning the manipulation of the needles. In this which will follow, you will have access to the true technique of our master. This part is therefore directed more specifically to the professionals. The personal technique that it transmits to us is perhaps a little different from the ancient techniques, but it has the merit of being very simple to understand and especially to help us obtain very convincing results. And it is mainly the result of the therapeutic experience of more than twenty generations of practitioners from father to son! Let us look at this, step after step.**

The depth of the Insertion

At the level of the choice of the length of the needles, the practitioner should know first what is the depth that it will apply and from there, choose

En pratique the needle which should be the better. If he knows that the point he will prick is only 0.5 Cun, why choose a needle of 1.5 cun? In a general way, the taking of the needles of 1.5 cun is more difficult than that of 1 Cun. (Cun is a unit of length Traditional Chinese. The reference is the width of a thumb which makes 1.5 Cun, either +/ - 20 mm.)

To prick points such as 36E, 34VB, it must use a depth higher. For these reasons, it is necessary to use of needles 2.3 Cun. To prick of persons with a strong overweight, it will be necessary to choose a needle longer.

If we take the example of 4IM in the text, it is said that to prick this point, it uses an average depth of 0.5 Cun. But this is theoretical. It must be understood that the depth that we must use experimental remains; it is at the time of the spades that one decides to depth. The depth of the Needles depends in particular on the reactions of the patient, but also and especially the moment where we seized the energy.

Technique of work of the needle

In a general way, it does not take the needles at the level of the body. The best outlet is located between the handle and the needle.

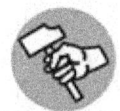

Fundamental, in the majority of cases it will be appropriate to prick perpendicular to the surface of the skin. If there are points that we must bite in

En pratique oblique, the hand must then be put in the direction of the needle. This is not the needle which changes position in the hand, but the hand that is positioned in relation to the point.

It is necessary to use the strength of the wrist and not the force of the fingers. When Spades with the strength of the wrist, the needle does not move, whereas if it stings with the fingers, the needle moves, and there is a risk of the twist.

After Piqué, attention should be paid to the time when the Qi arrives. When it feels that the Qi is arrived, it stops the penetration of the needle, and this is the proper depth. We often compare the Qi in the Tide: there are times where she is high and moments where it is low. For these reasons, there are times where there spades superficially, and other where there spades more deeply.

The Qi is influenced by several factors, such as the emotional states, the ingested food, the type of work and the Xith Qi, the perverse energy. When

À retenir the Qi is high, the depth is not important, but when the Qi is low, the depth is important. The good depth is entered when the Qi is arrived. When it is there, we do penetrates more the needle.

When the practitioner has short needles, and that it does not happen to have a good depth, a few tips:

"In the choice of points, it is better to prick in this case the location next to the OS. If one takes 4GI for example, in a general way, it puts the needle in the middle where is located the flesh. But when one knows that the needle is not long enough, it is rather toward the side of the OS. This does not mean that it piques the OS, but we spades just to the side of the OS.

"Often, to prick the point 30VB, point at the level of the buttock (where spades the nurse), it must use the needles of 5 Cun. But we do not find them often. You can only use the needles of 3 cun or 2.5. In this case, it is necessary to use this technique: the patient is asked to lie on the side, the leg of the Below is right, one above is bent and it spades where is located the hollow. This is the correct position. So when we did not of needles long enough, it must prick at the place where is located the OS in the articulation between the two OS.

"There is another method. When you must use a needle of 1.5 cun and that it was only a needle to 1, we withdraw the needle just a little, it leaves a time, and then either we turn, either move the needle toward the top or bottom. But of course, the ideal is to have the right needle.

In a general way, it must leave a space between the body of the needle and the handle by report to the skin. It must not be push the needle up to the level of the handle. In effect, the latter risk of be absorbed in part by the QI who arrives. In this case, the patient felt a pain. For these reasons, it must always leave a small distance between the needle and the handle.

When the Qi is not there, it must turn a little the needle by small up-and-coming during a time, and when one feels that it arrives, the needle is a little absorbed. There, we leave the needle.

A lot of acupuncturists do not know recognize the time of the arrival of the Qi. Often these people leave the needles in the body of the patient without the handle, because leaving the needles, the qi can happen by the suite, but this is not a good method. Often, in this case, the qi can arrive 10, 15, or 20 minutes after.

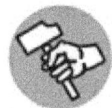

A good acupuncturist must have experience on the arrival of the Qi. It must feel the time where the Qi arrives, it is very important. If we let the Qi En pratique arrive all alone, or if we let the needle as this, without knowing the time of the arrival of the Qi, one loses the opportunity for toning or to disperse. Because

430

it is at this time, when the Qi arrives, that we can do the techniques Bu or Xie, sedation or toning.

Duration of the poncture

Between the penetration of the needle and the output of the needle, there is between a breathing and seven breaths, regardless of the technique of toning or sedation. Leave the needles is not so important. What is important is the way to leave the needles between one or seven breaths.

We cannot say that the fact to leave the needles longer or to remove more quickly gives the best effects. The important thing is the manipulation and the feeling of the needle.

If we let the needles a little longer, it gets only a moderate effect, either in toning or sedation. Therefore, when we speak of toning-sedation balanced, this will be on the duration of the poncture that this will come into play.

Order of the poncture

In a general way, for toning, one chooses the points close to the location of the disease. To disperse, one chooses points distant. (We will return there.)

However, to obtain good results, it must know how to manipulate and change the order of points. There are three points which we must make Attention:

En pratique

It is the Practitioner that is positioned in relation to the patient. Let us take an example. When we must use points such as 36E (to the knee), 14DM (on top of the back), 6CC (on front-arm). When it is a pathology of type fullness, Shi, one begins by the points to distance, and then subsequently, the points near. It then asks the patient to lie on your back to reach the 36th and the 6cc. Then it will on the side for the 14DM. Whereas if it is a disease of type Xu, we first take the points near and then the points at a distance.

The second point is also important. When spades the points on the back, it is better to avoid asking the patient to lie on the chest. This is the lateral decubitus position which is the best. It puts a cushion between the two legs, for well stall the patient. This is to raise a little the thigh. The muscles will then be perfectly released. On the chest, the muscles of the back are more contracted. It is difficult to penetrate the needles and the point is more difficult to find.

When the patient is in lateral decubitus, to take the point, it traces of first the vertebral column. Indeed, some people have the column diverted to the right or to the left. This position also allows you to more easily find the muscle, which is located at the side of the column. Often in this position, you can find a hollow that is located at the side of the column and there, we pressed easier the needles.

Therefore, in this position, it may sting vertically the points of the back, because it sees the muscles. They are not contracted and you can easily find the hollow that is located between the two muscles.

But the position on the side is not absolute.

As regards the problems of distal points or close, it must decide according to the state of the patient. If the patient has really very afraid of being bitten, it must be especially prick the points which are located to the members, that is to say to the hand or foot. For a patient who is very tense, in general, it is necessary to avoid prick the points such as 20VB (in the neck) or 14DM (on top of the back), because these are places that are a little dangerous.

And if, despite everything, has headaches , one tries to avoid piercing these places, because it is afraid to the patient and it would be frightened. When the patient is tense, it must not prick the points which are intended to his illness. It spades rather the point Shen Men, 7C (wrist) or Yang Ling Quan, 34VB (at the knee): these two points are very good for the people nervous.

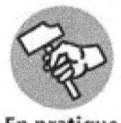

The Sesame of the acupuncturist
I applied the method which will follow, as all the faithful students of my master, for more than
En pratique thirty years with this feeling very deep of pure energy sharing.

When spades, attention should be paid to the finger which supports. When it is well supported on the skin, and that is a concentrated, one begins to bite. In principle, it pierces the skin quickly. Once the needle has crossed the skin, it pushes the needle in depth, all gently, up to the time where one feels that the needle is a bit tense or a little absorbed, it stops. Either for the toning or sedation, one stops to push the needle when one feels that the Qi is arrived.

For toning, Bu, it continues to maintain the needle, when the Qi is come, up to the time where one feels that the Qi is sufficiently arrived. At this time, it loose the needle. After having dropped the hand, it leaves in general the needle between one and seven breaths of the patient. If we must apply the moxa, we can leave the needle a little longer. If we must tone more Using Moxa, we leave the needle in place a dozen minutes. In the contrary case, it begins to remove the needle, following the breathing of a patient, but very gently. In principle, the Qi happens all gently and then massively. When the Qi is arrived massively, we can already withdraw the needle. For these reasons, there is no need to leave the needle even more. The fact to leave the needle depends mainly on the location where you spades.

To disperse Xie, it leaves the Qi arrive all gently, then massively. When one feels that the Qi is completely arrived, one enters a little more in depth the needle and then aspen the needle, up to the time where one feels that the needle is completely tense. There, we loose.

We loose the needle for toning, when the Qi is barely arrived. To disperse, we loose the hand when the QI is completely arrived. After this, we leave the needle between three and seven breaths. If it is believed that one must leave the needle during three breaths, we must first have the impression that the needle is completely tense, as soon as the first breath. At the second respiration, either one rotates the needle, either we the aspen, we made a to-and-fro movement vertical. It depends on our need. After the second respiration, we loose the hand and then it turns a last time the needle and it is located here, to the third breathing. At the end of the third, it begins to highlight the needle gently.

433

However, there are two kinds of dispersion: for the great dispersion, one uses a little more force, that is to say, it aspen, or it turns a little more the needles. For the small dispersion, it moves less the needles.

To make a sedation toning-balanced, Bing Bu, Bing Xie, it pushes the needle, one expects the Qi. When it arrives, it continues to turn the needles up to the time where the Qi arrives massively. At this time, there is the loose hand. After this, we leave the needle between three and seven breaths, and then you go out the needle by turning very gently.

In each of these three techniques, it penetrates and it fate gently all the needle and, after that, we must make a massage. All of this pertains to the personal experiences of Pr Leung that he has asked us to apply in our practice. Otherwise, you can always use the old techniques.

Appendix B
The method of choice
Of the points according to the
Pr Leung Kok Yuen

NOu will see the criteria which, from everything that has been asked the chapter dedicated to acupuncture (chapitre 13**), will enable the practitioner to establish the right formula to treat his patient. Two groups of points will be the basis of this method.**

The mode of employment
We have in effect of the so-called points "major" which are divided into three parts:
" The points near;
" The median points;
" The Distal points.
And the additional points which are often for specific use.

The rule is that the main points must be used. The additional points are not necessarily mandatory. They will be able to increase the effect of the En pratique formula, but it will then be necessary to take account of the Constitution of the subject at the time of the poncture.

I remind you that the Pr Leung Kok Yuen insisted on the fact that we should use that few points to each treatment. Between five and seven in average. And especially pay attention to the first sessions where, to be schematic, this "moved" at the level of energy.

You will see that with this method, if the pathology is really benign, a single point is sufficient. Then we let me add depending on the severity.

For the main points, we have seen that:
" The points near were therefore near the home of the disease;
" The distal points were them away, most of the time on the hands and feet;
" The median points them are especially vertebral or on the of the May.

As regards the order of poncture, there will tweak always the main points first. And then, depending on the case, the additional points.

For the main points :

"When you is located in front of a Syndrome Xu, of weakness, it will tweak the points near First, the median points then, and the distal points at the end.

"Before a syndrome Shi, in excess, it spades the distal points first, the median points and then the points close.

"If it was decided to make a moxibustion with the acupuncture, we will begin by the Acupuncture and then the moxas.

The 57 points of the Pr Leung Kok Yuen

The Pr Leung we thus has given a list of 57 points with which we are going to have to learn to juggle perfectly. Most of these points are found elsewhere in the different series of points seen previously.

Table B-1 The 57 points of the Pr Leung Kok Yuen.

HAND	11p, Shao Shang 9P, Tai Yuan 1IG, Shao Ze	Points to particular purpose
WRIST	5C, Tong Li 6CC, Nis Guan 7P, binds that 4GI, He GI 4IG, Wan Gu 6IG, Yang Lao	Distal points
ELBOW	3CC, that Ze 5P, Chi Ze 3C, Shao Hai 11GI, that Chi	Distal points
Shoulder	15GI, Jian Yu	Median point
FOOT	1F, Da Dun	Particular Purpose

436

	1RN, Yong Quan	
Foot, kick	6RN, Zao Hai 3F, Tai Chong 44E, Nis Ting	Distal points
LEG	39VB, Xuan Zhong 6RT, San Yin Jiao 57V, Cheng Shan	Distal points
KNEE	36E, zu San Li 34VB, Yang Ling Quan 40V, Wei Zhong 9RT, Yin Ling Quan	Distal points
HIP	30VB, Huan Tiao	Distal Point
The head	26DM, Shui Gou 24DM, Shen Ting 20DM, Bai Today 20VB, Feng Shi 14Dm, Da Zhui	The first two to particular purpose The other: median points
BACK	13V, EIF SHU 14V, Jue Yin SHU 15V, Xin Shu 18V, Gan SHU 19V, Dan SHU 20V, Pi SHU 21V, Wei SHU	Points near
LOMBES	22V, San Jiao SHU 23V, shen shu 25V, Da Chang Shu 27V, Xiao Chang Shu 28V, Pang Guang SHU	Points near 4DM, the mid-point

	4DM, Ming Men	
Chest, Abdomen	1P, Zhong Fu 25E, Tian SHU 12RM, Zhong WAN 13F, Zhang Men 14RM, Ju that 4WD, Guan Yuan 3WD, Zhong Ji 25VB, Jing Men 17RM, Tan Zhong 5WD, shi men 24VB, Ri Yue 14F, Qi Men	Points near

Will later in the Method

It should be first of all to differentiate a disease of type Xu, weakness, or type Shi, fullness. It can, for example, at first glance, consider that a malaria is a disease Shi. But when it becomes chronic, it is a disease Xu.

Then we will decide on the policy of the treatment. Is it that we are going to treat the Ben, the root of the disease, or only relieve the apparent manifestation. For example, if one is in front of a symptom or an acute illness, there will be a temptation, which is logical, to deal first with the Biao, the symptom, for then, later, in return to the root.

You may find in front of three cases of figure:

"If you are located in the presence of a pathology of which the cause is well identified and that the evolution symptomatic is normal, we are not taking care of the symptoms to treat. There is concern about the Ben, the root, for more efficient results and more durable and most of the time we have at our disposal of pre-established treatments.

"If the cause of the disease and the pathological changes are not clear, and that it has not to our provision of effective treatments pre-established, it can use only a palliative

treatment symptomatic, in particular if the symptoms are sudden and dangerous.
" Finally, we can sometimes make both a curative treatment, in s interesting to the root, at the Ben, the disruption of the Palliative and, treating the Biao. In order to avoid that there is an antagonism between the points to prick, it must first of all avoid take too much and it should be the prick in the order.

It is from these three criteria that we will choose our treatment.

To summarize

Table To predominance Xu

If we are in the presence of a table to predominance Xu, we will take as the criteria for the choice of points:
" Nearest for benign disease.
" We will add a mid-point for a disease more serious.
" We will add a mid-point and the distal points for diseases to very strong symptomatology.
" In all ways, there will be more points close to that of distal points.

With regard to the procedure of treatment, you will take the points near first and the distal points then. In addition, we will take the points of the top of the body before those on the bottom.

With respect to the operating mode, the stimulation will be light on the points near. It will be average or slight on the Distal points. This will be the most often moxas.

Table predominantly Shi

If we are in the presence of a table of predominantly Shi, we will take as the criteria for the choice of points:
" The distal point for benign disease.
" We will add a mid-point to a more serious illness.
" And if the illness is more important, in addition to the mid-points, one will add points relatives.

439

"Of all the ways, the distal points will be more numerous than the points near.

"To obtain a drainage strong, it will use or the distal points associated on a same meridian, or an association top-down, hands and feet.

With regard to the procedure of treatment, we will take the distal point in first, then the near point if there is place. Emphasis will be placed on the points of the bottom of the body first and then the points of the top.

With respect to the operating mode, there will be a strong stimulation on the distal points and an average stimulation on the points means and relatives.

We are going to take a concrete example taken from this general rule.

If we find ourselves in front of a gastritis, a inflammatory pain at the level of the stomach. It can be chronic or acute.

If we find ourselves in front of a chronic case which can therefore be considered as Xu:

"In a case Benin, it will use the 12RM which is therefore the near point.

"We may add the point Mu which is the 17V, which will serve to tonify the Yin and the Yang.

"If the pathology is a little more serious, there will be append the 21Vb, which will be the mid-point.

"In the cases even more important, there join the 44E as the distal point or the 36E.

For a case of acute gastritis, therefore Shi:

"If the case is Benin, we can be satisfied with the 44E, which is the distal point.

"For a case a little more acute, there join the 17V, the point MU or the 20VB considered as point median.

"If the case is much more acute, one will add the 21V, point near, and the 36E, point associated with the same meridian, with the 44E or the 6CC if account is taken of the theory of the association top-bottom.

There is a nursery rhyme that has given us our master: "For cases Xu, points near, stimulation slight, for cases Shi, distal points, strong stimulation. "

440

The method applied to different pathologies

The diseases can be divided into:
" Disease of the trunk;
" Diseases of the hands and feet;
" Diseases of the zang-fu, organs;
" Diseases of the whole body.

Table B-2 disease of the trunk.

	Take	Examples
Case Xu CHRONICLE	Of the points close and median as main points. In complementary point and in the case of need, there piochera according the case among the five distal points which are: - For the abdominal area, the 36E; - For the area of the loin and back, the 40V (formerly referred to as 54V); - For the area of the head and neck the 7P; - For the area of the mouth and face, the 4GI; - And finally for the area of the chest and flanks, 6Cc. Therefore, according to the degree of gravity of the disease, it will take more points near and Median. And in function of the affected area, it will complement by an action of drainage with points of general action. Therefore, according to the degree of gravity of the	*In case of weak abdominal muscle or more precisely in the case of hernia, we will take as points: - The 25E, point close; - The 4WD, point close; - The 4DM, mid-point; - The 36e, additional point. *In case of muscle atrophy des Lombes: - The 23V near point; - The 4DM mid-point; - The 40V additional point. *In case of dizziness: - The 23DM, near point;

441

	disease, it will take more points near and Median. And in function of the affected area, it will complement by an action of drainage with points of general action.	- The 20VB mid-point; - The 7P additional point. In the case of paresis or facial paralysis: - The 6E in near point; - The 20VB in mid-point; - The 4E in near point; - The 4IM in additional point. *In case of chronic pain of the chest and flank: - The 1P in near point; - The 14DM in mid-point; - The 6CC in additional point.
Case Shi Acute	It will consider the points to general action as Distal points. - For the abdominal area, the 36E; - For the area of the loin and back, the 40V Ex 54V; - For the area of the head and neck, the 7P; - For the area of the mouth and face, the 4GI; - Finally to the area of the chest and flanks, 6Cc.	*In case of muscle spasm of the abdomen, acute hernia by example, we will take: - The 36E, as remote point; - The 4DM, mid-point; - The 6WD, near point.

Then, following the general rule, we will take the median points and relatives as complementary points.

Depending on the severity, it will take one or several additional points.

*In case of lumbago, the 40V as remote point.

*In case of the ills of teeth: the 4IM as remote point to which we can add the 7E or the 6E.

*For Intercostal neuralgia prior as the Zona:
- The 6cc as distal point;
- The 14DM as mid-point.

The rhyme said: "take in addition to the five points to general action".

Table B-3 localized diseases of the hands and feet.

	Take	Examples
Case Xu CHRONICLE	It will take a point above the affected area on the same meridian. For the additional points, we will use: - The 30VB for the foot; - The 15IM for the hand; - The 14DM or the	For example, in the case of a blockage of the atrial, we will take the 5C and 3C. In the case of a blockage at the level of the elbow, we will take the 15IM and the 10TF.

	4DM for the median points.	
Case Shi Acute	It will take a point below the affected area on the same meridian. Then, choose between: - The 30VB for the foot; - The 15IM for the hand; - The14DM or - The 4DM for the median points.	For example, in cases of inflammation of the elbow joint, we will take the 15IM and the 5p. In the case of sciatica, the 40VB as remote point, the 30VB, mid-point and the 36V as near point. The rhyme said: "take points on the same meridian, point the top to a state Xu, point at the bottom for a State Shi".

Table B-4 localized disease to the Zang (solid organs) and to the FU (hollow organs).

Case Xu CHRONICLE	In the first, take as points near the points Shu back, the points MU or the points of the affected area. Secondly, select among the four median points: O The 20DM, Ba today; O The 20VB, Feng Shi; O The 14Dm, Da Zhui; O The 4DM, Ming men. Thirdly, choose the distal points to be in relationship with the meridians. For example, in the case of lung disease, points of the meridian of the lung; either among the points the most used by experience. For example, the 6RT for the genital organs. The fourth point is the following: O for the diseases above the diaphragm, respiratory organs, heart, brain, cervical column and dorsal, one uses a distal point on the hand to

444

action of drainage.

O For diseases under the umbilicus, component urinary or reproductive, one uses a distal point on the foot.

O for a disease in the middle, between the diaphragm and the umbilicus, one uses a distal point on the hand or foot.

Case Shi Acute	The first four points are identical. There is just a difference for diseases of the environment where it uses simultaneously a distal point of the hand and foot, while in the case Xu, it was or at the level of the hand or at the level of the foot.

Examples of pathologies types

We are going to see a lot of examples. For each pathology, there will be three or four levels of severity.

Diseases of the respiratory organs (the nose, the pharynx, larynx, lung, trachea)

" The distal points: the 7p, 5p and 14DM ;
" The median points: the 20Vb, the 1P, the 13V and 23DM ;
" The points near: the 20GI, the 22RM.

Table B-5 diseases of the respiratory organs.

Case Xu CHRONICLE	In the case of chronic asthma: O The 13V (or the 12V); O The 14DM+13V; O The 13V+14Public DM+7P; O The 13V+1P+14Public DM+7P. In the case of pulmonary	O The 13V+14Public DM+7P; O The 13V+1P+14Public DM+7P or yet O The 13V+1P+14Public DM+5P. For a chronic rhinitis: O The 23DM, or O The 20GI+20VB, or O The 20GI+20VB+7P, or O The 20GI+20VB+7P+23DM.

445

	tuberculosis: **O** The 17V+43V; O The 17V+14Public DM ;	
Case Shi Acute	In the case of acute angina: **O** The 7P or the 4GI; O The 7P+20VB; O The 7P+20VB+22RM; O The 7P+5P+20VB+22RM. In the case of acute bronchitis: O The 7P, or O The 7P+14Public DM, or	**O** The 7P+14Public DM+12V; O The 7P+5P+14Public DM+1P. In the case of acute rhinitis: O The 4IM or the 7p, or O The 4GI+20VB; O The 7P+20VB+20IM or O The 7P+20VB+20GI+5P.

Diseases of the Circulatory System

"The distal points: the 6cc, the 11GI, the 40V Ex 54V;
"The median points: the 14DM and the 20VB;
"The points near: the 15V, the 43V (ex 38), 14rm and the 17V.

Table B-6 diseases of the circulatory system.

Case Xu CHRONICLE	Cardiac arrhythmia: according to the degree of severity: O The 17 (or 14JM); O The 17V +20VB; O The 17V+20VB+6CC and finally O The 17V+14Public RM+20VB+6CC.	In the event of Hypotension: O The 43V (or the 15V); O The 15V+20VB; O The 15V+20VB+6CC and finally O The 15V+43V+20VB+6CC.
Case Shi	In case of hypertension	In the case of angina:

Acute	O The 11IM (or 40V); O The 11GI+20VB (or 14DM); O The 11GI+14Public DM+15V and finally O The 11GI+14Public DM (or 20VB) + 6CC+ 43V.	O The 6cc; O The 6cc+20VB; O The 6cc+20VB+15V and finally O The 6cc+20VB+15V+11IM.

Diseases of the nervous system, brain and spinal cord

" The distal points: the 5C and 3C;
" The median points: the 20DM, the 14DM and the 20VB;
" The points near: the 43V (ex 38), the 15V, the 17RM, the 8WD, the 26DM, the 24DM and the 13F.

Table B-7 diseases of the nervous system, brain and spinal cord.

Case Xu CHRONICLE	In case of cerebral softening: O The 24DM ; O The 24DM+20DM (or 20VB); O The 24DM+14Public DM+5C; O The 20DM+26DM+14Public DM+3C.	In the case of chronic hysteria: O The 13F; O The 13F+20VB or 14DM ; O The 13F+14Public DM+5C; O The 13F+14Public DM+3C+43V.
Case Shi Acute	In the event of access maniac: O The 5C; O The 5C+14Public DM ; O The 5C+14Public DM+26DM ; O The 5C+14Public DM+26DM+3C.	In cases of epilepsy: O The 5C; O The 5C+20VB (for the wind); O The 5C+20VB+12RM; O The 5C+20VB+15V+3C.

447

Diseases of the digestive system (Estomac-Rate)

"The distal points: 44E, 36E, 6CC;
"The median points: 20VB;
"The points near: 12RM, 8WD, 17V, 18V, 20V, 21V.

Table B-8 diseases of the digestive system (Estomac-Rate).

Case Xu CHRONICLE	In the case of the indigestion by fatigue: O The 12RM; O The 12rm+The 20VB; O The 12RM+20VB+36E; O The 12RM+20VB+36E+17V.	In the case of gastric ptosis: O The 12rm or the 8RM in moxa; O The 12RM+20VB; O The 8RM+20VB+44E; O The 12RM+20VB+36E+21V.
Case Shi Acute	In the case of acute gastritis, spasms in the stomach, nerve pain of the stomach: **O** The 36E or 6cc; **O** The 36th+20VB; **O** The 36th+20VB+12RM; **O** The 36th+44E or the 6cc+20VB+21V/	In the case of vomiting, nervous: **O** The 6cc or the 44E; **O** The 6cc+20VB; **O** The 6cc+20VB+12RM ; **O** The 6cc+36E+20VB+17RM or 22RM.

Diseases of the digestive system (Foie-Vésicule bile)

"The distal points: 3F, 34VB, 6tf;
"The median points: 4DM and 20VB;
"The points near: 14F, 13F, 18V, 19V, 24VB and 9DM.

Table B-9 diseases of the digestive system (biliary Foie-Vésicule).

Case Xu CHRONICLE	In the case of jaundice:	O The 9DM+20VB+3F; O The

448

	O The 9DM ;	9DM+20VB+3F+14Public
	O The 9DM+20VB.	F.
Case Shi Acute	In the case of inflammation of the vb: O The 3F or 6tf; O The 3F or 6TF+20VB; O The 3F or 6TF+20VB+19V.	In the event of nerve pain of the liver: O The 3F; O The 34VB or 6TF+4DM ; O The 3F+6TF+4DM+14Public F.

Diseases of the digestive system (large Intestin-Intestin hail)

" The remote points: 57V, 36E;
" The median points: 4DM;
" The points near: 10RM, 8WD, 25E, 6WD, 4WD, 25V, 27V.

Table B-10 diseases of the digestive system (large Intestin-Intestin hail).

Case Xu CHRONICLE	In the case of ENTERITIS CHRONIC: O The 25E; O The 25th+4DM ;	O The 8WD (moxa to salt) +4DM+57V; O The 25th +8 RM (moxa) +4DM+36E.
Case Shi Acute	In the case of acute enteritis outbreak: O The 57V; O The 57V or 36E +4DM ; O The 57V+4DM+25E; O The 57V+4DM+25E+36E.	In the case of entérodynie with intestinal pains: O The 36E; O The 36th+4DM ; O The 36th+4DM+25E; O The 36th+57V+4DM+25E.

Diseases of the urinary system (Rein-Vessie)

" The remote points: 6RN, 9rt;
" The median point: 4DM;
" The points near: 23V+28V+4RM+3RM+28E+25VB.

Table B-11 diseases of the urinary system (Rein-Vessie).

Case Xu CHRONICLE	In the case of weakness of the bladder: O The 3WD; O The 3RM+4DM ; O The 3RM+4DM+9rt; O The 3RM+4DM+6RN+28V.	In the case of bedwetting: O The 3WD; O The 3RM+4DM ; O The 3RM+4DM+6RN; O The 3RM+28V+4DM+6RN.
Case Shi Acute	In the case of acute nephritis: O The 6RN; O The 6RN (or the 9rt) +4DM ; O The 6RN+4DM+23V; O The 6RN+9Rt+4DM+23V.	In the event of a spasm of the bladder: O The 6RN (or the 9rt); O The 6RN (or the 9rt) +the 4DM; O The 6RN + the 4DM +3WD; O The 6RN+9Rt+4DM+3RM.

Diseases of the reproductive system

" The remote points: 6RT, 9rt;
" The median points: 4DM, 23V;
" The points near: 6WD, 4WD, 3WD, 29E, 25vb, 32V + points extra: Bai-Lao or if Liao and Wei Bao in the inguinal fold.

Table B-12 diseases of the reproductive system.

Case Xu CHRONICLE	In the case of spermatorrhée:	O The 3RM+4DM+6rt; O The

	O The 23V; O The 4RM+L4DM ; O The 4WD+4DM+6rt; O The 4WD+4DM+6Rt+23V. In the case of vaginal discharge: O The 29E; O The 29th+4DM ;	3RM+32V+4DM+6Rt. In the case of delay of menses: O The 29E; O The 4WD+4DM ; O The 4WD+4DM+6rt; O The 23V+4DM+4RM+6Rt.
Case Shi Acute	In the case of orchitis : O the 6rt; O The 6RT+4DM ; O The 6RT+4DM+29E; O The 6RT+4DM+29E+9Rt.	In the case of nerve pain in the uterus and dysmenorrhea: O the 6rt; O The 6RT+4RM; O The 6RT+4DM+4RM; O The 6RT+9Rt+4DM+4RM.

Diseases in the whole of the body

In cases Xu, of weakness:
" Points near: 16DM, 12DM, 13DM, 9DM ;
" Median points: 20DM, 20vb, 14DM, 4DM;
" Distal points: 10RT, 11GI, 4GI, 36E.
With the distal points and midpoints, make a action of drainage in the top and bottom, namely: for the violations at the bottom, take the points of the top. For the offenses at the top, take the points of the bottom. In the dangerous diseases, it will use the points to special purpose. Example:
" In case of collapse, we will take the 16DM in point near + the 20DM in mid-point and the 15IM as a point to special use.
" For vertigo with sluggish: The 20VB and the 4DM in mid-point and the 4IM in distal.

451

In cases Shi, excess

The method is the same as that for the cases Xu, except that for the dangerous diseases, we can make bleeding the special points. Example:

" In case of insolation: the 12 points Tsing and the 11IM in bleeding + 14dm.

" In case of hyperthermia: The 1RN, the 11GI, 14DM, 12DM.

" In the event of widespread dermatosis: 10RT, 11GI, 14DM, 12DM. If the symptoms are severe, add a point on affected area.

" For a cold with fever Very important: the 1GI, 4GI, 14DM, 20VB.

The whole of the examples that we have just to see will allow you to take ownership of the method. Then very quickly, you will learn how you-even, according to the pathologies, to create your own formula. This technique of choice of points in acupuncture-Moxibustion is obviously applicable in the techniques of digitoponcture.

Appendix C

Glossary

Ba gang: the eight rules : Yin-Yang, internal (Li)-External (Biao), Han (cold)-RE (hot), weakness (Xu)-fullness (SHI).

Ke cycle: control cycle.

Shen cycle: cycle of begetting.

Dao de Jing : written in 600 av. J.-C. and assigned to Lao Tseu.

Dao Yin: is to implement certain techniques for lead, guide the blood and energy.

Fu: The six hollow organs (IG, IM, Is., VB, bladder, three households).

Huang Di Neijing : Book founder of the MTC dating back 2 500 years.

Hun: The spiritual soul, under the emblem of the liver, the Yang original.

Jin Kui Yao : Breviary of the **luggage compartment of gold** of zhang zhong Jing, beginning of the third century.

Jin ye: liquids, foster care.

Jing Luo: meridians comprising the 12 meridians Jing May, and 15 Luo vessels connecting to the Jing Main.

Jing qi: The battery of the body that governs the software five bodies.

Ku Qi: energy of the food bowl pulled by the spleen.

Lao Tseu : Founder of Taoism.

Ling Qi: energy very subtle from the sky.

Ming Men: small flame of the oil lamp, starter of all the metabolism of the body.

Nan Jing : classical difficulties (220-280), Comment of the **Nei Jing.**

Po: the soul from the body, under the emblem of the lung, the Yin original.

Qi: the energy located upstream of the matter.

Qi Gong: The mastery of the Qi, of the vital energy.

Qi Zi: blockage or stagnation of energy in the body.

Qian Jin Fang: prescription worth a thousand pieces of gold of Sun If Miao (end of the viith century).

San Bao: the three treasures that are the Jing, gasoline, the Qi, the energy and the Shen, the Spirit.

San Jiao: the three homes.

Shang Han Za Bing: Treaty of febrile diseases of zhang zhong Jing (Year 160).

Shen: the spirit, the mind under the emblem of the heart.

Shen Ming: The vitality.

Tai Ji: symbol of the one. Everything is in the process of becoming. Contains all the potentialities.

Tan: Generic term meaning the waste, substances that the organization has not had the strength to eliminate.

Wen Zhen: the interrogation.

Wu Ji: The zero métaphyisque.

Wu Xing: The five elements (wood, fire, earth, metal, water).

Xie Qi: perverse energy.

Xue Wei: Point of acupuncture.

Yang Qi: energy of the air drawn by the lung.

Yi Jing: dating back to more than 5 000 years, this book poses the bases of any Chinese culture.

Yi Shi: the conscience, a mixture of the Innate (The Shen) and of the knowledge acquired.

Yin-Yang : in relation with the number 2. The principle of duality inherent to life.

Yu Xue: stagnation of blood, blood stasis.

Yuan Qi: fundamental IQ of the start of the life, stored in the kidney, oil lamp.

Zang: the five solid organs (F, P, C, RT, Rn).

Zhen qi: The original Qi which maintains the vitality, derived from the energy bequeathed by our ancestors and that coming from the sky and the earth.

Zheng Qi: all the physiological Qi allowing for the proper functioning of the body.

Zhong Qi: Qi of the center, energy of the average household.

Appendix D

Useful addresses

A few good schools of MTC

" The CATC, The College Therapeutic arts Chinese: https://www.catc.fr/

" The CEDRE, the collective of study, development and research in ethnomedicine: http://www.cedre.org/

" The Institute ChuZhen: http://www.chuzhen.com/

" Sinologique circle of the West: http://www.chine.org/

For the practice of Qi Gong

" The IEQG, the institute of Qi Gong directed by Yves Réquéna: http://www.ieqg.com/

A practitioner to side of among you?

" The UFPMTC, the French Union of Traditional Chinese Medicine: https://www.ufpmtc.fr/

A practitioner in bodily techniques according to the principles of the MTC (Shiatsu)

" The French Institute of Shiatsu: https://www.shiatsu-institut.fr/

The moxas, equipment of acupuncture

" Planeta Verde: https://www.planetaverd.net/

" Sinolux: https://www.sinolux.lu

The sites of the teaching of the author

" http://www.jeanpelissier.com/ For the news of the quarter, the new courses and conferences free.

" https://boutique.jeanpelissier.com/ For all courses in the MTC.

" http://blog.jeanpelissier.com/ For the blog on the nutraceuticals.

" https://www.jeanpelissier.net/ For the subscription to the Cahiers de sinobiologie.

" You can contact the author at the following e-mail address: Pelissier.j@wanadoo.fr

Executive Summary

456

A few good schools of MTC
For the practice of Qi Gong
A practitioner to side of among you?
A practitioner in bodily techniques according
to the principles of the MTC (Shiatsu)
The moxas, equipment of acupuncture
The sites of the teaching of the author

www.ingramcontent.com/pod-product-compliance
Lightning Source LLC
Chambersburg PA
CBHW060818170526
45158CB00001B/14